CURRENT CLINICAL UROLOGY

ERIC A. KLEIN, MD, SERIES EDITOR
PROFESSOR OF SURGERY
CLEVELAND CLINIC LERNER COLLEGE OF MEDICINE HEAD
SECTION OF UROLOGIC ONCOLOGY
GLICKMAN UROLOGICAL AND KIDNEY INSTITUTE
CLEVELAND, OH

For further volumes:
http://www.springer.com/series/7635

Howard B. Goldman
Editor

Complications of Female Incontinence and Pelvic Reconstructive Surgery

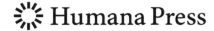 Humana Press

Editor
Howard B. Goldman, MD
Glickman Urologic and Kidney Institute
The Cleveland Clinic
Center for Female Pelvic Medicine
and Reconstructive Surgery
Cleveland, OH, USA

ISBN 978-1-61779-923-5   ISBN 978-1-61779-924-2 (eBook)
DOI 10.1007/978-1-61779-924-2
Springer New York Heidelberg Dordrecht London

Library of Congress Control Number: 2012942910

Printed on acid-free paper

Humana Press is a brand of Springer
Springer is part of Springer Science+Business Media (www.springer.com)

To my wife Suri for her support and encouragement.

To all of my mentors and students who all continue to teach me.

Preface

I am honored and pleased to write a preface for the textbook on *Complications of Female Incontinence and Pelvic Reconstructive Surgery*. At a time when the subspecialty of female pelvic medicine and reconstructive surgery is in its infancy, I feel having such a resource available to pelvic surgeons is extremely beneficial. Dr. Goldman has invited internationally respected contributors to provide their experience and expertise regarding the avoidance and management of surgical complications related to a variety of female pelvic floor surgeries. As the majority of the surgeries we perform on our female patients are done for quality of life symptoms, it has become apparent that we need to do a better job reporting and managing the untoward outcomes that can sometimes occur after these interventions. This book brings these potential complications to the forefront.

It will be of great use for both general urologists and gynecologists who perform pelvic floor surgeries as well as current and future specialists in female pelvic medicine and reconstructive surgery.

Cincinnati, OH, USA   Mickey Karram, MD

Preface

Surgery for incontinence, pelvic organ prolapse, and other disorders of the female pelvic floor has evolved in the past two decades as the specialty of Female Pelvic Medicine and Reconstructive Surgery has incorporated expertise from the fields of urology, gynecology, and colorectal surgery. Today, more surgeons are better equipped to treat disorders of the female pelvic floor than ever before. Unfortunately complications of surgery, whether intraoperative or postoperative, are inevitable even for the most experienced and highly skilled surgeon. Whether it is an unexpected finding in the operating room or an undesirable outcome of surgery, the Female Pelvic Surgeon must be equipped to prevent and manage a variety of complications.

While there are several excellent texts devoted to indications for surgery and the technical aspects of surgical procedures "Complications of Female Incontinence and Pelvic Reconstructive Surgery" fills a need by providing readers with a comprehensive review of the prevention and management of common and not so common complications of female pelvic surgery. Dr. Howard Goldman has assembled a group of highly experienced authors from all three disciplines of Female Pelvic Medicine and Reconstructive Surgery. These authors offer in-depth descriptions of three critical areas: prevention, evaluation, and management of complications. They present practical information and surgical tips based on years of experience and a thorough review of the relevant literature. In addition, a look at the table of contents shows that complications from all types of reconstructive procedures are covered.

I believe that "Complications of Female Incontinence and Pelvic Reconstructive Surgery" will be a great complement to the libraries of those of us who treat female pelvic disorders. Whether one is just starting a career or is highly experienced, this book is a welcome addition.

Cincinnati, OH, USA   Victor W. Nitti, MD

Contents

Contributors

Patricia C. Alves-Ferreira, PT Department of Colorectal Surgery A30, Cleveland Clinic, Cleveland, OH, USA

Matthew D. Barber, MD, MHS Obstetrics, Gynecology and Women's Health Institute, Cleveland Clinic, Cleveland, OH, USA

Jerry Blaivas, MD Department of Urology, Weill Medical College of Cornell University, New York, NY, USA

Dorota Borawski, MD SUNY Downstate Medical Center and the Institute for Bladder and Prostate Research, Brooklyn, NY, USA

Benjamin M. Brucker, MD Department of Urology, New York University Langone Medical Center, New York, NY, USA

Roger R. Dmochowski, MD, FACS Department of Urologic Surgery, Vanderbilt University School of Medicine, Nashville, TN, USA

Shay Erisson, MD Urogynecology Service, Department of Obstetrics and Gynecology, Technion-Israel Institute of Technology, Haifa, Israel

Farzeen Firoozi, MD Center for Pelvic Health and Reconstructive Surgery, The Arthur Smith Institute for Urology, Garden City, NY, USA

Alienor S. Gilchrist, MD Department of Urology, Medical University of South Carolina, Charleston, SC, USA

David A. Ginsberg, MD Department of Urology, Keck School of Medicine of USC, Los Angeles, CA, USA

Howard B. Goldman, MD, FACS Center for Female Pelvic Medicine and Reconstructive Surgery, Center for Quality and Patient Safety, Glickman Urologic and Kidney Institute, The Cleveland Clinic, Cleveland, OH, USA

Lerner College of Medicine, Case Western Reserve University, Cleveland, OH, USA

Alex Gomelsky, MD Department of Urology, Louisiana State University Health Sciences Center, Shreveport, Shreveport, LA, USA

Brooke Gurland, MD, FACS Department of Colorectal Surgery A30, Cleveland Clinic, Cleveland, OH, USA

Sender Herschorn, BSc, MDCM, FRCSC Division of Urology, Sunnybrook Health Sciences Centre, University of Toronto, Toronto, ON, Canada

Michael Ingber, MD Department of Urogynecology, Saint Clare's Health System, Denville, NJ, USA

Department of Urology, Weill Cornell Medical College, New York, NY, USA

Mickey Karram, MD Division of Female Pelvic Medicine & Reconstructive Surgery, The Christ Hospital, University of Cincinnati, Cincinnati, OH, USA

Department of Obstetrics/Gynecology, University of Cincinnati, Cincinnati, OH, USA

Melissa Kaufman, MD Department of Urological Surgery, Vanderbilt University School of Medicine, Nashville, TN, USA

Laura Chang-Kit, MD Department of Urological Surgery, Vanderbilt University School of Medicine, Nashville, TN, USA

John J. Knoedler, MD Department of Urology, Mayo Clinic, Rochester, MN, USA

Michelle Koski, MD Department of Urology, Medical University of South Carolina, Charleston, SC, USA

Deborah J. Lightner, MD Department of Urology, Mayo Clinic, Rochester, MN, USA

Lior Lowenstein, MD, MS Urogynecology Service, Department of Obstetrics and Gynecology, Technion-Israel Institute of Technology, Haifa, Israel

Courtenay K. Moore, MD Glickman Urological and Kidney Institute, Cleveland Clinic, Cleveland, OH, USA

Elizabeth R. Mueller, MD, MSME, FACS Division of Female Pelvic Medicine and Reconstructive Surgery, Departments of Urology and Obstetrics/Gynecology, Loyola University Chicago Stritch School of Medicine, Maywood, IL, USA

Alana Murphy, MD Glickman Urological and Kidney Institute, Cleveland Clinic, Cleveland, OH, USA

Sunshine Murray, MD Department of Urology, UT Southwestern Medical Center, Dallas, TX, USA

Victor W. Nitti, MD Department of Urology, New York University Langone Medical Center, New York, NY, USA

Ray Rackley, MD Department of Urology, Cleveland Clinic, Cleveland, OH, USA

Shlomo Raz, MD Division of Pelvic Medicine and Reconstructive Surgery, University of California Los Angeles, Los Angeles, CA, USA

Lisa Rogo-Gupta, MD Division of Pelvic Medicine and Reconstructive Surgery, University of California Los Angeles, Los Angeles, CA, USA

Eric S. Rovner, MD Department of Urology, Medical University of South Carolina, Charleston, SC, USA

Kamran P. Sajadi, MD Division of Urology, Oregon Health and Science University, Portland, OR, USA

Ellen R. Solomon, MD Obstetrics, Gynecology and Women's Health Institute, Cleveland Clinic, Cleveland, OH, USA

Sandip P. Vasavada, MD Center for Female Urology and Reconstructive Pelvic Surgery , Cleveland Clinic Main Campus, Cleveland, OH, USA

Glickman Urological and Kidney Institute, Cleveland Clinic, Cleveland, OH, USA

Blayne K. Welk, MD, FRCSC Division of Urology, Sunnybrook Health Sciences Centre, University of Toronto, Toronto, ON, Canada

J. Christian Winters, MD Department of Urology, Louisiana State University, New Orleans, LA, USA

Philippe E. Zimmern, MD Department of Urology, UT Southwestern Medical School, Dallas, TX, USA

Dani Zoorob, MD Division of Female Pelvic Medicine & Reconstructive Surgery, The Christ Hospital, University of Cincinnati, Cincinnati, OH, USA

Department of Obstetrics/Gynecology, University of Cincinnati, Cincinnati, OH, USA

Taxonomy of Complications of Pelvic Floor Surgery

Roger R. Dmochowski, Alex Gomelsky, and Laura Chang-Kit

Introduction

The etymology of the word "taxonomy" is from the Greek *taxis*, meaning orderly arrangement, and *nomos*, meaning law. Steadman's Medical Dictionary defines "taxonomy" as the systemic classification of living things or organisms, and, more recently, the term has come to mean any specialized method of classifying objects or events. In the scientific community, taxonomies have proven to be highly efficient structures for organizing vast amounts of content. Taxonomy, as it relates to surgical complications, is a relatively novel concept. Intuitively, the idea to organize complications for ease of comparison and to assist in risk stratification is a noble one. However, if improperly designed, classification systems may be cumbersome to use and may not be widely adopted. In this chapter, we explore the details behind taxonomy development in the surgical and urological literature and assess their potential for implementation in pelvic reconstruction procedures.

R.R. Dmochowski, MD, FACS (✉) • L. Chang-Kit, MD
Department of Urologic Surgery,
Vanderbilt University School of Medicine,
A-1302 Medical Center North,
Nashville, TN 37232, USA
e-mail: roger.dmochowski@Vanderbilt.edu

A. Gomelsky, MD
Department of Urology, Louisiana State University
Health Sciences Center, Shreveport,
Shreveport, LA, USA

The Need for Taxonomy of Complications

Complications are an essential aspect of performing surgery. They are usually multifactorial and may accompany even the least-invasive and routine procedures. Complications reported in the surgical literature can also serve as vital outcome measures and valuable quality indicators. Traditionally, however, the reliability of reporting complications has been inconsistent. Martin et al. developed a list of ten critical elements of accurate and comprehensive reporting of surgical complications [1]. These criteria included providing the methods of accruing data, duration of follow-up, outpatient information, definition of complications, mortality rate and causes of death, morbidity rate and total complications, procedure-specific complications, severity grade, length-of-stay data, and risk factor included in the analysis. Out of 119 articles reporting outcomes in 22,530 patients that underwent pancreatectomy, esophagectomy, and hepatectomy, no article reported all ten criteria and only 2% reported nine of ten. The most commonly unmet criteria were outpatient information (22%), definitions of complications provided (34%), severity grade used (20%), and risk factors used in analysis (29%). Reporting of complications in the urologic literature has been similarly inconsistent. In a MEDLINE search encompassing 109 studies and nearly 150,000 patient-outcomes following radical uro-oncologic

H.B. Goldman (ed.), *Complications of Female Incontinence and Pelvic Reconstructive Surgery*,
Current Clinical Urology, DOI 10.1007/978-1-61779-924-2_1, © Springer Science+Business Media, LLC 2013

surgical procedures, Donat found that only 2% of the studies met 9–10 of the ten established criteria for surgical complication reporting [2]. The most commonly underreported criteria were complication definitions in 79%, complication severity and/or grade in 67%, outpatient data in 63%, comorbidities in 59%, and the duration of the reporting period in 56%. Certainly the disparity in the quality of complication reporting makes it nearly impossible to compare the morbidity of surgical techniques and outcomes.

Depending on the type of procedure and definition of complication, the prevalence of complications in reconstructive pelvic surgery varies significantly. In a retrospective review of 100 consecutive reconstructive cases, Lambrou et al. reported a complication prevalence of 46%, which included 13 intraoperative complications and 33 postoperative complications [3]. The readmission rate for complications was 15%. The number of procedures per patient was an independent risk factor for intraoperative blood loss, while blood loss was an independent risk factor for perioperative complications. The prevalence of complications in midurethral sling (MUS) surgery appears to also vary significantly [4]. In a systematic review and meta-analysis of randomized, controlled trials (RCTs) comparing various MUS procedures, Novara et al. reported bladder penetration rates ranging from 0 to 24%. Rates of hematoma formation, bladder erosion, and vaginal extrusion were 0–16.1%, 0–13.1%, and 0–5.9%, respectively. Postoperative urinary tract infections (UTIs) were reported in up to 17.8% of women, while the rates of postoperative storage lower urinary tract symptoms (LUTS) and voiding LUTS were 0–41.3% and 0–55.1%, respectively. It must also be noted that a large portion of the evaluated RCTs had no available data for several of the complication categories mentioned above. Likewise, in a meta-analysis of surgical procedures for repair of pelvic organ prolapse (POP), Maher et al. noted that the impact of surgery on associated bladder, bowel, and sexual function symptoms was poorly reported in 40 RCTs reporting on over 3,700 women [5]. When reported, complications such as intraoperative blood loss and the rates of persistent, worsened,

or de novo LUTS varied widely, making comparisons of studies even more challenging.

The reporting of complications in surgery, and reconstructive pelvic surgery in particular, may be inconsistent for several reasons. First, a complication by one surgeon's consideration may not be seen as one by another surgeon and, thus, may not be consistently reported. Second, specific cutoff values for outcome criteria such as estimated blood loss and postvoid residual volume are not universally agreed upon, further complicating the reporting of these sequelae. Third, studies in the past have often focused on anatomic outcomes, such as resolution of stress urinary incontinence and improved POP grade following repair. It appears that only in the last several years surgeons have developed an increasing appreciation of subjective outcomes, or those having a significant impact on quality of life (QoL). Similarly, the acceptance of subjective complications such as pelvic pain and dyspareunia continues to evolve.

The connection between quality and health care delivery has recently taken a forefront in the public eye. The Office of the Inspector General Work Plan for Fiscal Year 2011 describes at least seven items focusing on quality data for hospitals and providers, such as readmissions, adverse events, and responses to adverse events. Likewise, Title III of the Patient Protection and Affordable Care Act of 2010 (PPACA) is entitled "Improving the Quality and Efficiency of Health Care." The name summarizes the framework in which quality is considered as part of health care reform and becomes intimately connected with payment. Despite the obvious Federal focus on quality improvement initiatives, there appear to be obstacles to reporting of complications. Studies have shown that physicians often underreport the incidence of serious complications associated with surgery [6, 7]. Another study found that the reporting of complications associated with MUS placement in the U.S. Food and Drug Administration (FDA) manufacturer and user faculty device experience (MAUDE) database significantly exceeded the complications reported in published literature [8]. One reason for underreporting may be that there is a clear lack of centralized registries of complications. Another may be that surgeons may view the reporting of complications as a stigma and may fear public embarrassment or professional retribution. Regardless of the potential reasons, it is clear that it becomes increasingly difficult for surgeons to learn from the experiences of others without accurate estimates and sources of complications. It also makes the process of informed consent even more tenuous.

Existing Classification Systems of Complications

As the classification of complications in pelvic reconstructive surgery is thus far in its infancy, valuable information may be gleaned from the general surgery literature. Clavien et al. first developed a distinction between three types of negative outcomes: complications, failure to cure, or sequelae [9]. Complications were defined as any deviation from the normal postoperative course, which also took into account asymptomatic complications such as arrhythmias and atelectasis. A sequela was defined as an "after-effect" of surgery that was inherent to the procedure. Failure to achieve a cure meant that the original purpose of the surgery was not achieved, even if the surgery was executed properly and without complications. What came to be known as the Clavien classification took into consideration only complications, and not treatment failures or sequelae.

The initial Clavien classification consisted of four severity grades and the current, modified classification is composed of five grades [10]. Grade I is any deviation from the normal postoperative course without the need for any pharmacological treatment or surgical, endoscopic, and radiological intervention. The allowed therapeutic regimens include replacement of electrolytes, physiotherapy, and medications such as antiemetics, antipyretics, analgesics, and diuretics. Wound infections that are opened at the bedside also fall into this grade. Complications falling into grade II require pharmacological

treatment with medications other than such allowed for grade I complications. The requirement for transfusion of blood products and total parenteral nutrition also constitutes a grade II complication. Grade III complications require surgical, endoscopic, or radiological intervention. This category is subdivided into IIIa (not under general anesthesia) and IIIb (under general anesthesia). Grade IV complications are life-threatening and require intermediate or intensive care management. Central nervous system complications such as brain hemorrhage, ischemic stroke, and subarachnoid bleeding are included in this category, while transient ischemic attacks are not. This category is also subdivided into IVa (single-organ dysfunction, with or without dialysis) and IVb (multiorgan dysfunction). Death of a patient is a grade V complication. The suffix "d" (for "disability") is added to the respective grade of complication if the patient suffers from a complication at the time of discharge. This label indicates the need for a follow-up to fully evaluate and stage the complication.

The key to ranking the complications using the modified Clavien system is the intricacy of the treatment used to correct the complication [10]. The authors validated this classification in over 6,300 patients undergoing elective surgery in their institution over a 10-year period. The complexity of surgery was estimated according to a modification of an established graduation and the authors found that the classification of complications significantly correlated with the duration of the hospital stay, a surrogate marker of outcome. A strong correlation was also found between the complexity of surgery (and assumed higher complication rates) and outcome of surgery as assessed by the novel, modified classification. The authors then conducted an international survey to access acceptability and reproducibility of the classification. Over 90% of the surgeons queried found the classification to be simple, reproducible, and logical. These surgeons stated that they would support the introduction of the classification into their clinical practice.

The modified Clavien classification has thus far been employed in classifying complications in several urologic surgical applications, including radical cysto-urethrectomy, percutaneous nephrolithotomy, live donor nephrectomy, laparoscopic radical prostatectomy, and ureteroscopy [11–15]. To date, the modified Clavien classification has not been rigorously evaluated in the milieu of pelvic reconstructive surgery.

Recently, a classification of complications directly related to the insertion of prostheses (meshes, implants, tapes) or grafts in female pelvic floor surgery has been introduced [16]. This report combined the input of members of the Standardization and Terminology Committees of two International Organizations, the International Urogynecological Association (IUGA) and the International Continence Society (ICS) and a Joint IUGA/ICS Working Group on Complications Terminology, and was assisted at intervals by many expert external referees. An extensive process of 11 rounds of internal and external review took place with exhaustive examination of each aspect of the terminology and classification. The decision-making process was conducted by collective opinion (consensus). The classification is based on category, time, and site classes and divisions. The category (C) is stratified by location of compromise (vagina, urinary tract, bowel or rectum, skin or musculocutaneous system, and hematologic or systemic compromise) and symptom severity (asymptomatic, symptomatic, presence of infection, and abscess formation). The timing of complication (T) is subdivided into four groups (intraoperative to 48 h, 48 h to 2 months, 2–12 months, and >12 months), while the site of complication (S) includes vagina (at or away from the suture line), due to trocar passage, other skin or musculoskeletal site, and intra-abdominal location. Additionally, grades of pain may be assigned as a subclassification of complication category. The subjective presence of pain by the patient only may be graded from a–e (asymptomatic or no pain to spontaneous pain). Each complication is assigned a CTS code consisting of three or four letters and four numerals and should theoretically encompass all conceivable scenarios for describing insertion complications and healing abnormalities.

The Challenge of Implementing a Classification System of Complications

Inherent to the definition of taxonomy is that the classification system should reduce complexity by suggesting a logical and hierarchical representation of categories. The classification should likewise provide a means for organizing and accessing vast quantities of data in an intuitive manner. Unfortunately, the adoption of classification systems in pelvic reconstructive surgery has not, to date, been encouraging. The Pelvic Organ Prolapse Quantification (POP-Q) system is a prime example.

While classification systems for pelvic organ support have existed since the 1800s, no system has gained consistent and widespread acceptance [17]. Over the past 20 years, the POP-Q has become the first and only classification system to be recognized by the ICS, the American Urogynecologic Society (AUGS), and the Society of Gynecologic Surgeons (SGS) [18]. This system has been extensively studied and excellent inter- and intraobserver reliability have been demonstrated [19, 20]. Although the POP-Q is arguably the only universally accepted classification system for grading the severity of POP, it has not been universally adopted. As of 2006, the POP-Q has been used clinically by only 40% of the members of ICS and AUGS, the groups that acknowledge this system as the classification standard for POP [21]. Some of the reasons given by clinicians surveyed for not consistently employing the POP-Q were that the system is too confusing, overly time-consuming, and that it was not being used by their colleagues [21]. While some of these reasons are not supported by literature [19], it remains that even the most rigorous and well-conceived classification systems may not achieve widespread use owing to concerns regarding simplicity of use. Since, Swift et al. have validated a simplified POP-Q system to address the concerns that the traditional POP-Q is not a "user-friendly" classification system [22].

Table 1.1 Common complications in pelvic reconstructive surgery

Time	General	Specific	Reoperation
Perioperative	Acute bleeding		Hematoma drainage
	Transfusion		
	Organ injury		Repair organ injury
	Pneumonia, atelectasis		
	Ileus		
	Arrhythmia, MI, CVA, PE, DVT, death		
Postoperative <30 days	MI, CVA, PE, DVT, death	UTI	
	Incisional pain	Wound infection	I&D wound
	Pelvic pain	AUR	Sling revision
	PSBO	Leg pain	
		Storage LUTS	
		Voiding LUTS	
		Extrusion	Sling/mesh revision
		Erosion into GU tract	
Postoperative >30 days	Incisional pain	Storage LUTS	Sling/mesh revision
	Pelvic pain	Voiding LUTS	
		Dyspareunia	
		Extrusion	
		Erosion into GU tract	
		Leg pain	

MI myocardial infarction; *CVA* cerebrovascular accident; *PE* pulmonary embolism; *DVT* deep vein thrombosis; *UTI* urinary tract infection; *I&D* incision and drainage; *AUR* acute urinary retention; *PSBO* partial small bowel obstruction; *LUTS* lower urinary tract symptoms; *GU* genitourinary

Table 1.2 Proposed pelvic reconstructive surgery modification of the Clavien system

Grade	Description	Examples
I	Deviation from normal course (no need for additional intervention)	Trocar bladder puncture, replaced; no formal repair Perioperative antipyretics Postoperative pelvic floor exercises
II	Pharmacological intervention (other than for Grade I)	Antibiotics for UTI or wound infection; antimuscarinics Transfusion of blood products Analgesics for incisional, pelvic, or leg pain
III	Short- or long-term complication, no operative intervention	De novo or worsened storage LUTS De novo or worsened voiding LUTS Incisional, pelvic, or leg pain
IV	Operative intervention required IVa: Intraoperative/immediately postoperative IVb: Postoperative, office IVc: Postoperative, operating room	 Repair organ injury (bladder, ureter, colorectal, vascular); endovascular embolization for bleeding Incision and drainage wound infection; partial excision extruded sling/mesh Sling/mesh incision/revision/excision; urethrolysis; laparotomy for small bowel obstruction; InterStim
V	Life-threatening event or demise Va: Single-organ dysfunction Vb: Multiorgan dysfunction Vc: Death	 DVT, PE, MI, CVA/CNS

UTI urinary tract infection; *LUTS* lower urinary tract symptoms; *DVT* deep vein thrombosis; *PE* pulmonary embolism; *MI* myocardial infarction; *CVA* cerebrovascular accident; *CNS* central nervous system event; *InterStim* sacral neuromodulation

The novel classification system proposed by IUGA/ICS, while comprehensive, may be cumbersome to use and does not immediately appear to reduce the complexity of organizing complications. Furthermore, the CTS classification does not leave room for reporting the presence of de novo or worsened storage or voiding LUTS commonly associated with surgery for stress urinary incontinence. The modified Clavien classification, while simpler to integrate, appears to be constructed for grading surgical procedures with a significant prevalence of postoperative intervention, reoperation, and morbidity. It can certainly be argued that, since pelvic reconstructive surgery is often performed in otherwise healthy individuals, it is associated with an overall low prevalence of significant morbidity. Thus, the modified Clavien classification may not be sensitive enough to classify the complications typically associated with pelvic reconstructive surgery.

Complications in urologic pelvic surgery may be classified as general or specific, by their temporal relationship to the surgery itself and by their relationship to a technique or specific material used in the procedure. These are summarized in Table 1.1. Taking into account these complications, we propose a modification of the Clavien classification constructed specifically for complications associated with pelvic reconstructive surgery (Table 1.2).

Conclusions

A taxonomy for the classification of complications in pelvic reconstructive surgery would be a valuable instrument for reporting outcome measures and quality indicators. While both the modified Clavien classification and the recent IUGA/ICS classification contain valuable components, at present, a single, comprehensive, user-friendly system does not exist. The determination of an optimal classification system would lead to an improved ability of surgeons to communicate with each other and compare data.

References

1. Martin II RC, Brennan MF, Jaques DP. Quality of complication reporting in the surgical literature. Ann Surg. 2002;235:803–13.
2. Donat SM. Standards for surgical complication reporting in urologic oncology: time for a change. Urology. 2007;69:221–5.
3. Lambrou NC, Buller JL, Thompson JR, et al. Prevalence of perioperative complications among women undergoing reconstructive pelvic surgery. Am J Obstet Gynecol. 2000;183:1355–60.
4. Novara G, Galfano A, Boscolo-Berto R, et al. Complication rates of tension-free midurethral slings in the treatment of female stress urinary incontinence: a systematic review and meta-analysis of randomized controlled trials comparing tension-free midurethral tapes to other surgical procedures and different devices. Eur Urol. 2008;53:288–304.
5. Maher C, Feiner B, Baessler K, et al. Surgical management of pelvic organ prolapse in women. Cochrane Database Syst Rev. 2010;(4):CD004014.
6. Cullen DJ, Bates DW, Small SD, et al. The incident reporting system does not detect adverse drug events: a problem for quality improvement. Jt Comm J Qual Improv. 1995;21:541–8.
7. Sanborn KV, Castro J, Kuroda M, Thys DM. Detection of intraoperative incidents by electronic scanning of computerized anesthesia records: comparison with voluntary reporting. Anesthesiology. 1996;85:977–87.
8. Deng DY, Rutman M, Raz S, Rodriguez LV. Presentation and management of major complications of midurethral slings: are complications underreported? Neurourol Urodyn. 2007;26:46–52.
9. Clavien P, Sanabria J, Strasberg S. Proposed classification of complication of surgery with examples of utility in cholecystectomy. Surgery. 1992;111:518–26.
10. Dindo D, Demartines N, Clavien P-A. Classification of surgical complications: a new proposal with evaluation in a cohort of 6336 patients and results of a survey. Ann Surg. 2004;240:205–13.
11. Elshal AM, Barakat TS, Mosbah A, et al. Complications of radical cysto-urethrectomy using modified Clavien grading system: prepubic versus perineal urethrectomy. BJU Int. 2011;108:1297–300.
12. Tefekli A, Ali Karadag M, Tepeler K, et al. Classification of percutaneous nephrolithotomy complications using the modified Clavien grading system: looking for a standard. Eur Urol. 2008;53:184–90.
13. Kocak B, Koffron AJ, Baker TB, et al. Proposed classification of complications after live donor nephrectomy. Urology. 2006;67:927–31.
14. Gonzalgo ML, Pavlovich CP, Trock BJ, et al. Classification and trends of perioperative morbidities following laparoscopic radical prostatectomy. J Urol. 2005;174:135–9.

15. Rioja J, Mamoulakis C, Sodha H, et al. A plea for centralized care for ureteroscopy: results from a comparative study under different conditions within the same center. J Endourol. 2011;25:425–9.

16. Haylen BT, Freeman RM, Swift SE, et al. An International Urogynecological Association (IUGA)/International Continence Society (ICS) joint terminology and classification of the complications related directly to the insertion of prostheses (meshes, implants, tapes) and grafts in female pelvic floor surgery. Neurourol Urodyn. 2011; 30:2–12.

17. Scanzoni FW. Senkung und Vorfall des uterus und der scheide. In: Scanzoni FW, editor. Lehrbuch der Krankheiten der Weiblichen Geschlechstorgane. 5th ed. Vienna: Braumueller; 1875. p. 654–64.

18. Bump RC, Mattiasson A, Bo K, et al. The standardization of terminology of female pelvic floor dysfunction. Am J Obstet Gynecol. 1996;175:10–7.

19. Hall AF, Theofrastous JP, Cundiff GC, et al. Interobserver and intraobserver reliability of the proposed International Continence Society, Society of Gynecologic Surgeons, and American Urogynecologic Society pelvic organ prolapse classification system. Am J Obstet Gynecol. 1996;175:1467–71.

20. Kobak WH, Rosenberger K, Walters MD. Interobserver variation in the assessment of pelvic organ prolapse. Int Urogynecol J Pelvic Floor Dysfunct. 1996;7:121–4.

21. Auwad W, Freeman R, Swift S. Is the pelvic organ prolapse quantification system (POP-Q) being used? A survey of the members of the International Continence Society (ICS) and the American Urogynecology Society (AUGS). Int Urogynecol J Pelvic Floor Dysfunct. 2004;15:324–7.

22. Swift SE, Morris S, McKinnie V. Validation of a simplified technique for using the POP-Q pelvic organ prolapse quantification system. Int Urogynecol J Pelvic Floor Dysfunct. 2006;17:615–20.

General Complications of Pelvic Reconstructive Surgery

2

Ellen R. Solomon and Matthew D. Barber

Assessing Perioperative Risk

Before a patient undergoes pelvic reconstructive surgery, the risk of potential complications should be carefully assessed and addressed with the patient. Complications may occur during or after the procedure and it is imperative to recognize high-risk patients and minimize risk from surgery before a patient is brought to the operating room. The lifetime risk of a woman undergoing prolapse or incontinence surgery by the age of 80 is 11.1% [1]. The prevalence of perioperative complications among women undergoing reconstructive pelvic surgery has been reported to be as high as 33% [2]. There are a multitude of factors which are found to increase perioperative risk. A large retrospective cohort study including 1,931 women who had undergone prolapse surgery found an overall complication rate of 14.9% [3]. The complications identified included infection, bleeding, surgical injuries, pulmonary, and cardiovascular morbidity. These complications were associated with medical comorbidities (odds ratio 11.2) and concomitant hysterectomy (odds ratio 1.5). Risk factors for complications after pelvic reconstructive surgery are listed in Table 2.1.

E.R. Solomon, MD • M.D. Barber, MD, MHS (✉)
Obstetrics, Gynecology and Women's Health Institute,
Cleveland Clinic, Cleveland Clinic Main Campus,
Mail Code A81, 9500 Euclid Avenue,
Cleveland, OH 44195, USA
e-mail: barberm2@ccf.org

Obesity is an increasingly important risk factor for perioperative complications. The prevalence of obesity continues to rise in industrialized countries [4]. With obesity, there is an increase in comorbid conditions including incidence of cardiac disease, type two diabetes, hypertension, stroke, sleep apnea, and some cancers [5]. One study of obese and overweight women found that obese women had significantly increased estimated blood loss and operative time [6]. In a retrospective cohort study from 2007, obese patients who underwent vaginal surgery were matched to patients who were of normal weight and perioperative comorbidities and complications were analyzed. This study found that there was no difference in perioperative complications between obese and nonobese patients; however, there was a higher rate of surgical site infection in the obese population [7].

In obese women undergoing hysterectomy, the abdominal approach results in significantly higher rates of wound infection than those receiving a vaginal hysterectomy [8]. Overall, vaginal surgery appears to be a safer approach for obese women [9]. It is important to assess BMI when planning route of surgery and to consider the increased risks with this population.

Age is also an important factor to consider when assessing perioperative risk. The median age of patients who undergo pelvic reconstructive surgery is 61.5 years [10]. Increasing age corresponds with increasing medical comorbidities including chronic illness, hypertension, coronary heart disease, diabetes, pulmonary

H.B. Goldman (ed.), *Complications of Female Incontinence and Pelvic Reconstructive Surgery*,
Current Clinical Urology, DOI 10.1007/978-1-61779-924-2_2, © Springer Science+Business Media, LLC 2013

Table 2.1 General risk factors of pelvic reconstructive surgery

Risk factors
Age
Central nervous system disease
Coronary heart disease
Diabetes
Hypertension
Obesity
Peripheral artery disease
Pulmonary disease

disease, and central nervous system disease [11]. A retrospective cohort study of 264,340 women undergoing pelvic surgery found that increasing age is associated with higher mortality risks and higher complication risks. Specifically, elderly women (>age 80) were found to have increased risk of perioperative complications compared with younger women [12]. In this same study, elderly women who underwent obliterative procedures (e.g., colpocleisis) had a lower risk of complications compared to patients who underwent reconstructive procedures for prolapse. In a prospective study of 2-year postoperative survival, survival was worse among 80-year-olds who experienced a postoperative complication [13]. In a retrospective chart review of patients ≥75 years old, 25.8% of patients had significant perioperative complications including significant blood loss, pulmonary edema, and congestive heart failure. Independent risk factors that were predictive of perioperative complications in this patient population included length of surgery, coronary artery disease, and peripheral vascular disease [14]. When choosing to perform a prolapse or incontinence procedure on an elderly patient, it is important to review the patient's comorbidities.

Cardiac risk factors also impact postoperative morbidity in pelvic surgery. In a retrospective cohort study by Heisler et al. [15], perioperative complications were increased in patients with a history of myocardial infarction or congestive heart failure, perioperative hemoglobin decrease greater than 3.1 g/dL, preoperative hemoglobin less than 12.0 g/L, or history of prior thrombosis. In a retrospective analysis of cardiac

comorbidities in pelvic surgery by Schakelford et al. [16], hypertension and ischemic heart disease were statistically significant risk factors for perioperative cardiac morbidity. It is important to ensure that a patient's cardiac status is optimized prior to proceeding with surgery [17]. In a retrospective cohort study of 4,315 patients undergoing elective major noncardiac surgery, predictors of major cardiac complications included high-risk types of surgeries, history of ischemic heart disease, history of congestive heart failure, history of cerebrovascular disease, preoperative treatment with insulin, and a serum creatinine of ≥2.0 mg/dL [18]. To further decrease cardiac morbidity in patients undergoing surgery, it has also been shown that continuing beta blockers in the perioperative period in patients with chronic beta blockade will decrease cardiovascular mortality [19]. Consultation with the patient's primary care physician or cardiologist prior to surgery is often warranted in patients with cardiac disease.

In conclusion, when considering pelvic reconstructive surgery, it is important to examine and evaluate the whole patient, including her medical comorbidities in order to appropriately assess her perioperative risk. This knowledge will help determine whether or not surgery is appropriate and, when appropriate, what route of surgery and procedure may be best for the individual patient. In high-risk patients, the vaginal route is often the lowest risk approach. In elderly patients no longer interested in sexual activity, obliterative procedures should be considered because of their quick surgical times and low risk of complications relative to reconstructive procedures.

Venous Thromboembolism

Deep venous thrombosis (DVT) and pulmonary embolism (PE), jointly referred to as venous thromboembolism (VTE), are among the leading causes of preventable perioperative morbidity and mortality. In the perioperative period, the risk of death after VTE is approximately 3–4% [20]. During surgery, the combination of epithelial damage, venous stasis, and hypercoagulability, collectively referred to as Virchow's triad, increases the risk of any patient undergoing surgery. Many pelvic reconstructive surgeries require the dorsal lithotomy position and steep Trendelenberg; positions that exacerbate the risk of venous stasis. The postoperative risk of VTE may be elevated up to 1 year after the initial procedure has been performed, but is highest in the immediate perioperative period [21].

The risk of VTE has been well studied in the general surgery, urology, and gynecologic oncology population. However, there have been few studies that address the risk of VTE in women undergoing pelvic reconstructive surgery. The data that does exist suggests that the risk of VTE is low after pelvic reconstructive procedures and that sequential compression devices used in the perioperative period are adequate prophylaxis in the majority of patients. In a retrospective cohort study of 1,104 patients who underwent prolapse and/or incontinence procedures by Solomon et al. [22], the incidence of VTE was found to be 0.3% (95% confidence interval, 0.1–0.8). Risk factors assessed for VTE among this patient population included histories of malignancy, breast cancer, hormone replacement therapy, oral contraceptive use, history of tamoxifen use, history of clotting disorder, decreased mobility in the perioperative period, and perioperative central line placement. There were no significant risk factors associated with VTE in this population. The only thromboprophylaxis used in this population were sequential compression devices placed before surgery and used until the patient returned home.

In another retrospective cohort study of 1,356 patients undergoing sling and/or prolapse procedures, the rate of VTE was 0.9% in women who had a sling alone and 2.2% in women who had concomitant prolapse surgery ($P=0.05$) [23]. While this study gives rise to concern of concomitant procedures, it remains unclear if any of the patients received thromboprophylaxis during this study, and therefore it is difficult to assess actual patient risk. In a retrospective review by Nick et al. [24], the incidence of DVT was assessed among patients who underwent laparoscopic gynecologic surgery and found to be 0.7% in this population.

A number of risk factors for VTE have been suggested for women undergoing pelvic surgery. In a retrospective review of 1,232 patients who underwent surgery for gynecologic conditions in Japan, it was found that malignancy, history of VTE, age greater than 50, and allergic-immunologic disease were all statistically significant risk factors for VTE [25]. However, this study only found three episodes of VTE in patients with benign disease making it significantly underpowered for this patient group. In a questionnaire study by Lindqvist et al. [26] that included 40,000 women, it was found that moderate drinkers and women who engaged in strenuous exercise most days were at half the risk of VTE compared to women who were heavy smokers and lead sedentary lifestyles (increased risk of 30%).

In a retrospective review of gynecologic surgery patients, 1,862 patients given VTE prophylaxis with intermittent compression devices alone, the incidence of VTE was 1.3%. The risk factors associated with VTE were diagnosis of cancer, age over 60, anesthesia over 3 h. Patients with two or three of these variables had a 3.2% incidence of developing VTE vs. 0.6% in patients with zero or one risk factor [27].

The question of which thromboprophylactic modality is best in the perioperative period is difficult to answer for women undergoing pelvic reconstructive surgery. As mentioned previously, in the study by Solomon et al. [22], the rate of VTE among patients who underwent pelvic reconstructive surgery was 0.3% where the only thromboprophylaxis used was sequential compression devices placed during the perioperative period. The American College of Obstetricians and Gynecologists [28] follow the recommendations provided by the American College of Chest Physicians from the Seventh ACCP Conference on Antithrombotic and Thrombolytic Therapy, published in 2004. The recommendations place patients into four risk categories including low, moderate, high, and highest risk (Table 2.2). The ACCP has updated its recommendations for prophylaxis in all surgical patients. Most female pelvic reconstructive surgery patients fall into the "high" risk category; however, because the rate of VTE is so low in this population, it is unknown

Table 2.2 American College of Chest physicians risk for venous thromboembolism in patients undergoing surgery

Level of risk	Definition[a]	Recommended prevention strategy
Low	Minor surgery	No specific thromboprophylaxis besides early and frequent mobilization
Moderate	Major surgery includes most general, open gynecologic and urologic cases	LMWH, LDUH bid or tid, fondaparinux, or mechanical thromboprophylaxis
High	Major surgery, or patients with additional VTE risk factors[b]	LMWH, fondaparinux, oral vitamin K antagonist, or mechanical prophylaxis; alternatively, one may consider combination of chemical and mechanical prophylaxis

Modified with permission from Geerts et al. [97]
Adapted from Solomon [96]
Bid twice daily; *LDUH* low-dose unfractionated heparin; *LMWH* low-molecular-weight heparin; *tid* three times daily; *VTE* venous thromboembolic events
[a]Descriptive terms are purposely left undefined to allow individual clinician interpretation
[b]Additional risk factors include major trauma or lower extremity injury, immobility, cancer, cancer therapy, venous compression (from tumor, hematoma, arterial anomaly), previous VTE, increasing age, pregnancy and postpartum period, estrogen-containing oral contraceptive or hormone replacement therapy, selective estrogen receptor modulators, erythropoiesis-stimulating agents, acute medical illness, inflammatory bowel disease, nephritic syndrome, myeloproliferative disorders, paroxysmal nocturnal hemoglobinuria, obesity, central venous catheterization, and inherited or acquired thrombophilia

which form of thromboprophylaxis is the best method to use. In a study performed by Montgomery and colleagues, a prospective randomized trial was performed to assess thromboprophylaxis using SCDs vs. fractionated heparin on urological laparoscopic patients. In both groups, the rate of VTE was 1.2%, but the rate of hemorrhagic complications was significantly higher in the fractionated heparin group (9.3%). As of now, there are no specific guidelines for thromboprophylaxis for patient undergoing pelvic reconstructive procedures. *When operating on women who have multiple risk factors for VTE, it would be judicious to consider chemothromboprophylaxis. Otherwise, without inciting risk factors, sequential compression devices may be the only thromboprophylaxis needed.*

It is essential to be able to recognize the symptoms of VTE in the postoperative patient. While many patients who have VTE may be asymptomatic, the symptoms of dyspnea, orthopnea, hemoptysis, calf pain, complaints of calf swelling, chest pain, and tachypnea may signify a thrombotic event [29]. The physical signs that suggest VTE include hypotension, tachycardia, crackles, decreased breath sounds, lower extremity edema, tenderness in lower extremities, and hypoxia [30]. Although the signs and symptoms of VTE are well known, it is difficult to rule out

VTE by clinical diagnosis alone. A systematic review evaluating the D-dimer test used in combination with clinical probability to rule out VTE found that the D-dimer test is a safe and relatively reliable first-line test to use. After a 3-month follow-up, only 0.46% of patients were later diagnosed with PE [31]. However, D-dimer test is not useful in pregnant patients, the elderly, and hospitalized patients due to decreased specificity [32].

Compression ultrasonography is a noninvasive, easy, and cost-effective procedure for the diagnosis of DVT in the lower extremities. The sensitivity and specificity for detecting DVT using compression ultrasonography in symptomatic patients is 89–96%, although the sensitivity is decreased in patients with calf DVT or asymptomatic patients [33]. Compression ultrasonography may also be used in conjunction with other diagnostic tests if PE is suspected [34]. If compression ultrasound is negative but patient remains symptomatic, venography may be used to further rule out DVT [35].

Indicated imaging for patients presenting with signs and symptoms of PE include ventilation perfusion scanning (V/Q), computed tomography (CT) pulmonary angiography, and spiral CT of the chest. The V/Q scan was the imaging modality of choice for decades; however, due to lack of ease of use and potential for indeterminate testing, CT has become the modality of choice [33]. CT angiography has specificity of 96% as well as 83% sensitivity [29]. This has become the gold standard for PE diagnosis. CT looking for PE may vary across centers due to type of CT used and radiologist's ability to make the diagnosis.

It is important to start anticoagulation immediately once VTE has been diagnosed; furthermore, if there is high suspicion for PE, anticoagulation may be started even before the diagnosis is confirmed. Acute PE should be treated initially with a rapid onset anticoagulant which may be followed by treatment with a vitamin K antagonist for at least 3 months [31]. For rapid onset anticoagulation, patients may be started on IV unfractionated heparin, subcutaneous unfractionated heparin, subcutaneous low molecular weight heparin, and subcutaneous fondaparinux. The American College of Chest Physicians recommends using subcutaneous low molecular weight heparin for the initial treatment of acute, nonmassive, PE. If the patient has decreased kidney function, morbid obesity, or is pregnant, IV unfractionated heparin may be used due to its shorter duration and titratability [36]. Once anticoagulation therapy has been established, the patient may continue on subcutaneous therapy or can be bridged to warfarin for at least 3 months. Warfarin may be more acceptable to patients because of its oral route and ease of use; however, warfarin requires continuous monitoring and titration [37]. If the patient has contraindications to anticoagulation therapy, an inferior vena cava (IVC) filter can be considered.

Pulmonary Complications

Postoperative pulmonary complications are a frequent cause of morbidity and mortality. Postoperative pneumonia, atelectasis, pneumothorax, and respiratory failure are postoperative complications that increase length of stay and are more common than postoperative cardiac complications [38]. The incidence of postoperative pulmonary complications in gynecologic patients has been reported to be between 1.22 and 2.16% [39]. There are multiple risk factors that may increase pulmonary complications in the postoperative surgical patient. In a prospective randomized trial of patients who underwent non-thoracic, on multivariate analysis four risk factors for postoperative pulmonary complications were age greater than 65, positive "cough test", perioperative nasogastric tube, and duration of anesthesia (procedures lasting longer than 2.5 h) [40]. A retrospective review of patients undergoing gynecologic laparoscopy found that operative time greater than 200 min and age greater than 65 contributed to hypercarbia. Predictors of the development of pneumothorax included pneumoperitoneum CO_2 pressure greater than 50 mmHg and operative time greater than 200 min [41].

Surgical approach is also a contributing factor for the development of a postoperative pulmonary complication. A study of patients undergoing abdominal surgery found that age greater than 60, smoking history within the past 8 weeks, body mass index greater than or equal to 27, history of cancer, and incision site in the upper abdomen or both upper/lower abdominal incision were identified as independent risk factors for postoperative pulmonary complications [42].

In a prospective randomized control trial involving 994 patients by Xue et al. [43], patients were divided into three groups (1) elective superficial plastic surgery, (2) upper abdominal surgery, and (3) thoracoabdominal surgery. It was found that the incidence of hypoxemia in the postoperative period was closely related to the operative site, where upper abdominal and thoracoabdominal sites gave the greatest risk. When evaluating this study, patients undergoing pelvic reconstructive surgery would most likely fall into the low-risk category similar to elective superficial plastic surgery, with a low risk of hypoxemia in the postoperative period.

Another risk factor associated with postoperative pulmonary complications is smoking. In a prospective cohort study of patients referred for nonthoracic surgery, the risk for postoperative pulmonary complications was increased by age of greater than 65 years or more and smoking of 40 pack-years or more [39]. In a retrospective review performed on 635,265 patients from the American College of Surgeons National Surgical Quality Improvement Program database, current smokers had increased odds of postoperative pneumonia and unplanned intubation [44]. Pulmonary complications significantly decrease after 8 weeks of smoking cessation [45]. Chronic obstructive pulmonary disease patients are at increased risk of having postoperative pulmonary complications. Preoperative pulmonary function tests may help to identify patients with increased pulmonary risk [46]. Patients with COPD were found to be 300–700 times more likely to have a postoperative pulmonary complication in a prospective cohort study [39]. Nasogastric intubation instead of orogastric intubation increases risk of pneumonia in this patient population as well [47].

Sleep apnea is an additional risk factor for postoperative pulmonary complications. Obstructive sleep apnea is defined as partial or complete obstruction of the upper airway during sleep [48]. The prevalence of sleep apnea is around 5% [49]. In an additional study evaluating the prevalence of sleep apnea in the general surgery population, 22% of surgical patients were found to have obstructive sleep apnea [50]. Therefore, we can hypothesize that obstructive sleep apnea is a prevalent and important risk factor for postoperative pulmonary complications in our population as well. In a retrospective cohort study of orthopedic and general surgery patients by Memtsoudis et al. [51], 51,509 patients with sleep apnea who underwent general surgery procedures were assessed for postoperative pulmonary complications. It was found that patients with sleep apnea developed pulmonary complications more frequently than their matched controls. Due to relaxation of the pharyngeal muscles from anesthetic agents, sedatives, and opioids, patients with obstructive sleep apnea may have increased airway collapse in the postoperative period [52]. The supine position that occurs during surgery and in the postoperative period may worsen obstructive sleep apnea [53]. Anesthesia may also blunt the hypercapnic and hypoxic

respiratory drive as well as the arousal response. In a study performed by Bolden et al. [54], the frequency of postoperative hypoxemia was measured in OSA patients in the postoperative period where 16% of the patients studied found multiple measured postoperative desaturations.

To avoid hypoxemia in OSA patients, it is necessary to encourage patients to bring in their home continuous positive airway pressure (CPAP) machines or to order home CPAP settings for the hospital machines. Careful evaluation of the patient is essential to preventing postoperative complications. If a patient is suspected to have OSA but has not been diagnosed, it is useful to place the patient under continuous pulse oxygen saturation monitoring for the first 24 h after surgery [48].

Atelectasis and hypoxemia are common after surgery especially surgeries that involve the abdomen or thorax. Early on, atelectasis may result from soft tissue edema from the upper pharynx due to intubation and tongue manipulation. Later, especially in patients who have undergone abdominal surgery, there is decreased ability to take in deep breaths or cough due to postoperative pain. Postoperative patients have decreased functional residual capacity [55]. These factors lead to hypoventilation. Diagnosis of atelectasis may be made clinically and/or via imaging tests. Atelectasis may present as postoperative fever, decreased breath sounds at the lung bases, and can be found on chest-X-ray or CT.

Pre- and postoperative incentive spirometry are the most common prevention and treatment intervention for atelectasis. Incentive spirometry used in the perioperative period enhances postoperative functional residual capacity and reminds patients to continue to take in large breaths. If patient becomes hypoxic from atelectasis, bronchoscopy may be performed to remove secretions from the airway [56]. Continuous positive airway pressure (CPAP) can be used in the postoperative period and has also been shown to decrease intubation in patients who are at high risk of hypoxemia from atelectasis after abdominal surgery [57].

Postoperative pneumonia is a common postoperative pulmonary complication. Hospital-acquired pneumonia refers to pneumonia that develops after 48 h in the hospital. Diagnosing postoperative pneumonia can be difficult. Infiltrates from atelectasis, pulmonary edema, and acute lung injury can all look identical to pneumonia on chest X-ray. Diagnosis should be suspected if patient has new onset fever, purulent sputum, leukocytosis, hypoxemia, and infiltrate on chest X-ray (American Thoracic Society, 2002) [58]. In a prospective case series of patients presenting with postoperative pneumonia within 14 days of surgery, 61% of patients developed pneumonia within the first 5 days postoperatively. The most common etiologic agents were *Staphylococcus aureas*, *Streptococci*, and *Enterobacter* [59].

Treatment of postoperative pneumonia should begin with broad spectrum antibiotics given the polymicrobial nature of hospital-acquired pneumonia. Recommendations by the American Thoracic Society and the Infectious Disease Society of America include coverage for aerobic bacteria as well as anaerobic coverage. Most hospitals have guidelines for treating hospital-acquired pneumonia based on regional microbial infection.

Urinary Tract Infection

Urinary tract infections (UTIs) are one of the most common infections seen in the postoperative period. The incidence of UTIs rises with increasing age. Eighty percent of UTIs are caused by bladder instrumentation, with catheter-associated UTI (CAUTI) being most common [60]. The rate of bacteriuria after undergoing an anti-incontinence procedure has been estimated to be between 17 and 85% [61]. Reconstructive pelvic surgery almost always involves bladder instrumentation via cystoscopy and/or catheter placement, thereby increasing the risk of UTI in these patients. Additional risk factors for UTI include inefficient bladder emptying, pelvic relaxation, neurogenic bladder, asymptomatic bacteriuria, decreased ability to get to the toilet, nosocomial infections, physiologic changes, and sexual intercourse, all seen commonly in the reconstructive pelvic surgery population [62]. Development of a

fever in the postoperative period after female pelvic reconstruction should warrant a urinary tract evaluation; however, it is rare that lower UTI causes fever in itself.

There have been multiple trials evaluating risk of UTI after urogynecological procedures including the SISTEr trial of Burch vs. autologous sling for treatment of stress urinary incontinence, where the reported rate of UTI was 48% in the sling cohort and 32% in the Burch cohort during the first 24 months of follow-up [63]. In a case–control study of women undergoing surgery for stress urinary incontinence and/or pelvic organ prolapse, 9% of women developed UTI and the risk of UTI was significantly increased by previous history of chronic or multiple UTIs, prolonged duration of catheterization, and increased distance between the urethra and anus [64].

Signs and symptoms of UTI in women are varied. Common cystitis symptoms include frequency, urgency, nocturia, dysuria, suprapubic discomfort, hematuria, and occasional mild incontinence. Fever, chills, general malaise, and costovertebral angle tenderness are associated with upper UTI [61]. There are multiple ways to diagnose UTI. Urine dipstick testing can detect the presence of leukocytes, bacteria, nitrates, and red blood cells. It also measures glucose, protein, ketones, blood, and bilirubin. In the office, the dipstick test can be used as a rapid diagnostic test. It can measure leukesterase, nitrates, hematuria, and pyuria. In the setting of leukocytosis, and/or nitrites and hematuria, the sensitivity to detect UTI is 75%, but the specificity is 66% with a positive predictive value of 81% and a negative predictive value of 57% [65]. The most important predictor of UTI measured by microscopy is leukocytosis; however, leukocytosis alone is not sufficient to diagnose UTI [66]. The gold standard to diagnosing UTI is a urine culture. The traditional diagnosis of UTI by culture is greater than 100,000 colony forming units/mL (CFU); however, many women may have asymptomatic bacteriuria. In a study performed by Schiotz [67], 193 women who underwent gynecologic surgery and had a Foley catheter for 24 h were assessed for bacteriuria; 40.9% of

Table 2.3 American Urological Association recommended antimicrobial prophylaxis for urologic procedures

Procedures	Organisms	Antimicrobials of choice	Alternative antimicrobials	Duration of therapy
Vaginal surgery and/or slings	E. coli, Proteus sp., Klebsiella sp., Enterococcus, skin flora, and Group B Strep.	First/second-generation cephalosporin	Ampicillin/sulbactam	≤24 h
		Aminoglycoside + metronidazole or clindamycin	Fluroquinolone	

Modified from AUA Best Practice Guidelines [71]

patients had asymptomatic bacteruria, while only 8.3% of patients actually developed UTI. In contrast, those with fewer than 100,000 CFU but symptoms of UTI can also be appropriately diagnosed as having a UTI.

The most common pathogen causing complicated and uncomplicated UTI is E. coli. The definition of complicated UTI is associated with a condition that increases the risk of acquiring infection or failing first-line treatment. Many patients with pelvic floor disorders with UTI may fit into the complicated category because they are status/postcatheterization and procedures [68]. Other uropathogens include Klebsiella, Pseudomonas, Enterobacter, Enterococcus, and Candida. The initial therapy for treatment of UTI traditionally has been Trimethoprim-Sulfamethozole (TMP-SMX) if the resistance in the population is less than 20%. However, due to empiric treatment of UTIs in the past, resistance for TMP-SMX and amoxicillin is high and has been reported to be up to 54% for TMP-SMX and 46% for penicillins. Nitrofurantoin has been well studied and is an additional agent used frequently to treat UTIs. It is a cost-effective agent that may be used in the setting of fluroquinolone and TMP-SMX resistance [69]. *When treating a postoperative reconstructive patient, it is important to evaluate the antimicrobiogram in the specific hospital setting and to prescribe accordingly.*

It is clear that patients who undergo female pelvic reconstructive procedures require antibiotics prophylaxis at the time of the procedure [70]. The American Urologic Association Best Practice Guidelines [71] recommend antibiotic prophylaxis for vaginal surgery to prevent both postoperative UTI and postoperative pelvic infection (Table 2.3). A prospective randomized trial by

Ingber et al. [72] found that patients who were given single-dose antibiotic therapy for midurethral slings had a low rate of postoperative UTI (5.9%). An additional prospective randomized control trial found that patients who received multiple doses of antibiotics in the perioperative period had decreased postoperative febrile morbidity and significantly decreased hospital stays than patients who did not receive antibiotics [73]. What is unclear is the need for prophylactic antibiotics beyond the perioperative period in patients who will require prolonged catheterization. In a randomized, double blind controlled trial by Rogers et al. [70], 449 patients who underwent pelvic organ prolapse and/or stress urinary incontinence surgery and had suprapubic catheters placed were given either placebo or nitrofurantoin monohydrate daily while the catheter was in place to assess rate of UTI. The study found that there was a significant decrease in positive urine cultures, as well as symptomatic UTI at suprapubic catheter removal with nitrofurantoin prophylaxis; however, there was no difference in symptomatic UTIs at the 6–8 week postoperative visit. Little data exists on the role of prophylactic antibiotics for patients with postoperative indwelling transurethral catheters.

Surgical Site Infections

Infection complicating pelvic surgery can occur in three different settings (1) fever of unknown origin, (2) operative site infection, and (3) infection remote from surgery. The pathological source of most surgical site infections is from bacteria located on the skin or in the vagina. Skin flora is usually aerobic gram positive *cocci*, but may include gram negative, anaerobic, and/or fecal flora if incisions are made near the perineum and groin [74]. Pelvic reconstructive surgery almost always involves the vagina and perineum and therefore places all of our patients at increased risk for surgical site infections. Other patient comorbidities that may increase the risk of surgical site infections include advanced age, obesity, medical conditions, cancer, smoking, malnutrition, and immunosuppressant use [75, 76]. Other risk factors for surgical site infection include poor hemostasis, length of stay, length of operative time, and tissue trauma. Specific risk factors for obese patients include increased bacterial growth on skin, decreased vascularity in the subcutaneous tissue, increased tension on wound closure due to increased intra-abdominal pressure, decreased tissue concentrations of prophylactic antibiotics, and a higher prevalence of diabetes with poor glucose control and longer operating time [77]. In a retrospective chart review of patients who underwent midline abdominal incisions, patients with increased subcutaneous fat were 1.7 times more likely to develop a superficial incisional infection [78]. In a prospective study of 5,279 patient who underwent hysterectomy, it was found that obese patients who underwent abdominal hysterectomy were five times more likely to have wound infection. Route of surgery was an additional risk factor for infection with the highest risk in patients who underwent abdominal hysterectomy. Patients who underwent laparoscopic or vaginal hysterectomy were more likely to have remote pelvic infections compared with abdominal hysterectomy [76].

Use of synthetic mesh may be an additional risk factor for surgical site infection. There have been multiple case studies describing mesh infection. In one retrospective case study of patients who had undergone abdominal sacrocolpopexy, 27% of patients who underwent hysterectomy at the time of sacrocolpopexy became infected requiring mesh removal vs. 1.3% of patients in the same study that had undergone sacrocolpopexy alone [79]. In an additional case series of 19 women who had undergone intravaginal slingplasty with synthetic mesh, 6 women had infected mesh that had to be removed [80]. In randomized trials comparing native tissue vaginal repair to transvaginal mesh placement using wide-pore [81] polypropylene, the risk of infection appears to be low in some trials and elevated in others [82]; however, many of these studies are small and are not adequately powered to detect differences in infectious morbidity.

Diagnosis of surgical site infection includes pain and tenderness at the operative site and fever. Fever is defined as a temperature of greater than 38 °C on two or more occasions occurring at least 4 h apart [83]. Skin erythema, induration, and/or drainage of purulent or serosanguinous fluid may be visualized on examination. On pelvic exam, there may be pelvic, vaginal cuff, or parametrial tenderness. There may be a leukocytosis on complete blood count [82]. If pelvic abscess is suspected, ultrasound, CT scan, or MRI may be used for diagnosis. Ultrasound is a cost-effective way to image a patient with a suspected abscess. The sensitivity and specificity of pelvic ultrasound to look for pelvic abscess is 81% and 91%, respectively [84]. Computed tomography may be used to diagnose pelvic abscess when the diagnosis by ultrasound is equivocal. However, computed tomography increases exposure to ionizing radiation which may be problematic in younger patients.

Patients with superficial wound cellulitis may be treated with oral therapy. If there is evidence of a wound seroma or hematoma, a small portion of the wound may be opened and/or evacuated. It is important to probe the wound to insure the fascia is intact [85]. It may be necessary to remove staples and sutures in the infected area. Admission is recommended if a patient is febrile, has signs of peritonitis, has failed oral agents, has evidence of a pelvic or intra-abdominal abscess, is unable to tolerate oral intake, or has laboratory evidence of sepsis [82]. Patients requiring admission should receive broad spectrum parenteral antibiotics. Pelvic abscess may need drainage via opening of the vaginal cuff, CT, or ultrasound-guided drainage [86]. A vaginal cuff abscess may necessitate opening part of or, in some cases, the entire cuff to allow for sufficient drainage. If mesh has been placed, it may need to be removed if

Table 2.4 Recommended antibiotic prophylaxis by American College of Obstetrics and Gynecology

Procedures	Antibiotic	Dose (single dose)
Hysterectomy, female pelvic reconstructive procedures, procedures involving mesh	Cefazolin[a] Clindamycin plus gentamicin or quinolone or aztreonam Metronidazole plus gentamicin or quinolone	1 or 2 g IV 600 mg IV with 1.5 mg/kg or 400 mg IV 1 g IV 500 mg IV with 1.5 mg/kg or 400 mg IV

Modified from ref. [74]

IV intravenously; *g* grams; *mg* milligrams

[a]Alternatives include cefotetan, cefoxitin, cefurtoxime, or ampicillin-sulbactam

directly involved with the infection in order to achieve adequate resolution.

Prevention of wound infection is paramount to the practice of reconstructive pelvic surgery. Good surgical technique, hemostasis, and gentle tissue handling may decrease risk of infection [84]. There have been multiple studies that suggest perioperative cleansing the vagina with saline increases infection rate [87, 88]. Currently, there is no evidence to suggest that cleansing the vagina with any preparation reduces postoperative infection.

The use of prophylactic antibiotics is an imperative strategy for lowering surgical site infection. Antibiotics should be given within 30 min of incision time to allow for the minimal inhibitory concentrations (MIC) of the drug to be in the skin and tissues at time of incision. Recommendations for prophylactic antibiotic regimens from the AUA and ACOG are listed in Tables 2.3 and 2.4. Cephalosporins are commonly used in pelvic surgery because of their broad antimicrobial spectrum with Cefazolin, the most commonly used agent [73]. Patients who are morbidly obese with BMI greater than 35 should receive increased dosing of antibiotics [74]. Procedures lasting longer than 3 h and blood loss greater than 1,500 cc require redosing of antibiotics.

Nerve Injury

Intraoperative nerve injury is a preventable iatrogenic complication. Injury to nerves in the upper and lower extremities, while uncommon, may occur during laparotomy, robotic, laparoscopic, and vaginal procedures. In a prospective cohort study of women who underwent elective gynecologic surgery, the overall incidence of postoperative neuropathy was 1.8% [89]. Brachial plexus injury has a reported incidence of 0.16% [90]. Risk factors for developing nerve injuries during surgery include increased operating room time, patient positioning, and history of smoking [91]. Stretching or direct compression of the nerve results in ischemia, and when prolonged, necrosis can develop [92]. With muscle relaxants given during anesthesia, patients are unable to reposition themselves from nonphysiologic positions, and risk of nerve damage increases. With nerve compression, blood flow to the nerve is decreased, therefore operating room time is a critical factor for nerve injury. The longer a patient is incorrectly positioned, the worse the nerve injury. With the development of robotic surgery, it has been theorized that brachial plexus injuries may become more common [93]. Most robotic procedures require steep Trendelenberg positioning, and depending on the operator, may require longer operating room times. Other risk factors include history of diabetes, alcoholism, and history of herpes zoster [94].

Nerve injuries to the upper extremity mostly occur from overstretching or compression of the brachial plexus or the ulnar nerve. Brachial plexus injury may result in both sensory and/or motor injury. Risk factors for brachial plexus injury includes Trendelenberg positioning, longer operating room time, use of shoulder braces, abduction of the arm ≥90°, and unequal shoulder support [89]. Patients with brachial plexus injury may present with numbness of the first, second, and third digits and the radial side of the fourth digit. Patients may experience motor deficits that involve the shoulder, wrist, arm, and hand.

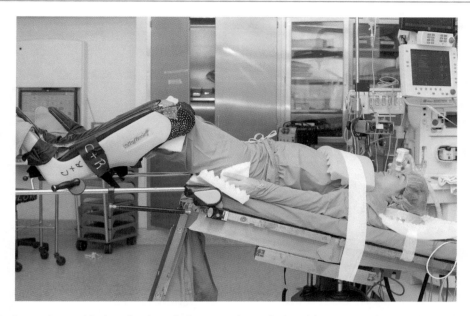

Fig. 2.1 Appropriate positioning of patients for laparoscopic or robotic pelvic reconstructive procedures with padding and taping to prevent neurologic injury

In severe cases, patients may experience Erb's palsy or Klumpke's paralysis [92]. Patients with ulnar nerve injury may present with the sensory loss of the lateral hand, with loss of sensation in the fourth and fifth digits.

Management of brachial plexus injury includes physical therapy, analgesics, nonsteroidal anti-inflammatory medications, physical therapy, and neuroleptic medications. Prevention of brachial plexus injury includes utilizing the minimum amount of Trendelenberg positioning, decreasing operating room times as much as possible, avoiding abduction or extension of the upper extremities, and avoiding shoulder braces [92]. For robotic and laparoscopic surgeries, we recommend padding and tucking the patient's arms to her sides, using a "thumbs up" hand position with the patient's palms facing her thighs to avoid overabduction. To avoid sliding down the operating room table while in Trendelenberg, placing the patient on an egg crate mattress that is taped to the operating room table and then padding the patient's chest with additional foam and tape the foam down to the operating room table can be helpful (Fig. 2.1).

Common lower extremity nerve injuries associated with female pelvic reconstructive medicine include femoral, lateral femoral cutaneous, obturator, sciatic, and common peroneal nerve injuries. Risk factors for lower extremity nerve injuries include ill positioning of the lower extremities using stirrups, lithotomy position, slender patients, smokers, Trendelenberg position, and operating room time greater than 4 h [95]. In laparoscopic and vaginal surgeries, the femoral nerve may be injured due to stretch encountered from the lithotomy position. The lateral cutaneous femoral nerve is one of the most common nerves injured from lithotomy position and injury is caused from compression and stretching under the inguinal ligament, most likely from prolonged flexion of the lower extremities. The obturator nerve may be injured from prolonged flexion of the legs in the lithotomy position. Sciatic nerve injury is less common in the dorsal lithotomy position; however, it may be caused by overflexion of the hip with abduction and external rotation. The common peroneal nerve can be injured via direct pressure on the nerve when legs are touching the pole of

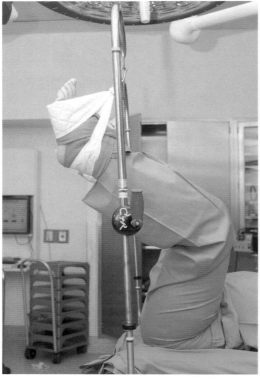

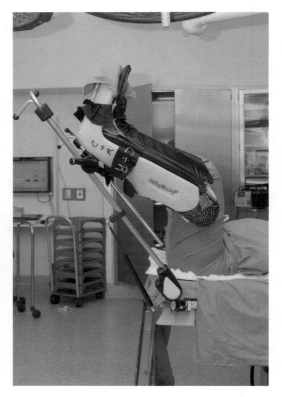

Fig. 2.2 Appropriate positioning of the lower extremities for dorsal lithotomy position using candy cane stirrups

Fig. 2.3 Appropriate positioning of the lower extremities for dorsal lithotomy position using Boot stirrups

Table 2.5 Motor and sensory defects associated with lower extremity neuropathy

Nerve	Motor function	Sensation
Femoral	Hip flexion and knee extension	Anterior and medial thigh, medial calf
Lateral femoral cutaneous	N/A	Anterior, and lateral thigh
Sciatic	Foot dorsiflexion and eversion	Foot, toes
Obturator	Thigh adduction and internal rotation	Medial aspect of the thigh
Common peroneal	Foot dorsiflexion and eversion	N/A

N/A not applicable

the candy cane stirrups—boot stirrups may aid in decreasing risk of injury to this nerve [94].

To prevent lower extremity neuropathies caused by female pelvic reconstructive surgery, it is necessary to utilize correct positioning of the lower extremities. Whenever possible, avoid candy can stirrups as they offer little support and may cause undue hip abduction and external rotation. When positioning the lower extremities in boot stirrups, make sure the heel of the patient's foot fits directly into the boot. Padding the lateral

aspect of the knee avoids injury to the peroneal nerve. When placing patient in high lithotomy, the knee should be flexed 90–120°, hip flexion should be less than 60°, and abduction of the thighs should be no greater than 90° (Figs. 2.2 and 2.3). Nerve injuries from reconstructive pelvic surgery are minimized when the patient's extremities are positioned correctly.

Diagnosis of postoperative neuropathy should include a thorough musculoskeletal and neurological exam (Table 2.5). Patient may also experience pain, numbness, and tingling in dermatomes of the nerve routes. EMG and MRI are procedures that may further aid in diagnosis. Treatment includes oral analgesics, nonsteroidal anti-inflammatory medications, low-dose anti-depressants, neurologic medications including gabapentin and pregabalin, and physical therapy, especially for prolonged neuropathies. Surgery and steroid injections may be used for severe cases [94].

References

1. Olsen AL, Smith VJ, Bergstrom JO, Colling JC, Clark AL. Epidemiology of surgically managed pelvic organ prolapse and urinary incontinence. Obstet Gynecol. 1997;89:501–6.
2. Lambrou NC, Buller JL, Thompson JR, Cundiff GW, Chou B, Montz FJ. Prevalence of perioperative complications among women undergoing reconstructive pelvic surgery. Am J Obstet Gynecol. 2000;183:1355–60.
3. Handa VL, Harvey L, Cundiff GW, Kjerulff KH. Perioperative complications of surgery for genital prolapse: does concomitant anti-incontinence surgery increase complications? Adult Urol. 2004;65:483–7.
4. National Task Force on the Prevention and Treatment of Obesity. Overweight, obesity, and health risk. Arch Intern Med. 2000;160:898–904.
5. Must A, Spandano J, Coakley EH, Field AE, Colditz G, Dietz WH. The disease burden associated with overweight and obesity. JAMA. 1999;282:1523–9.
6. Rogers RG, Lebkuchner U, Kammerer-Doak DN, Thompson PK, Walters MD, Nygaard IE. Obesity and retropubic surgery for stress incontinence: is there really an increased risk of intraoperative complications? Am J Obstet Gynecol. 2006;195:1794–8.
7. Chen CCG, Collins SA, Rodgers AK, Paraiso MFR, Walters MD, Barber MD. Perioperative complications in obese women vs normal-weight women who undergo vaginal surgery. Am J Obstet Gynecol. 2007;197:98.e1–8.
8. Pitkin RM. Vaginal hysterectomy in obese women. Obstet Gynecol. 1977;49:567–9.
9. Isik-Akbay EF, Harmanli OH, Panganamamula UR, Akbay M, Gaughan J, Chatwani AJ. Hysterectomy in obese women: a comparison of abdominal and vaginal routes. Obstet Gynecol. 2004;104:710–4.
10. Luber KM, Boero S, Choe JY. The demographics of pelvic floor disorders: current observations and future projections. Am J Obstet Gynecol. 2001;184:1496–503.
11. Toglia MR, Nolan TE. Morbidity and mortality rates of elective gynecologic surgery in the elderly woman. Am J Obstet Gynecol. 2003;189:1584–9.
12. Sung VW, Weitzen S, Sokol ER, Rardin CR, Myers DL. Effect of patient age on increasing morbidity and mortality following urogynecologic surgery. Am J Obstet Gynecol. 2006;194:1411–7.
13. Kawalpreet M, Bacchetti P, Leung JM. Prognostic significance of postoperative in-hospital complications in elderly patients. I. Long term survival. Anesth Analg. 2003;96:583–9.
14. Stepp KJ, Barber MD, Yoo EH, Whiteside JL, Paraiso MFR, Walters MD. Incidence of perioperative complications of urogynecologic surgery in elderly women. Am J Obstet Gynecol. 2005;192:1630–6.
15. Heisler CA, Aletti GD, Weaver AL, Melton LJ, Cliby WA, Gebhart JB. Improving quality of care: development of a risk-adjusted perioperative morbidity model for vaginal hysterectomy. Am J Obstet Gynecol. 2010;202:137.e1–5.
16. Schakelford DP, Hoffman MK, Kramer PR, Davies MF, Kaminiski PF. Evaluation of peroperative cardiac risk index values in patients undergoing vaginal surgery. Am J Obstet Gynecol. 1995;173:80–4.
17. Potyk D, Raudaskoski P. Peroperative cardiac evaluation for elective non cardiac surgery. Arch Fam Med. 1998;7:164–73.
18. Lee TH, Marcantonio ER, Mangione CM, Thomas EJ, Polanczyk CA, Cook EF, et al. Derivation and prospective validation of a simple index for prediction of cardiac risk of major noncardiac surgery. Circulation. 1999;100:1043–9.
19. Shammash JB, Trost JC, Gold JM, Berlin JA, Golden MA, Kimmel SE. Perioperative beta-blocker withdrawal and mortality in vascular surgical patients. Am Heart J. 2001;141:148–53.
20. Colwell CW, Collis DK, Paulson R, McCutchen JW, Bigler GT, Lutz S, et al. Comparison of enoxaparin and warfarin for the prevention of venous thromboembolic disease after total hip arthroplasty. J Bone Joint Surg Am. 1999;81:932–9.
21. Sweetland S, Green J, Liu B, et al. Duration and magnitude of the postoperative risk of venous thromboembolism in middle aged women: prospective cohort study. BMJ. 2009;339:1–8.
22. Solomon ER, Frick AC, Paraiso MFR, Barber MD. Risk of deep venous thrombosis and pulmonary embolism in urogynecologic surgical patients. Am J Obstet Gynecol. 2010;203:510.e1–4.
23. Anger JT, Weingberg AE, Gore JL, Wang Q, Pashos MJ, Leonardi LV, et al. Thromboembolic complications of sling surgery for stress urinary incontinence among female Medicare beneficiaries. Urology. 2009;74:1223–6.
24. Nick AM, Schmeler KM, Frumovitz MM, Soliman PT, Spannuth WA, Burzawa JK, et al. Risk of thromboembolic disease in patients undergoing laparoscopic gynecologic surgery. Obstet Gynecol. 2010;116(4):956–61.
25. Suzuki N, Yoshioka N, et al. Risk factors for perioperative venous thromboembolism: a retrospective study in Japanese women with gynecologic diseases. Thromb J. 2010;8:1–9.
26. Lindqvist PG, Epstein E, Olsson H. The relationship between lifestyle factors and venous thromboembolism among women: a report from the MISS study. Br J Haematol. 2008;114:234–40.
27. Clarke-Pearson DL, Dodge RK, Synan I, McClelland RC, Maxwell GL. Venous thromboembolism

prophylaxis: patients at high risk to fail intermittent pneumatic compression. Obstet Gynecol. 2003; 101(1):157–63.

28. ACOG Committee on Practice Bulletins No. 84: prevention of deep vein thrombosis and pulmonary embolism. 2007;84(2 Pt 1):429–40.

29. Okadome M, Saito T, et al. Postoperative pulmonary embolism including asymptomatic cases in gynecologic oncology. Int J Gynecol Cancer. 2010;20: 655–63.

30. Stein PD, Beemath A, Matta F, et al. Clinical characteristics of patients with acute pulmonary embolism: data from PIOPED II. Am J Med. 2007;120: 871–9.

31. Cate-Hoek AJT, Prins MH. Management studies using a combination of D-dimer test results and clinical probability to rule out venous thromboembolism: a systematic review. J Thromb Haemost. 2005;3: 2465–70.

32. Agnelli G, Becattini C. Acute pulmonary embolism. N Engl J Med. 2010;363:266–74.

33. Qaseem A, Snow V, et al. Current diagnosis of venous thromboembolism in primary care: a clinical practice guideline from the American Academy of Family Physicians and the American College of Physicians. Ann Intern Med. 2007;146:454–8.

34. Moores LK, King CS, Holley AB. Current approach to the diagnosis of acute nonmassive pulmonary embolism. Chest. 2011;140:509–18.

35. Krivak TC, Zorn KK. Venous thromboembolism in obstetrics and gynecology. Obstet Gynecol. 2007; 109:761–77.

36. Desciak MC, Martin DE. Perioperative pulmonary embolism: diagnosis and anesthetic management. J Clin Anesth. 2011;23:153–65.

37. Ansell J, Hirsch J, Hylek E, Jacobson A, Crowther M, Gualtiero P. Pharmacology and management of the vitamin K antagonists: American College of Chest Physicians Evidence-Based Clinical Practice Guidelines (8th edition). Chest. 2008;133:160S–98.

38. Lawrence VA, Hilsenbeck SG, Mulrow CD, Dhanda R, Sapp J, Page CP. Incidence and hospital stay for cardiac and pulmonary complications after abdominal surgery. J Gen Intern Med. 1995;10:671–8.

39. Pappachen S, Smith PR, Shah S, Brito V, Bader F, Koury B. Postoperative pulmonary complications after gynecologic surgery. Int J Obstet Gynecol. 2006;93:74–6.

40. McAlister FA, Bertsch K, Man J, Bradley J, Jacka M. Incidence of and risk factors for pulmonary complications after nonthoracic surgery. Am J Respir Crit Care Med. 2005;171:514–7.

41. Murdock CM, Wolff AJ, Van Geem T. Risk factors for hypercarbia, subcutaneous emphysema, pneumothorax and pneumomediastinum during laparoscopy. Obstet Gynecol. 2000;95:704–9.

42. Brooks-Brunn JA. Predictors of postoperative pulmonary complications following abdominal surgery. Chest. 1997;111:564–71.

43. Xue FS, Li BW, Zhang GS, Liao X, Zhang YM, Liu JH, et al. The influence of surgical sites on early postoperative hypoxemia in adults undergoing elective surgery. Anesth Analg. 1999;88:213–9.

44. Turan A, Mascha EJ, Roberman D, Turner PL, You J, Kurz A, et al. Smoking and perioperative outcomes. Anesthesiology. 2011;114(4):837–46.

45. Warner MA, Divertie MB, Tinker JH. Preoperative cessation of smoking and pulmonary complications in coronary artery bypass patients. Anesthesiology. 1984;60(4):380–3.

46. Doyle RL. Assessing and modifying the risk of postoperative pulmonary complications. Chest. 1999;115: 77S–81.

47. Ephgrave KS, Kleiman-Wexler R, Pfaller M, Booth B, Werkmeister L, Young S. Postoperative pneumonia: a prospective study of risk factors and morbidity. Surgery. 1993;114:815–21.

48. Adesanya AO, Lee W, Greilich NB, Joshi GP. Perioperative management of obstructive sleep apnea. Chest. 2010;138:1489–98.

49. Young T, Peppard PE, Gottlieb DJ. Epidemiology of obstructive sleep apnea. A population health perspective. Am J Respir Crit Care Med. 2002;165:1217–39.

50. Hwang D, Shakir N, Limann B, Sison C, Kaira S, Shulman L, et al. Association of sleep-disordered breathing with postoperative complications. Chest. 2008;133:1128–34.

51. Memtsoudis S, Liu SS, Ma Y, Chiu YL, Walz JM, Gaber-Baylis BA, et al. Perioperative pulmonary outcomes in patients with sleep apnea after noncardiac surgery. Anesth Analg. 2011;112:113–21.

52. Bolden N, Smith CE, Auckley D. Avoiding adverse outcomes in patients with obstructive sleep apnea (OSA): development and implementation of a perioperative OSA protocol. J Clin Anesth. 2009;21: 286–93.

53. Johnson MM, Conde MV. Overview of the management of postoperative pulmonary complications. In: Maneker S, editor. Waltham, MA, UpToDate; 2011.

54. Bolden N, Smith CE, Auckley D, Maraski J, Ramachangdra A. Perioperative complications during use of an obstructive sleep apnea protocol following surgery and anesthesia. Int Anesth Res Soc. 2007; 105:1869–70.

55. Wahba RM. Airway closure and intraoperative hypoxaemia: twenty-five years later. Can J Anaesth. 1996; 43:1144–9.

56. Barrett CR. Flexible fiberoptic bronchoscopy in the critically ill patient, methodology and indications. Chest. 1978;73:746–9.

57. Squadrone V, Coha M, Cerutti E, et al. Continuous positive airway pressure for treatment of postoperative hypoxemia. JAMA. 2005;293:589–95.

58. American Thoracic Society and the Infectious Diseases Society America. Guidelines for the management of adults with hospital-acquired, ventilator-associated, and healthcare-associated pneumonia. Am J Respir Crit Care Med. 2005;171(4):388–416.

59. Montavers P, Veber B, Auboyer C, Dupont H, Gauzit R, Korinek AM, et al. Diagnostic and therapeutic management of nosocomial pneumonia in surgical patients: results of the Eole study. Crit Care Med. 2002;30:368–75.

60. Lo E, Nocolle L, Classen D, et al. Strategies to prevent catheter-associated urinary tract infections in acute care hospitals. Infect Control Hosp Epidemiol. 2008;29:S41–50.

61. Nygaard IE, Kreder KJ. Complications of incontinence surgery. Int Urogynecol J. 1994;5:353–60.

62. Karram MM, Kleeman SD. Lower urinary tract infection. In: Walters M, Karram MM, editors. Urogynecology and reconstructive pelvic surgery. 3rd ed. Philadelphia: Mosby Elsevier; 2007. p. 413–24.

63. Albo ME, Richter HE, Brubaker L, Norton P, Kraus S, Zimmern PE, et al. Burch colposuspension versus fascial sling to reduce urinary stress incontinence. N Engl J Med. 2007;356:2143–55.

64. Sutkin G, Alperin M, Meyn L, Wiesenfeld HC, Ellison R, Zyczynski HM. Symptomatic urinary tract infections after surgery for prolapse and/or incontinence. Int Urogynecol J. 2010;21:955–61.

65. Little P, Moore MV, Turner S, Rumsby K, Warner G, Lowes JA, et al. Effectiveness of five different approaches in management of urinary tract infection: radomised controlled trial. BMJ. 2010;340:c199.

66. Komoroff AL. Urinalysis and urine culture in women with dysuria. Ann Intern Med. 1986;104:212–8.

67. Schiotz HA. Urinary tract infections and bacteriuria after gynecological surgery: experience with 24-hour Foley catheterization. Int Urogynecol J. 1994;5: 345–8.

68. Hooten TM, Stamm WE. Diagnosis and treatment of uncomplicated urinary tract infection. Infect Dis Clin North Am. 1997;11:551–81.

69. Mckinnell JA, Stollenwerk NS, Jung CW, Miller LG. Nitrofurantoin compares favorably to recommended agents as empirical treatment of uncomplicated urinary tract infections in a decision and cost analysis. Mayo Clin Proc. 2011;86(6):480–8.

70. Rogers RG, Kammerer-Doak D, Olsen A, Thompson PK, Walters MD, Lukacz ES, et al. A randomized, double-blind, placebo-controlled comparison of the effect of nitrofurantoin monohydrate macrocrystals on the development of urinary tract infections after surgery for pelvic organ prolapse and/or stress urinary incontinence with suprapubic catheterization. Am J Obstet Gynecol. 2004;191:182–7.

71. Wolf JS Jr, Bennett CJ, Dmochowski RR, Hollenbeck BK, Pearle MS, Schaeffer AJ. Urologic surgery antimicrobial prophylaxis best practice policy panel. J Urol. 2008;179(4):1379–90. Erratum in J Urol. 2008;180(5):2262–3.

72. Ingber MS, Vasavada SP, Firoozi F, Goldman HB. Incidence of perioperative urinary tract infection after single-dose antibiotic therapy for midurethral slings. Urology. 2010;76:830–4.

73. Bhatia NN, Karram MM, Bergman A. Role of antibiotic prophylaxis in retropubic surgery for stress urinary incontinence. Obstet Gynecol. 1989;74:637–9.

74. ACOG Committee on Practice Bulletins No. 104: antibiotic prophylaxis for gynecologic procedures. Obstet Gynecol. 2009;113(5):1180–9.

75. Walsh C, Scaife C, Hopf H. Prevention and management of surgical site infections in morbidly obese women. Obstet Gynecol. 2009;113:411–5.

76. Boesch CE, Umek W. Effects of wound closure on wound healing in gynecologic surgery. J Reprod Med. 2009;54:139–44.

77. Brummer THI, Jalkanen J, Fraser J, Heikkinine AM, Kauko M, Makinin J, et al. Prevention and management of surgical site infections in morbidly obese women. Hum Reprod. 2011;26:1741–51.

78. Lee JS, Terjimanian MD, Tishberg LM, Alawieh AZ, Harbaugh CM, Sheetz KH, et al. Surgical site infection and analytic morphometric assessment of body composition in patients undergoing midline laparotomy. J Am Coll Surg. 2011;213:237–44.

79. Mattox TF, Sanford EJ, Varner E. Infected abdominal sacrocolpopexies: diagnosis and treatment. Int Urogynecol J Pelvic Floor Dysfunct. 2004;15:319–23.

80. Baessler K, Hewson AD, Tunn R, Schuessler B, Maher CF. Severe mesh complications following intravaginal slingplasty. Obstet Gynecol. 2005;106: 713–6.

81. Hiltunen R, Nieminen K, Takula T, Heiskanen E, Merikari M, Niemi KI, et al. Low-weight polypropylene mesh for anterior vaginal wall prolapse. Obstet Gynecol. 2007;110:455–62.

82. Vakili B, Huynh T, Loesch H, Franco N, Chesson RR. Outcomes of vaginal reconstructive surgery with and without graft material. Am J Obstet Gynecol. 2005;193:2126–32.

83. Lazenby GB, Soper DE. Prevention, diagnosis, and treatment of gynecologic surgical site infections. Obstet Gynecol Clin North Am. 2010;37:379–86.

84. Moir C, Robins ER. Role of ultrasonography, gallium scanning, and computed tomography in the diagnosis of intraabdominal abscess. Am J Surg. 1982;143: 582–5.

85. Walters MD, Barber MD. Complications of hysterectomy. In: Karram M, editor. Hysterectomy for benign disease. Philadelphia, PA: Saunders Elsevier; 2010. p. 195–212.

86. Levenson RB, Pearson KM, Saokar A, Lee SI, Mueller PR, Hahn PF. Image-guided drainage of tuboovarian abscesses of gastrointestinal or genitourinary origin: a retrospective analysis. J Vasc Interv Radiol. 2011; 22(5):678–86.

87. Kjolhede P, Shefquet H, Lofgren M. Vaginal cleansing and postoperative infectious morbidity in vaginal hysterectomy. A register study from the Swedish National Register for Gynecological Surgery. Acta Obstet Gynecol Scand. 2011;90:63–71.

88. Kjolhede P, Shefqet H, Lofgren M. The influence of preoperative vaginal cleansing on postoperative infectious morbidity in abdominal total hysterectomy

for benign indications. Acta Obstet Gynecol. 2009;88: 408–16.

89. Bohrer JC, Walters M, Park A, Polston D, Barber MD. Pelvic nerve injury following gynecologic surgery: a prospective cohort study. Am J Obstet Gynecol. 2009;201:531.e1–7.

90. Romanowski L, Reich H, McGlynn F, Adelson MD, Taylor PJ. Brachial plexus neuropathies after advances laparoscopic surgery. Fertil Steril. 1993;60:729–32.

91. Warner MA, Warner DO, Harper CM, Schroeder DR, Maxon PM. Lower extremity neuropathies associated with lithotomy positions. Anesthesiology. 2000;93: 938–42.

92. Britt BA, Gordon RA. Peripheral nerve injuries associated with anesthesia. Can Anaesth Soc J. 1964;11:514–36.

93. Shveiky D, Aseff JN, Iglesia CB. Brachial plexus injury after laparoscopic and robotic surgery. J Minim Invasive Gynecol. 2010;17:414–20.

94. Parks BJ. Postoperative peripheral neuropathies. Surgery. 1973;74:348–57.

95. Barnett JC, Hurd WW, Rogers RM, Williams NL, Shapiro SA. Laparoscopic positioning and nerve injuries. J Minim Invasive Gynecol. 2007;14: 664–72.

96. Solomon. Venous thromboembolism in urogyneco-logic patients. Am J Obstet Gynecol.; 2010.

97. Geerts WH, Bergqvist D, Pineo GF. Prevention of venous thromboembolism: American College of Chest Physicians evidence-based clinical practice guidelines, (8th edition). Chest. 2008;133: 381s–453.

Complications of Anterior Compartment Repair

3

Alana Murphy and Courtenay K. Moore

Introduction

Transvaginal repair of anterior compartment prolapse was popularized by Kelly in the early twentieth century [1]. While this plication technique has generally fallen out of favor for the treatment of stress urinary incontinence (SUI), the same principles are utilized in contemporary anterior compartment repairs. In addition to a traditional colporrhaphy, the role of mesh in anterior compartment repair continues to evolve, with current evidence supporting superior anatomic results with mesh repairs but at the cost of higher complications rates. This chapter will focus on complications associated with anterior repairs. The specific complications associated with the use of mesh in vaginal surgery will be discussed in detail in another chapter.

Intra-operative and immediate postoperative complications associated with anterior compartment repairs are uncommon. However, potential anterior compartment repair complications include intra-operative hemorrhage and blood transfusion, genitourinary tract injury, onset of de novo SUI, and recurrent prolapse. Given the infrequent nature of these complications, there is

a paucity of literature focusing on intra-operative and immediate postoperative complications. In this regard, data on the immediate and shorter-term complications must be extracted from studies that focus primarily on long-term anatomical and functional outcomes. Utilization of this data is further complicated by the inclusion of concomitant procedures. Women with high-grade anterior compartment prolapse may require a simultaneous vault procedure to adequately address all aspects of pelvic floor support. While these additional procedures often have complication profiles similar to anterior repairs, the complication rates are often higher. This chapter will focus on the complications and complication rates only for anterior repairs.

Injury to the Lower Urinary Tract

The incidence of lower urinary tract injuries varies based on the type of vaginal surgery, ranging from 0 to 19.5/1,000 surgeries performed, with injuries occurring more commonly after surgery for reconstructive pelvic and incontinence surgery than other gynecological surgeries [2–4]. While injuries are uncommon, the consequences of unrecognized injuries can significantly increase patient morbidity.

Bladder Injuries

Bladder injury at the time of anterior colporrhaphy is very rare. Gilmour et al. conducted a systematic review of the literature from 1966 to

A. Murphy, MD • C.K. Moore, MD (✉)
Glickman Urological and Kidney Institute,
Cleveland Clinic, 9500 Euclid Avenue, Cleveland,
OH 44195, USA
e-mail: moorec6@ccf.org

H.B. Goldman (ed.), *Complications of Female Incontinence and Pelvic Reconstructive Surgery*,
Current Clinical Urology, DOI 10.1007/978-1-61779-924-2_3, © Springer Science+Business Media, LLC 2013

2004 and found the rate of bladder injuries during urogynecologic surgery excluding hysterectomies varied from 12.1/1,000 surgeries to 16.3/1,000 surgeries when intra-operative cystoscopy was performed [2]. Of those studies that performed intra-operative cystoscopy, 95% of bladder injuries were diagnosed and corrected intra-operatively compared to a 43% detection rate when cystoscopy was not performed, underscoring the importance of intra-operative cystoscopy.

While the majority of the studies on bladder injuries during urogynecological surgery include multiple concomitant procedures, several do report on the rate of bladder injury after anterior colporrhaphy alone. In a study by Kwon et al., of the 346 women who underwent traditional anterior colporrhaphy, there were no reported bladder injuries [5].

When comparing the rate of bladder injury among traditional anterior colporrhaphy and transvaginal mesh kits, two randomized controlled studies found there to be no difference in the rate of cystotomy with Weber et al. reporting no injuries and Hiltunen reporting one in the mesh group [6, 7]. A more recent randomized controlled study by Altman et al. found there to be a higher rate of cystotomy in the transvaginal mesh group vs. traditional anterior colporrhaphy, 3.5% vs. 0.5%; however, this did not reach statistical significance ($p = 0.07$) [8].

Immediate recognition of bladder injury during anterior compartment repairs is essential in reducing postoperative morbidity and potential fistula formation. As sited earlier, intra-operative cystoscopy increases the rate of intra-operative diagnosis and repair. *If an intra-operative cystotomy is detected, then the injury should be closed in two layers with absorbable sutures. If the planned anterior repair involved the use of mesh, it is our practice to abort the mesh procedure and perform a traditional anterior colporrhaphy.*

Should the injury be missed, depending on the duration of postoperative catheter drainage and the extent of the injury, the patient is at risk for developing a vesico-vaginal fistula requiring either prolonged catheter drainage or a transvaginal vesico-vaginal fistula repair.

Ureteral Injuries

Ureteral injuries occur infrequently after routine gynecological procedures, with patients undergoing complex reconstructive procedures for pelvic organ prolapse at an increased risk of ureteral injury [9]. Like bladder injuries, the incidence of ureteral injuries varies depending on the type of urogynecologic surgery, ranging from 2 to 11% [3, 10]. Women with pelvic organ prolapse are also at an increased risk of ureteric injury given the anatomic distortion caused by the prolapse itself, with 12–20% of women with symptomatic pelvic organ prolapse having moderate-to-severe hydronephrosis secondary to chronic obstruction from ureteral kinking [10].

The majority of the studies on ureteral injuries during gynecologic surgery do not separate the rate of injury by procedure. However, a study by Kwon et al. looked at the incidence of ureteral injury after anterior colporrhaphy alone [5]. Of the 346 procedures performed, there were 7 reported ureteral injuries (2.0%). There was no comment on the POP-Q staging of the women with ureteral injuries. All injuries were recognized at the time of surgery.

Diagnosis of Ureteral Injuries

Intra-operative Diagnosis

If a ureteral injury does occur, the ability to identify the injury at the time of the initial operation is paramount to avoid the permanent damage associated with unrecognized injuries. The single most controllable factor adversely affecting the outcome of ureteral injuries is delayed diagnosis. Studies have shown that intra-operative recognition and repair of ureteral injuries decreases postoperative morbidity and minimizes loss of renal function and need for nephrectomy. Early recognition also decreases the incidence of ureterovaginal fistulas as compared to postoperative diagnosis with delayed repair [11].

If a ureteral injury is suspected during abdominal surgery, direct inspection of the ureter is recommended. However, during vaginal surgery, direct visualization of the ureter is usually not feasible. Therefore, intra-operative cystoscopy has been recommended as a means to identify ureteral injuries during vaginal surgery while obviating the need for an abdominal incision. Five to 10 mL of intravenous indigo carmine dye is given intravenously prior to cystoscopy. Efflux of blue urine from both ureteral ostia assesses ureteral patency. By patiently observing and comparing to the opposite ureter, one may detect subtle sluggish flow which may suggest obstruction.

If fluoroscopy is available, another method of assessing ureteral patency is retrograde ureterography. If fluoroscopy is not available, a one-shot excretory urogram can be obtained 10 min after the administration of intravenous contrast material (1 mL/lb of body weight). Fluoroscopically, ureteral injuries present as urinary extravasation or obstruction.

Delayed Diagnosis

Most ureteral injuries are unsuspected and diagnosed postoperatively [12]. In a study by Meirow et al., the mean delay to diagnosis of patients sustaining ureteral injuries after gynecologic surgery was 5.6 days [13]. Undiagnosed ureteral injuries are associated with significant morbidity, the formation of ureterovaginal fistulas and potential loss of renal function [14]. The majority of patients present with fever, flank pain, continuous incontinence, pyelonephritis, ileus, peritonitis, or anuria. However, 5% of patients remain asymptomatic and are diagnosed at a later date secondary to a nonfunctioning or hydronephrotic kidney [12]. Delayed diagnosis is most often (66–76%) made by CT pyelography, excretory urography, or retrograde ureterography [15].

General Principles of Management

Immediate Intra-operative Management

The management of ureteral injuries depends on the time of diagnosis, location, nature, and extent of the injury. Injuries recognized intra-operatively must be treated immediately. Inadvertent ligation or kinking of the ureter should be treated by suture removal and repeat cystoscopy to ensure ureteral efflux. Typically, if recognized immediately, ureteric damage is minimal as these injuries include other tissue in the ligature [11]. If the extent of the ureteral injury is in question, at a minimum, ureteral stent placement is warranted [11]. For more severe injuries, when ureteral viability is unlikely, exploration and direct visualization of the ureter is recommended [16]. The involved ureter should be resected, debrided, and reanastomosed over a stent. If the diagnosis of an intra-operative ureteral injury is made during retrograde ureterography, attempts at retrograde stent placement should be made.

Delayed Management

The type of repair and the timing of delayed recognition injury repair are controversial. Postoperatively noted suture entrapment can be managed conservatively with immediate attempt at placement of a double-J ureteral stent or nephrostomy tube drainage if the suture is absorbable [17]. However, placement is only possible in 20–50% of patients [15]. In a study by Ghali, only 2 of 21 (19%) iatrogenic ureteral injuries identified postoperatively were able to be stented [15]. When stent placement is possible, as many as 73% of patients will *not* require open surgery.

While some have suggested stent placement or percutaneous nephrostomy as the first line of therapy, others recommend open repair. The traditional recommendation is that repair of iatrogenic ureteral injuries after urogynecologic surgery should not be undertaken for 3–6 months [18]. Yet, more recent studies suggest similar outcomes after immediate and delayed repairs [18].

Given that most injuries after vaginal surgery occur to the distal one-third of the ureter, open intervention often involves ureteral reimplantation or ureteroneocystostomy. Ureteroneocystostomy is used to repair distal ureteral injuries close to the bladder or in the intramural tunnel.

Hemorrhage

Hemorrhage is a rare complication of anterior compartment repair. During a traditional suture plication repair, proper dissection between the vaginal epithelium and the underlying vaginal muscularis (or the controversially named pubocervical fascia) will minimize blood loss and reduce the risk of postoperative hemorrhage. Judicious use of electrocautery during the anterior vaginal wall dissection can also be used to maintain hemostasis. A recent randomized controlled trial by Altman et al. included 389 women who underwent isolated anterior compartment repair [8]. Women with stage ≥2 prolapse were randomized to a repair using trocar-guided transvaginal mesh ($n=200$) or a traditional colporrhaphy ($n=189$). The two treatment groups did not differ significantly in terms of POP-Q stage or previous anterior compartment repairs. The traditional colporrhaphy group had a significantly lower mean estimated blood loss (EBL) (35.4 ± 35.4 mL) compared to the trocar-guided transvaginal mesh group (84.7 ± 163.5 mL, $p<0.001$). The study reported five cases (1.3%) of clinically significant intra-operative blood loss with all 5 patients having undergone trocar-guided transvaginal mesh placement: 4 patients (1.0%) had an EBL greater than 500 mL and 1 patient (0.3%) had an EBL greater than 1,000 mL and a subsequent retropubic hematoma. The authors did not provide data on transfusion rates. Due to its focus on anterior compartment repairs without concomitant pelvic floor procedures, the Altman study is a valuable addition to the limited body of literature that addresses the complications of isolated anterior compartment repairs.

Studies that included concomitant pelvic floor procedures also provide data regarding the low incidence of hemorrhage associated with anterior compartment repair [7, 19–21]. Weber et al. who performed the very first randomized study of anterior compartment repairs, comparing standard plication, plication with absorbable mesh, and ultra-lateral anterior colporrhaphy [6]. Subjects were excluded if they underwent any anti-incontinence procedure other than a suburethral plication. Subjects undergoing additional procedures for prolapse were included. Of the 109 women undergoing anterior compartment repair with concomitant pelvic floor procedures, 1 patient (0.9%) in the standard anterior colporrhaphy group required transfusion rate.

A more recent randomized controlled trial by Hiltunen et al., comparing anterior colporrhaphy with and without tailored mesh, included 201 women with pelvic organ prolapse [7]. Subjects were excluded from the study if they had gynecologic malignancies, apical prolapse mandating apical fixation, SUI, or their main symptomatic compartment was the posterior vaginal wall. Women could be included if they underwent concomitant vaginal hysterectomy, resection of an enterocele, culdoplasty, or posterior colporrhaphy without mesh. Women were randomized to traditional anterior compartment repair ($n=97$) or anterior compartment repair reinforced with mesh ($n=104$). A total of 29 patients (14%) underwent an isolated anterior compartment repair with no concomitant procedure. There was no difference in rates of previous vaginal surgery or concomitant hysterectomy between groups. All patients had vaginal packing in place for 20 h postoperatively. Although the mean EBL in the traditional repair group (114 ± 109 mL) was less than the mean EBL in the mesh group (190 ± 23 mL), the difference was not statistically significant ($p=0.004$). There was no statistically significant difference in clinically significant blood loss (EBL>400 mL) between the groups (3.1% vs. 9.6%, $p=0.07$). Two patients in total (1.0%) required blood transfusions (not specified which group they were in).

Careful attention should be paid during dissection of anterior vaginal wall and muscularis to minimize blood loss. Hemostasis can typically be attained using electrocautery. If electrocautery is insufficient, a figure-of-eight stitch with a 2-0 Vicryl suture can be used to oversew a small vessel. When closing the anterior vaginal wall incision, great care should be taken to achieve a secure hemostatic closure. A tight closure can provide an additional degree of hemostasis by allowing tamponade within the closed anterior compartment.

The low incidence of clinically significant blood loss affects our routine postoperative care pathway. Given that hemorrhage is a rare complication of anterior compartment repair, our practice is to not obtain routine postoperative lab work. If the patient undergoes a pelvic floor reconstruction that includes a concomitant hysterectomy, then we will obtain routine postoperative blood work and admit the patient for overnight observation. A vaginal pack is placed at the completion of the anterior compartment repair and removed after 1 h in the recovery room. If the patient is admitted for observation due to a concomitant pelvic floor procedure, then the vaginal packing is removed in the early morning of the first postoperative day. Vaginal packs are commonly used as a means to reduce postoperative hemorrhage, despite the lack of evidence in the literature. A recent abstract from Thiagamoorthy et al. reported the results of a randomized controlled trial assessing the effect of vaginal packing after a vaginal hysterectomy and/or pelvic floor repair [22]. Women were randomized to receive a vaginal pack ($n = 86$) or no vaginal pack ($n = 87$). A total of five patients were withdrawn from the no packing group due to intra-operative bleeding. The study demonstrated no significant difference in mean postoperative hemoglobin on the first postoperative day (11.75 g/dL vs. 11.94 g/dL, $p = 0.061$) and 6 weeks postoperatively (12.55 g/dL vs. 12.49 g/dL, $p = 0.884$) between the packing and the no packing group. Although the packing group had fewer postoperative hematomas ($n = 4$) compared to the no packing group ($n = 9$), the difference was not significant ($p = 0.098$). Despite the lack of statistical significance, all three clinically significant complications related to bleeding were in the no packing group. One patient returned to the operating room for hemorrhage and two patients required repeat admission for intravenous antibiotics to treat an infected pelvic hematoma. The data presented in the abstract supports our continued use of vaginal packing until additional data is available to influence our care pathway.

Hemorrhage recognized in the postoperative setting is rare after an anterior compartment repair. If a patient demonstrates a clinical sign of hemorrhage, such as significant transvaginal bleeding or tachycardia, a vaginal packing should be placed, vital signs closely monitored, and serial hematologic profiles checked until stable values are achieved. As demonstrated in the previously discussed studies, up to 1% of patients will require a transfusion after an anterior compartment repair. In cases of severe hemorrhage that are not responsive to transfusion or are associated with significant hemodynamic instability, angiography with selective embolization may be utilized to control the hemorrhage.

De Novo Stress Urinary Incontinence

De novo SUI should be included in the preoperative discussion of potential postoperative complications with greater emphasis in patients with high-grade anterior compartment prolapse. Women with severe anterior compartment prolapse may not experience SUI due to urethral kinking and SUI may not be detected by the patient or the physician until the prolapse is reduced or surgically repaired [23]. According to the International Continence Society (ICS), occult SUI is defined as SUI observed only after the reduction of coexistent prolapse [24]. Once any degree of urethral kinking is relieved with reduction of the anterior compartment prolapse, the mechanism of de novo SUI is likely multifactorial and may include urethral hypersuspension or intra-operative damage to the sphincter [25]. In addition to intra-operative factors, reduction of anterior compartment prolapse may unmask compromised periurethral support or frank intrinsic sphincter deficiency [26]. In order to minimize the risk of developing de novo SUI, each patient without subjective and/or objective evidence of SUI should be assessed for occult SUI before undergoing anterior compartment repair for high stage prolapse.

Proper assessment of occult SUI requires adequate reduction of the patient's anterior compartment prolapse. In the office setting, our practice is to perform a stress test after the anterior prolapse is reduced with half of a speculum. If SUI is not demonstrated in the office, the patient may then be referred for urodynamic evaluation with prolapse reduction. The most common techniques for prolapse reduction include a vaginal pack, pessaries, and a speculum. No general consensus exists regarding the best method for prolapse reduction. A study conducted by Mattox and

Bhatia demonstrated no difference in maximal urethral closure pressure whether a Smith-Hodge pessary, a ring pessary, or half of a Graves speculum was used for prolapse reduction [27]. Visco et al. found that rates of occult SUI differed based on method of prolapse reduction, which included a pessary, manual reduction, a forceps, a swab, and a speculum [28]. When interpreting urodynamic results, it is important to remember that each method of prolapse reduction may partially obstruct the urethra and lead to a false-negative occult SUI assessment.

Controversy continues to surround the management of women with either isolated occult SUI or no evidence of subjective or objective SUI with prolapse reduction. Should these women undergo a concomitant anti-incontinence procedure at the time of anterior compartment repair?

A study done by Chaikin et al. on 24 stress-continent women with stage III or IV pelvic organ prolapse (POP) found 14 patients (58.3%) to have occult SUI on preoperative urodynamics who subsequently underwent pubovaginal sling placement with concomitant anterior compartment repair [29]. The remaining ten patients (41.7%) had no occult SUI and underwent isolated anterior compartment repair. Two of the patients (14%) in the pubovaginal sling group had persistent postoperative SUI, while no patient in the group without occult SUI developed de novo SUI at a mean follow-up of 44 months.

Liang and colleagues reported on 79 stress-continent women with stage III or IV POP [30]. The patients were divided into three treatment groups based on the presence or absence of occult SUI on preoperative urodynamics. In group I, 32 patients with occult SUI underwent total vaginal hysterectomy (TVH), anterior/posterior (AP) repair, and a midurethral sling (MUS). In group IIa, 17 patients with occult SUI underwent TVH and AP repair with no anti-incontinence procedure. In group IIb, 30 patients without occult SUI underwent TVH and AP repair with no anti-incontinence procedure. Postoperatively, group I had three patients (9.4%) with subjective SUI and zero patients with objective SUI. Group IIa had 11 patients (64.7%) with subjective SUI and 9 patients (52.9%) with objective SUI on repeat urodynamics. Group IIb had 3 patients (10.0%)

with subjective SUI and zero patients with objective SUI. The data presented by both Chaikin and colleagues and Liang and colleagues suggests that the rate of de novo SUI is low in women with no subjective or occult SUI, while women with occult SUI appear to benefit from a concomitant anti-incontinence procedure.

The Colpopexy and Urinary Reduction Efforts (CARE) trial is the only randomized controlled trial addressing the role of an anti-incontinence procedure at the time of POP repair [31]. A total of 322 women with stage II or greater POP were randomized to abdominal sacrocolpopexy with Burch colposuspension ($n = 157$) or abdominal sacrocolpopexy alone (control group, $n = 165$). All women were considered stress continent, if they answered of "rarely" or "never" to six questions regarding SUI on the Medical, Epidemiological, and Social Aspects of Aging (MESA) questionnaire, despite preoperative urodynamics results. Three months postoperatively, one or more criteria for SUI were met by 23.8% of patients in the Burch group and 44.1% of patients in the control group ($p < 0.001$). When patients with occult SUI were excluded, de novo SUI was reduced from 38.2 to 20.8% in the control group vs. the Burch group ($p = 0.007$). A 2-year update of the CARE trial reported that the reduction in de novo SUI was durable with 32.0% of the Burch group and 45.2% of the control group meeting one or more criteria for SUI [32]. The CARE study also supports the utility of preoperative urodynamic testing in reportedly stress-continent women as a valuable tool to enhance preoperative counseling and planning. Examination of the preoperative urodynamic results revealed that 3.7% of women demonstrated urodynamic SUI without prolapse reduction and 6–30% of women demonstrated occult SUI when their prolapse was reduced (the range of occult SUI rates reflects the use of various methods for reducing prolapse). Regardless of whether or not they underwent Burch colposuspension, patients who demonstrated occult SUI were more likely to have postoperative SUI compared to women without occult SUI (Burch 32% vs. 21% ($p = 0.19$), controls 58% vs. 38% ($p = 0.04$)) [28]. Widespread application of the lessons learned in the CARE trial is limited by the use of the Burch procedure as the anti-incontinence procedure.

The literature also suggests that the rate of de novo SUI may be higher after anterior compartment repairs with mesh compared to traditional repairs. A study by Ek et al. randomized 50 women with stage ≥ 2 anterior compartment prolapse to a traditional repair ($n=27$) or a transvaginal trocar-guided mesh repair ($n=23$) [33]. All patients underwent preoperative urodynamics without prolapse reduction and postoperative urodynamics. Postoperatively, the rate of de novo SUI in the transvaginal mesh group (32%) was significantly higher compared to the traditional repair group (8%, $p=0.038$). In a similar fashion, a previous multicenter randomized controlled study by Altman reported that patients in the transvaginal mesh repair group were noted to have a statistically higher rate of de novo SUI compared to traditional anterior colporrhaphy (12.3% vs. 6.2%; $p=0.05$).

Transvaginal trocar-guided mesh repairs may result in a greater tendency towards hypersuspension of the anterior vaginal axis compared to a traditional repair with subsequent change in urethral pressure dynamics and increased de novo SUI. The more extensive dissection utilized in trocar-guided mesh repairs may also contribute to some degree to impairment of periurethral support and de novo SUI.

Our preference is to perform a concomitant anti-incontinence procedure in patients who demonstrate SUI preoperatively on physical exam or during UDS. Since anterior compartment repair alters the axis of the anterior vaginal wall and may affect the urethral axis, our practice is to perform an anti-incontinence procedure after the anterior compartment repair. If de novo SUI occurs in previously stress-continent women after anterior compartment repair, we perform an anti-incontinence procedure at a later date.

Summary

While complications during anterior compartment repairs are rare, they do occur. Attention to detail and an in-depth knowledge of pelvic anatomy can reduce the risk of complications and potential patient morbidities.

References

1. Kelly HA. Incontinence of urine in women. Urol Cutaneous Rev. 1913;XVII:291–3.
2. Gilmour DT, Das S, Flowerdew G. Rates of urinary tract injury from gynecologic surgery and the role of intraoperative cystoscopy. Obstet Gynecol. 2006;107: 1366–72.
3. Barber MD, Visco AG, Weidner AC, et al. Bilateral uterosacral ligament vaginal vault suspension with site-specific endopelvic fascia defect repair for treatment of pelvic organ prolapse. Am J Obstet Gynecol. 2000;183:1402–10; discussion 1401–10.
4. Harris RL, Cundiff GW, Theofrastous JP, et al. The value of intraoperative cystoscopy in urogynecologic and reconstructive pelvic surgery. Am J Obstet Gynecol. 1997;177:1367–9; discussion 1369–71.
5. Kwon CH, Goldberg RP, Koduri S, et al. The use of intraoperative cystoscopy in major vaginal and urogynecologic surgeries. Am J Obstet Gynecol. 2002;187:1466–71; discussion 1471–2.
6. Weber AM, Walters MD, Piedmonte MR, et al. Anterior colporrhaphy: a randomized trial of three surgical techniques. Am J Obstet Gynecol. 2001;185:1299–304; discussion 1304–6.
7. Hiltunen R, Nieminen K, Takala T, et al. Low-weight polypropylene mesh for anterior vaginal wall prolapse: a randomized controlled trial. Obstet Gynecol. 2007;110:455–62.
8. Altman D, Vayrynen T, Engh ME, et al. Anterior colporrhaphy versus transvaginal mesh for pelvic-organ prolapse. N Engl J Med. 2011;364:1826–36.
9. Liapis A, Bakas P, Giannopoulos V, et al. Ureteral injuries during gynecological surgery. Int Urogynecol J Pelvic Floor Dysfunct. 2001;12:391–3; discussion 394.
10. Handa VL, Maddox MD. Diagnosis of ureteral obstruction during complex urogynecologic surgery. Int Urogynecol J Pelvic Floor Dysfunct. 2001;12: 345–8.
11. Brandes S, Coburn M, Armenakas N, et al. Diagnosis and management of ureteric injury: an evidence-based analysis. BJU Int. 2004;94:277–89.
12. Visco AG, Taber KH, Weidner AC, et al. Cost-effectiveness of universal cystoscopy to identify ureteral injury at hysterectomy. Obstet Gynecol. 2001;97:685–92.
13. Meirow D, Moriel EZ, Zilberman M, et al. Evaluation and treatment of iatrogenic ureteral injuries during obstetric and gynecologic operations for nonmalignant conditions. J Am Coll Surg. 1994;178:144–8.
14. Rafique M, Arif MH. Management of iatrogenic ureteric injuries associated with gynecological surgery. Int Urol Nephrol. 2002;34:31–5.
15. Ghali AM, El Malik EM, Ibrahim AI, et al. Ureteric injuries: diagnosis, management, and outcome. J Trauma. 1999;46:150–8.
16. Assimos DG, Patterson LC, Taylor CL. Changing incidence and etiology of iatrogenic ureteral injuries. J Urol. 1994;152:2240–6.

17. Harshman MW, Pollack HM, Banner MP, et al. Conservative management of ureteral obstruction secondary to suture entrapment. J Urol. 1982;127: 121–3.

18. Ku JH, Kim ME, Jeon YS, et al. Minimally invasive management of ureteral injuries recognized late after obstetric and gynaecologic surgery. Injury. 2003;34:480–3.

19. Iglesia CB, Sokol AI, Sokol ER, et al. Vaginal mesh for prolapse: a randomized controlled trial. Obstet Gynecol. 2010;116:293–303.

20. Feldner Jr PC, Castro RA, Cipolotti LA, et al. Anterior vaginal wall prolapse: a randomized controlled trial of SIS graft versus traditional colporrhaphy. Int Urogynecol J Pelvic Floor Dysfunct. 2010;21: 1057–63.

21. Moore RD, Miklos JR. Vaginal repair of cystocele with anterior wall mesh via transobturator route: efficacy and complications with up to 3-year followup. Adv Urol. 2009;743–831.

22. Thiagamoorthy G, Khalil A, Leslie G. Should we pack it in? A prospective randomized double blind study assessing the effect of vaginal packing in vaginal surgery. In: Presented at international urogynecological association annual meeting; Lisbon, Portugal. 2011.

23. Bump RC, Fantl JA, Hurt WG. The mechanism of urinary continence in women with severe uterovaginal prolapse: results of barrier studies. Obstet Gynecol. 1988;72:291–5.

24. Haylen BT, de Ridder D, Freeman RM, et al. An International Urogynecological Association (IUGA)/International Continence Society (ICS) joint report on the terminology for female pelvic floor dysfunction. Neurourol Urodyn. 2010;29:4–20.

25. Zivkovic F, Tamussino K, Ralph G, et al. Long-term effects of vaginal dissection on the innervation of the striated urethral sphincter. Obstet Gynecol. 1996;87: 257–60.

26. Goepel C, Hefler L, Methfessel HD, et al. Periurethral connective tissue status of postmenopausal women with genital prolapse with and without stress incontinence. Acta Obstet Gynecol Scand. 2003;82:659–64.

27. Mattox TF, Bhatia NN. Urodynamic effects of reducing devices in women with genital prolapse. Int Urogynecol J. 1994;5:283.

28. Visco AG, Brubaker L, Nygaard I, et al. The role of preoperative urodynamic testing in stress-continent women undergoing sacrocolpopexy: the Colpopexy and Urinary Reduction Efforts (CARE) randomized surgical trial. Int Urogynecol J Pelvic Floor Dysfunct. 2008;19:607–14.

29. Chaikin DC, Groutz A, Blaivas JG. Predicting the need for anti-incontinence surgery in continent women undergoing repair of severe urogenital prolapse. J Urol. 2000;163:531–4.

30. Lo TS, Lin CT, Huang HJ, et al. The use of general anesthesia for the tension-free vaginal tape procedure and concomitant surgery. Acta Obstet Gynecol Scand. 2003;82:367–73.

31. Brubaker L, Cundiff GW, Fine P, et al. Abdominal sacrocolpopexy with Burch colposuspension to reduce urinary stress incontinence. N Engl J Med. 2006;354: 1557–66.

32. Richter HE, Goode PS, Brubaker L, et al. Two-year outcomes after surgery for stress urinary incontinence in older compared with younger women. Obstet Gynecol. 2008;112:621–9.

33. Ek M, Tegerstedt G, Falconer C, et al. Urodynamic assessment of anterior vaginal wall surgery: a randomized comparison between colporrhaphy and transvaginal mesh. Neurourol Urodyn. 2010;29: 527–31.

Posterior Compartment Repair

4

Benjamin M. Brucker and Victor W. Nitti

Introduction

Posterior compartment prolapse is a herniation of the posterior vaginal wall or anterior rectal wall into the lumen of the vagina. These defects may result from pudendal nerve damage or disruption of connective tissue and muscular attachments [1]. Many factors, including childbirth, aging, estrogen withdrawal, chronic abdominal straining, and heavy labor, weaken the pelvic floor and its associated support structures. Childbirth can cause stretching of the prerectal and pararectal fasciae with detachment of the prerectal fascia from the perineal body, allowing rectocele formation. In addition, childbirth damages and weakens the levator musculature and its fascia, attenuating the decussating prerectal levator fibers and the attachment of the levator ani to the central tendon of the perineum. The result is a convex sagging of the levator plate with a loss of the normal horizontal vaginal axis. The vagina becomes rotated downward and posteriorly, no longer providing horizontal support. These anatomic changes allow downward herniation of the pelvic organs along this new vaginal axis. There are also genetic factors that predispose women to this condition.

B.M. Brucker, MD (✉) • V.W. Nitti, MD
Department of Urology, New York University
Langone Medical Center, 150 East 32nd Street,
Second Floor, New York, NY 10016, USA
e-mail: Benjamin.brucker@nyumc.org

Posterior compartment prolapse is not uncommon. A cross-sectional study (Women's Health Initiative Hormone Replacement Therapy Clinical Trial) found that 18.6% of 16,616 women with a uterus had a rectocele on a baseline pelvic examination and 18.3% of 10,727 women who had undergone hysterectomy had a rectocele [2]. Rates of anterior prolapse (cystocele) were higher in both groups at 34.3% and 32.9%, respectively. Isolated posterior compartment defects are relatively unusual are seen most often in women after severe posterior tears associated with vaginal delivery or in women who have previously undergone correction of the anterior or apical compartment. More frequently, posterior compartment defects are associated with more global pelvic floor dysfunction and vaginal prolapse. Widening of the anogenital hiatus and damage to the urogenital diaphragm and central tendon further facilitates pelvic prolapse by preventing the normal compensatory narrowing of the vaginal opening. Varying degrees of perineal trauma and tears contribute to widening of the vaginal introitus. The repair of the relaxed or disrupted perineum and the repair of a rectocele are two distinct operative procedures, though they are often performed together.

Between the rectum and the vagina there is a layer of dense connective tissue. The homologous tissue in men was first described by Denonvillier. This was called the rectovesical septum and was later seen in female autopsies. This rectovaginal "fascia" is found from the posterior aspect of the cervix and cardial/uretrosacral complex cephelad, to the perineal body caudally. Laterally this reaches to the edges of the levator ani muscles [3].

There are several structures that provide support for the posterior vagina and rectum.

1. The rectovaginal septum lies between the rectum and the vagina. It extends caudad from the posterior cervix and the uterosacral/cardinal complex to the perineal body centrally and the levator fascia laterally on each side. The rectovaginal septum is densest distally where it is composed of dense connective tissue. Its midportion contains fibrous tissue, fat, and neurovascular tissue. Proximally it is mostly composed of fat cells.

2. The pararectal "fascia" lies between the rectovaginal septum and the rectum. It originates from the pelvic sidewalls and divides into fibrous anterior and posterior sheaths, which envelop the rectum. It also contains blood vessels, nerves, and lymph nodes that supply the rectum.

3. The levator ani consists of the paired ileococcygeus, puborectalis, and pubococcygeus muscles. These function to maintain constant basal tone and a closed urogenital hiatus. They also provide a reflex contraction in response to increases in intra-abdominal pressure. The puborectalis muscle acts as a sort of sling that causes the posterior vaginal wall to angulate about 45° from the vertical.

4. The perineal body is the central point between the urogenital and anal triangles. It contains interlacing muscle fibers from the bulbospongiousus and superficial transverse perineal muscles as well as and the anterior portion of the external anal sphincter. There is also a contribution from the longitudinal rectal muscle and the medial fibers of the puborectalis muscle.

There are several critical components of pelvic floor relaxation that are associated with rectocele formation. Loss of the normal horizontal axis of the levator plate and vagina, weakness of the urogenital and pelvic floor diaphragms, detachment of the levator ani from the central tendon of the perineum, and widening of the anogenital hiatus allow intra-abdominal forces to be transmitted directly to pelvic organs without normal underlying compensatory mechanisms. In addition, the rectovaginal septum becomes attenuated or disrupted, allowing intra-vaginal herniation of the rectum. Isolated breaks in the rectovaginal septum facilitate rectocele formation. There are several areas along the rectovaginal septum where breaks are commonly found. The most common site is a transverse separation immediately above the attachment of this septum to the perineal body, resulting in a low or distal rectocele (seen just inside the introitus). A midline vertical defect is equally common and most likely represents a poorly repaired or poorly healed episiotomy. Rarely, one can see lateral separation on one side. Defects can occur in isolation or in combination. Identification of specific defects is important when one is considering performing a site-specific posterior repair. Therefore, each of these components of pelvic floor relaxation must be addressed at the time of rectocele or posterior vaginal wall repair. Identification of this pathophysiology is critical when evaluating female patients with symptoms or signs of pelvic floor relaxation, including stress incontinence, cystocele and/or uterine prolapse. Maintenance of the normal horizontal vaginal axis is an important goal of surgical repair of pelvic floor relaxation, in order to allow compensatory mechanisms to be reestablished. Corrective surgery for posterior vaginal wall prolapse may include correction of the rectocele by reinforcement of the rectovaginal septum, prerectal and pararectal fasciae, repair of the levator muscle defect to restore the levator hiatus, restoration of the horizontal supporting plate of the proximal vagina, and repair of the perineum.

Up to 80% of rectoceles seen on physical examination are asymptomatic [4]. In cases of isolated rectoceles, or small rectoceles, with concomitant anterior and/or apical prolapse, that are asymptomatic any surgical intervention should be cautiously approached because of the potential complications that will be discussed below. However, when rectoceles are symptomatic surgical correction may be a very reasonable option. Symptoms associated with rectocele include constipation, incomplete rectal emptying, rectal pressure, vaginal bulge [5]. Some patients will also describe stool being trapped in the rectocele pocket and the need to apply perineal or vaginal pressure in order to facilitate take defecation, this is known as splinting.

Nonsurgical Therapies

Although it is not the intent of this chapter to discuss the evidence behind alternative therapies, these must be considered when trying to avoid surgical complications. This is because if nonsurgical therapies are successful the need for surgery may be obviated.

Observation, or watchful waiting, may be appropriate if the patient has little bother or minor symptoms from her posterior compartment laxity. A support device such as a pessary can also be considered in a woman with symptoms from pelvic organ prolapse. In the authors' experience, posterior compartment prolapsed symptoms can be difficult to treat with these devices. However, if the decision is made to trial a pessary, the process of fitting a pessary in a women with posterior compartment predominant prolapse should not be anymore difficult than fitting other women with anterior or apical prolapse [6]. If a woman derives symptomatic improvement, she can be taught how to remove and clean the pessary, or it can be changed on a regular basis in a physician's office. In either case, routine examination is necessary to ensure that there is no unwanted irritation or granulation tissue development.

Pelvic floor muscle rehabilitation can also be considered as a therapy for posterior compartment prolapsed. There is a paucity of data to support its use in preventing progression or improvement of rectocele specific symptoms. However rectoceles are often not isolated findings. The pelvic floor disorders that may coexist may be effectively addressed with nonsurgical options. For example, pelvic floor exercises are useful in the treatment of stress urinary incontinence. Women with concomitant disorders of the pelvic floor may favor the nonsurgical route for the treatment of the rectocele because the improvement in the symptoms of other conditions.

In summary, nonsurgical therapies should be discussed with all patients. Given the favorable side effect profile, there is no great downside to attempting these therapies if a women so desires. The nonsurgical options are also important in counseling patients that are poor surgical candidates secondary to medical comorbidities.

Surgical Approaches

Rectocele repairs can be approached via the abdominal, transanal, and transvaginal approach. Urologists and Gynecologists most often perform the repair transvaginally [1]. There is no definitive evidence that suggests which surgical approach is best. Surgeon's skills, patient's desires, anatomic and functional outcomes are all important to consider. As importantly, the potential unwanted outcomes, or complications, must be considered.

As we are considering potential complications, which vary based on each different surgical approach, some relative indications for the route of repair that is selected should be considered. The vaginal approach is useful if there is other genital prolapse, compromised anal sphincter function (and the surgeon would like to avoid anal dilation from the retractor utilized from the transanal approach), or a high rectocele is present (may not be able to be reached through a transanal approach) [7]. The transrectal approach is utilized if there is other perianal or rectal pathology that needs to be treated concurrently. These pathologies include redundant rectal mucosa, hemorrhoids, etc. A disadvantage of this transrectal approach is that the patient is placed in the prone jackknife position, and it can be difficult to perform a simultaneous perineorrhaphy if needed. The abdominal approach may be indicated in cases where a rectal prolapse is concomitantly noted. The abdominal approach has also become more popular with the widespread use of the robotic technology. This has lead to more publications describing the abdominal approach for rectocele repair [8].

A Cochran review in 2010 that suggested that for posterior vaginal wall prolapse, the vaginal approach was associated with a lower rate of recurrent rectocele or enterocele or both than the transanal approach (RR 0.24, 95% CI 0.09–0.64) [9]. The review noted a higher postoperative narcotic use and blood loss in this vaginal repair group.

In addition to the approach used, there are other questions that remain. Should a surgeon utilize mesh or graft material? Are traditional repairs vs. site-specific repairs more appropriate? The chapter will address some of the more common complications, and in doing so may help answer some of these questions, or at least inspire future investigation to those questions that remain unanswered. Technique selection and operative plan are always the first step to consider when aiming to minimize and manage complications.

Complications of Posterior Repair

Hemorrhage

Excessive bleeding or hemorrhage is a complication of rectocele repair regardless of the surgical approach. The rectovaginal septum and pararectal fascia are rich in blood vessels. In cases where the tissue is "loose or disrupted," as it often is in cases of posterior prolapse, these vessels have a tendency to retract after they are cut, making identification difficult. This complication should be considered during the preoperative evaluation, intra-operatively and in the postoperative management of patients. Blood loss to a more mild degree is relatively unavoidable result when surgical repair is selected. The surgeon's role, however, should be aimed at preventing hemorrhage by attempting to be aware during all phases of patient care.

Avoidance

Avoidance of excessive bleeding or hemorrhage starts with the preoperative evaluation. A thorough history and physical exam can help identify any bleeding diatheses or hereditary bleeding problems that may require further workup. Taking the time to review medication and dietary supplement that the patient is taking can identify agents that may contribute to intra-operative and postoperative bleeding. Stopping antiplatelet agents approximately 7 days prior to surgery will reduce the risk of bleeding. These agents include medications such as aspirin, NSAIDs, clopidogrel, and supplements such as fish oil. Stopping these medications must be weighed against potential adverse outcomes arising from the relative hypercoagulable state. Consultation is recommended in cases where the safety to stopping antiplatelet agents is in question. This is especially important in patients with coronary artery disease, veinocclusive disease, history of cerebral vascular accidents. A recently published study suggests higher adverse outcomes (2.4 times more likely to experience acute coronary syndrome or death) during the first 90 days of discontinuing clopidogrel therapy compared to days 91–180 [10]. A general rule is that the risk of bleeding must be weighed against the risk of adverse outcomes resulting from stopping these medications, i.e., thrombocclusion [11, 12].

Care must also be taken as well with other medications that affect the clotting cascade. Medications such as Coumadin/warfarin should also prompt consultation to decide on appropriate perioperative management.

Preoperative lab tests can help identify patients with bleeding diatheses especially if it is suggested by history. Depending on institutional regulations, surgeon's preference, and patient's history, PT/INR/PTT and platelet counts can be evaluated preoperatively.

Physical examination is also very important in attempting to avoid surgical bleeding complications. Inspection for prior surgical scars, as well as signs of potential vascular abnormalities, should be routine. This information can aid in selection of which approach is most appropriate, as well as the need for other preoperative evaluations. For example, vulvar varicosities (though rare) may lead a surgeon to evaluate the patient with imaging to rule out aberrant vasculature or pelvic congestion syndrome. In a patient with abnormal vasculature, blind passage of trochars (i.e., those found in mesh repairs) should be used with extreme caution [13].

Identification of Hemorrhage

Surgeons have various techniques at their disposal to treat patients with rectoceles. With each technique there are differences in expected blood loss. The tactics to avoid or identify hemorrhage also differ. Good surgical techniques should aim to establish excellent intra-operative hemostatic control. This should also reduce the risk of excessive "oozing" in the postoperative period. Obviously, stopping bleeding by controlling injured vessels is preferred over managing bleeding from uncontrolled vessels. Good visualization can help achieve this goal. This is provided by suction, irrigation, lap pads and lights, etc. In cases where pneumoperitoneum is utilized (i.e., laparoscopy, with or without robotic assistance) inspection after intra-abdominal pressure has been decreased to physiologic levels is helpful to identify any bleeding areas that may be masked by the affects of the positive pressure that pneumoperitoneum provides. Other general intra-operative considerations (use of electrocautery, suturing technique, etc.) will not be further discussed here.

Abdominal approaches to the repair of pelvic organ prolapse routinely required dissection and identification of the sacral promontory. The presacral venous plexus that runs on the anterior aspect of the sacrum can result in significant bleeding that can be difficult to control using conventional measures such as suturing, clipping or electrocautery. Especially when patients are in the lithotomy position, the hydrostatic pressure can increase 2–3 times that of the inferior vena [14]. Intra-operative management of presacral bleeding with the use of hemostatic matrix (FloSeal; Baxter Healthcare Corporation, Fremont, CA) and an absorbable hemostat (Surgicel Fibrillar; Ethicon, Somerville, NJ) has been advocated by some as first line treatment for presacral bleeding if it is encountered intra-operatively [15]. More traditionally, things like long periods of compression, sterile thumbtacks or the use of a fat bolster have also been utilized.

Another question is whether the use of robotic assistance decreases the risk of bleeding compared to pure laparoscopy. A recent study compared the abdominal techniques (robotic assisted and pure laparoscopic) for the repair of a rectocele. The laparoscopic group had a higher intra-operative blood loss compared to the robotic group (mean, 45 ± 91 mL vs. 6 ± 23 mL; $p = 0.048$), however the authors acknowledge that this is likely not clinically significant [8].

Stapled Transanal Rectal Resection (STARR) can be used for the treatment of internal rectal prolapse, as well as rectocele. Postoperative bleeding is not rare following a stapled hemorrhoidopexy, as it occurs in about 5% of cases [16]. The bleeding usually occurs at the level of the endorectal suture line. After a stapled rectal resection, reinforcing this staple line with a hand sewn suture has been suggested to decrease this risk of hemorrhage [17]. Careful inspection is important to identify any bleeding vessel after a procedure such as this.

At least one study compared intra-operative blood loss across rectocele repair techniques. There was less intra-operative blood loss from the STARR group compared to standard vaginal rectocele repair (transvaginal rectocele repair, 108 mL vs. STARR, 43 mL; $p = 0.0015$) [18]. However, the study showed a higher complication rate from the transanal resection group (STARR 61.1% vs. transvaginal rectocele repair 18.9%, $p = 0.0001$). The complication of postoperative bleeding, for example, was three times higher in the STARR group. Obviously a single outcome such as intra-operative blood loss must not be the only driving factor for selecting an appropriate procedure.

Utilizing the vaginal approach for an isolated posterior prolapse repair does not allow for a substantial space for blood to accumulate without the surgeon being aware. In cases where it is difficult to identify specific site of bleeding, temporary packing can be very useful. This not only allows the patient's innate clotting cascade to begin to work, but it also allows the surgical staff to obtain equipment necessary to assist in visualization. Lighted retractors (i.e., Miyazaki retractor) (see Fig. 4.1) can be quite useful in the vaginal surgery if visualize of bleeding is difficult. Although mentioned above, hemostatic agents

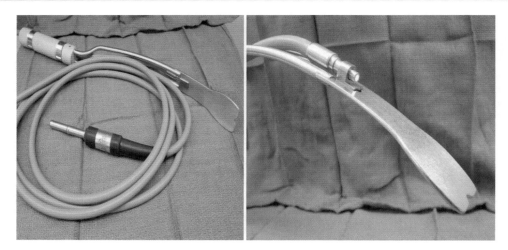

Fig. 4.1 The Miyazaki retractor is shown here. This retractor has a fiber optic light on the end that is useful when the surgeon is working in a narrow space and visualization is poor

such as FloSeal (Baxter Healthcare Corporation, Fremont, CA) can also be effective in vaginal surgery if specific sites of bleeding cannot be identified or traditional methods are unsuccessful at stopping bleeding.

Vasoconstrictive agents (such as lidocaine with epinephrine or pitressin) are used by some surgeons during the vaginal dissection. Not only can this help, but the vasoconstriction can also potentially minimize intra-operative blood loss. The down side of this technique is that bleeding vessels may be "hidden" while the epinephrine is active and become problematic postoperatively. There is also the question of the distortion of tissue plans if a site-specific repair is selected. Surgeon preference is unfortunately all that is available to base the decision on the use vasoactive agents on.

If extensive dissection is carried out during a vaginal repair, or if there is a high suspicion that postoperative bleeding may occur, placing of a vaginal packing while the patient is still anesthetized allows for a tighter packing with less discomfort to the patient. The packing can be removed the next morning if patients are staying overnight or in the recovery room prior to discharge if patients are set to be discharged the same day.

If a vaginal repair is selected and uses blind passage of trocars or anchoring sutures (such as are seen in "mesh kits") appropriate identification of landmarks, intimate knowledge of anatomy, as well as high suspicion of anatomic variations are extremely important to minimize the risk of vessel injury.

Treatment of Hemorrhage After Posterior Repair

It is important to identify postoperative hemorrhage in a timely manner so treatment and resuscitation can prevent other unwanted complications. Good communication with recovery room staff and education of recovery room staff are necessary to help identify patients who may require intervention. Monitoring heart rate, blood pressure, and inspecting surgical incisions or pads should be a standard part of the recovery room protocol in the immediate postoperative period.

Patients who are hemodynamically stable, but that are noted to have excessive oozing from the surgical site should have a vaginal packing placed in order to help tamponade bleeding vessels and minimize the potential space for blood loss. Aside from packing gauze, other compressive devices have utilized balloons (i.e., Foley catheters) to allow for appropriate pressure. These maneuvers are not applicable to abdominal repairs, as the potential space is often too large to contain and cannot be effectively compressed.

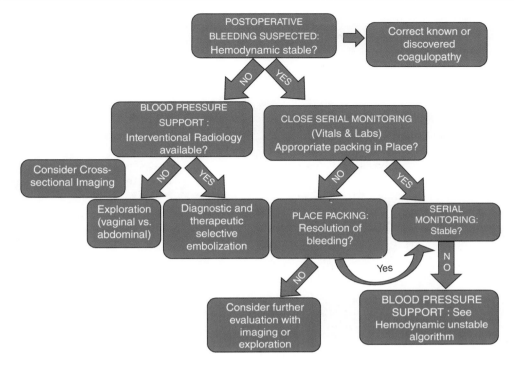

Fig. 4.2 Bleeding flow chart

When conservative measures of fluid resuscitation and packing are not sufficient more invasive measures may be necessary. This is especially true if a patient become hemodynamically unstable. Traditionally these patients were reexplored in order to identify bleeding vessels and obtained hemostatic control. This can be effective; however one must carefully make this decision to reexplore. Bleeding that has slowed from tamponade (intrinsic or iatogenic) now become brisker or uncontrolled after clot evacuation relieves pressure on the vessel or vessels.

Another option for uncontrolled bleeding is the use of selective embolization of bleeding vessels. Depending on availability and expertise, super-selective embolization may be successfully performed [19, 20].

The use of cross-sectional imaging (i.e., CT scan) before re/exploration and/or intravascular intervention can be considered, however it should not be done if it will delay definitive treatment in a patient who is hemodynamically

unstable and a bleeding source is suspected. A flow chart (Fig. 4.2) is provided as a reference for clinicians to use if postoperative bleeding is suspected. The assessment and managing of bleeding complications from posterior compartment repairs must obviously be managed in an individual manor based on clinical scenario and available recourses.

Dyspareunia

Sexual function is a very complex process that involves many organs of the female pelvis. Further, there is an intricate interaction with the central nervous system, hormonal axis, peripheral nerves, blood vessels, etc. Women with pelvic organ prolapse may present with varying degrees of sexual dysfunction and one of the aims of the pelvic organ prolapsed surgery is to restore function. Another aim is to avoid creating (or worsening) any sexual dysfunction. In spite of best efforts, painful intercourse, or dyspareunia, is a potential complication of any pelvic organ prolapsed repair and this section will focus on this potential outcome from posterior prolapse repair.

Preoperative Selection

It is very important when taking a history preoperatively to assess a patient's sexual activity and current function, because dyspareunia (pain with intercourse) is another potential complication of posterior compartment repair. There are numerous questionnaires that can be utilized to objectively classify a woman's sexual function both pre and postoperatively. For example, the Sexual History Form and the Female Sexual Function Index are validated measures [21, 22]. Some questionnaires are for general sexual function and others have been validated specifically in the pelvic organ prolapse population. This preoperative assessment is important to help counsel the patient on the appropriate repair. It is also useful so that there is a baseline to compare postoperative outcomes against if results are not satisfactory.

When levatorplasty is performed it is believed that the de novo dyspareunia is a result of the pressure atrophy of the included muscle, and the subsequent scaring that takes place [23]. However it has been suggested that dyspareunia is associated with posterior colporrhaphy even if there is no concomitant levatorplasty or synthetic material used.

A cohort study of women who underwent anti-incontinence surgeries and pelvic organ prolapsed repairs looked at those women who had a posterior repair and those that did not. Although bother groups had improvements postoperatively in their Pelvic Organ Prolapse-Urinary incontinence Sexual Function Questionnaire (PISQ) score the women that did not have posterior repairs were noted to have a lower incidence of dyspareunia than those who had posterior repairs [24]. Another study compared site-specific repairs to a more traditional posterior colporrhaphy and found the site-specific repair had a higher recurrence rate, with similar rates of dyspareunia and bowel symptoms [25].

Women with rectoceles can present with dyspareunia, along with other aspects of sexual dysfunction. As noted above, in many cases after posterior repair there is an improvement in some of the sexual function domains. A selective group of 68 women with sexual dysfunction, all arranged to undergo fascial suture rectocele repairs, were noted to have dyspareunia as a presenting symptom in 86%. After the repair, patients showed significant improvement in desire ($p > 0.001$), satisfaction ($p > 0.0001$), and pain ($p > 0.0001$) domains. There was no significant changes in arousal ($p = 0.0897$), lubrication ($p = 1$), or orgasm ($p = 0.0893$). Only one patient experienced *de novo* dyspareunia. This was attributed to a postoperative infection resulting in excessive scar tissue of the posterior wall of the vagina. The follow-up was 6 months [26].

Another option that the surgeon has if a transvaginal repair is performed is the use of an absorbable mesh. After randomization to synthetic absorbable mesh (polyglactin 910) to reinforce a posterior colporrhaphy vs. a nonmesh repair no difference in rectocele recurrence rates was seen. Unfortunately this randomized study did not consider functional outcomes such as dyspareunia. They did not report any erosions, now defined as extrusions [27].

The use of biologic graphs has also been considered and there is some data considering sexual function. This study was a comparison of posterior colporrhaphy, site-specific repair and site-specific repair with porcine small intestine submucosa graft [28]. There was no difference in postoperative sexual function (PISQ-12 and asking "Do you feel pain during intercourse?"). There were also no differences in quantity of life measures or bowel function. Perioperative and postoperative morbidity also did not show a difference, albeit the study was underpowered to discern differences in these events. Importantly, however, they reported a lower failure rate of traditional repair techniques compared to the site-specific repair with porcine small intestine submucosa graft for rectoceles. This study suggests that sexual complications are not any different based on repair type, but biologic agents did have higher failure rates.

Permanent meshes are also used in prolapse repair. One study that looked at posterior repair with permanent mesh (composite polyglactin 910-polypropylene) with 3-year follow-up found de novo dyspareunia in 27% of women [29]. With the long-term follow-up they discovered that there was actually no improvement from baseline in preoperative dyspareunia. This was in contrast to previously published short-term results showing an improvement. The combination of persistent dyspareunia and de novo dyspareunia the prevalence of dyspareunia was a staggering 60%. The repair described in the study avoided a rectovaginal placation, and trimming of vaginal wall. Presumably these maneuvers (that they avoided) could result in vaginal narrowing, and ultimately dyspareunia. The "extrusion" rate was 30% and the recurrence rate was 22%.

A prospective study of monofilament polypropylene meshes for posterior repair reported a statistically significant increase of dyspareunia from 6% preoperatively to 69% postoperatively (mean follow-up 17 months) [30]. In this study, the surgeon dissected laterally to the rectal pillars, performed a placation of the rectovaginal fascial tissues, and secured the mesh. Excess vaginal wall was also trimmed prior to closing the posterior vaginal wall.

Traditionally, colorectal surgeons prefer the transanal repair of rectocele. A randomized study compared the transanal with a transvaginal rectocele repair and although none of the subjects reported de novo dyspareunia, 27% reported improvement of sexual function, slightly in favor to the transanal repair [31]. The higher recurrence rates from the transanal approach are noted in the sections above.

Surgeon and patient factors ultimately factor into the type of repair performed, however if a vaginal approach is elected, based on the available studies, we would caution if considering the use of biological agents or permanent mesh (in posterior repairs) given the high incidence recurrence and dyspareunia, respectively. Further the International Urogynecological Association Grafts Roundtable [32] (that convened in 2005) suggested the following patient factors as relative contraindications for the use of biomaterials in

pelvic floor reconstructions: pelvic irradiation, severe urogenital atrophy, immunosuppression, active infection, and comorbidities such as poorly controlled diabetes, morbid obesity, and heavy smoking and we would agree with this relative contraindication for the use in posterior repairs. It is our opinion that because the data of the use of mesh in the posterior compartment would not support its routine use (no significant reduction in recurrence rate with a higher complication rate) we reserve it for the rare case when the rectovaginal septum is completely obliterated.

Intra-operative

There are no good studies that prospectively evaluate specific surgical techniques that should be used to decrease risk of dyspareunia. However expert opinion would suggest avoiding excessive tightening of the posterior vaginal during a rectocele repair. If a concomitant perineal body repair is needed it is also important to avoid excessive tightening of the introits as this can contribute significantly to sexual dysfunction after surgery. The surgeon's fingers can be used intra-operatively to calibrate the vagina to an appropriate size. Some advocate calibrating the vagina to 2–3 fingers breaths, which should prevent anatomic difficulties with vaginal penetration in women who are interested in resuming this type of sexual activity [33].

The use of mesh to augment posterior repairs was discussed above as a potential contributor to postoperative dyspareunia. If the surgeon and patient elect to use a permanent mesh selecting the appropriate type of mesh is an intra-operative decision that can help minimize morbidity. Macroporous, monofilament, polypropylene mesh (type I) has been found to have the most favorable biocompatibility profile of the synthetics meshes that are currently available. The lack of interstices allows native collagen to growth in to the material and the large pores size allow for entry of macrophages and the body's other immune mediators [34].

Mesh also has been show to retract or contract after placement, and some have shown up to a 66% decrease in size [35]. This is important to remember that the mesh may contract when it is placed or tailored intra-operatively so as to avoid excessive tightening after this occurs. To date there is no clear evidence that this gradual decrease in mesh sized is associated with dyspareunia, but it is a potential explanation for those that believe that mesh augmentation of posterior compartment can worsen sexual outcomes.

Also, though mostly based on expert opinion, there are a few areas of surgical technique that should be considered when placing mesh posteriorly. Care must also be used to ensure the appropriate planes of dissection. Improper dissection can potentially lead to thinned vaginal wall that is used to cover the mesh and can increase the chance of mesh extrusions. Further, care must be used to ensure appropriate placement of mesh so that it does not bunch or role in the vagina. This can form areas of inflammatory reactions that can be uncomfortable for women, but can also be felt by male partners. Another potential cause of dyspareunia is vaginal narrowing that can occur secondary to excessive trimming of the vaginal wall. This also contributes to vaginal narrowing and also result in tenuous coverage of any foreign material utilized.

Posterior prolapse can also be addressed abdominally. Patients are often selected for an abdominal repair because of a predominance of apical decent. This should be remembered when reviewing the literature. The studies may include women with some degree of posterior prolapsed, but this is often not the predominant defect.

Dyspareunia is seen even with the abdominal approach. Sergent et al. [36] found that sacrocolopexy with polyester mesh had a de novo dyschezia rate of 1.7 and dyspareunia rate of 0.8%. Claerhout et al. utilized polypropylene mesh and found a rate of 5% and 19%, respectively [37]. A comparison of these two small studies is not meant to replace a large randomized studies (with the power to show differences in these domains), but rather to illustrate that different mesh types used abdominally may result in different dyspareunia rates.

We also recommend the use of copious irrigation and the use of perioperative antibiotics. These simple methods are meant to avoid infections. Infection has a host of complication

that we will not explicitly discuss here. However excessive scarring and inflammation may lead more directly to painful intercourse.

Postoperative Identification and Management

In order to identify dyspareunia postoperatively specific questions on patient's sexual function should be asked. Careful physical examination is also extremely useful to identify the specific cause of dyspareunia. Patient's bother and time from surgery must be considered when discussing potential treatments of this outcome. Palpation for tight bands of tissue, extrusions, tender pelvic muscles are all aspects of the physical exam that can help with the management of this complication.

If there is significant bother and a patient elects for therapy for dyspareunia conservative treatment options exist. Topical lubricants, vaginal estrogen, and even topical local anesthetics have been described to help lessen or alleviate some of the more mild symptoms. If physical examination reveals pain from palpation of the specific trigger points injections with local anesthetics and/or steroids can be considered. The use of systemic or local anxiolytics such as benzodiazepines has also been utilized to help relax pelvic floor muscles. Physical therapy with the optional use of dilators is another method that can help address symptoms.

The physical examination may also identify a discrete band of tissue attached to the vaginal wall that has been incorporated into levator ani muscles. If this is the case operative release of this tissue can help alleviate symptoms of pain during intercourse. Excessive narrowing of the vaginal introitus or canal may also require surgical intervention. Aside from the release of excessively tight and tissue, graft material may be necessary if there is a paucity of local tissue to reconstruct an adequate vaginal lumen.

Other therapies have also been studied for the treatment of dyspareunia. There is level III evidence to support the use of botulinum toxin in the treatment of severe refractory vaginismus. This comes from a study of 24 women were the etiology of vaginismus was not specified in the inclusion criteria. After failing other therapies these women were injected with 150–400 units of botulinum toxin type A into three sites on each side in the puborectalis muscle. After a mean follow-up of 12 months, none of the patients had recurrent vaginismus, and 75% were able to achieve satisfactory intercourse [38]. More specifically there are case reports describing the use of botulinum toxin in a postoperative patient who experienced de novo dyspareunia and vaginismus [39].

Rectal Injury

Injury to surrounding structures is always a potential complication of surgical intervention. The defect present in a rectocele is of the tissue between the vagina and rectum. This intimate relationship of the rectum and the rectocele defect make the rectum a potential source of inadvertent injury.

Preoperative Avoidance in Preparation

Once again, there are multiple ways to address posterior repairs, and when thinking about the approach, the chance of rectal injury deserves consideration. Depending on surgeon preference, and surgical approach, bowel prep may be used preoperatively. A bowel prep does not necessarily decrease the risk of rectal injury; however it does decrease the risk of gross contamination if in fact a rectal injury is made. Women with symptomatic rectoceles can have a significant of constipation and trapping of stool at baseline. In cases where women have excessive amounts of stool in the rectal vault, intra-operative rectal exam can be a more challenging proposition. An enema given preoperatively can be an effective way of cleaning out the rectal vault. Enemas are generally well tolerated and do not dehydrate patients the same way a full bowel prep would.

Patients that are undergoing intra-abdominal repairs of rectocele, may benefit from a modified bowel prep. The authors of this chapter have not found this particularly helpful in routine laparoscopic/robotic cases. Other laparoscopic surgeons have suggested this decreases distention

secondary to bulky stool or excessive bowel gas that can make dissection more challenging and interfere with visualization.

Intra-operative

Utilizing a drape or a draping technique that allows for digital rectal examinations during rectocele repair is very valuable to help avoid or recognize rectal injury during dissection and or suture/trocar placement. The finger allows the surgeon to ensure that the rectal wall is not violated. Further, after repair palpation via rectal exam, the surgeon can identify the presence of suture or mesh material that may have been inadvertently placed.

If an abdominal approach with laproscopic or robotic assistance is selected good basic laparoscopic technique should be observed. Use of these measures is aimed at minimizing risk of injury to hollow viscous organs. These practices include utilizing an OGT or NGT, and placement of a Foley catheter. We also avoid the use of nitrous oxide to prevent distention of the bowel. Decompression of bowel and bladder is especially important when gaining access to the abdominal cavity and thus these measures are not necessarily aimed at reducing rectal injury. However intra-operatively they allow for better visualization and can prevent inadvertent injury during dissection.

In a retrospective look at rectal injury during vaginal surgery Hoffman et al. found that over an 11-year period they had a 0.7% injury rate utilizing a vaginal approach for a variety of surgical indication including prolapse [40]. They felt that after reviewing the cases prevention of injury required careful sharp dissection, preliminary dissection on either side of the midline, and occasionally the insertion of a finger into the rectum. They suggest that Injection of sodium chloride solution or a dilute vasoconstrictor may also facilitate dissection. The authors of this chapter do not routinely utilize this technique during the posterior dissection because of the potential for distortion of the already thin tissue planes.

Preoperative use of estrogen in postmenopausal women can also be considered to thicken the vagina and this may facilitate dissection.

However this has not been investigated directly to make evidence-based recommendations.

Mesh prolapse repair kits may require placement via blind trocar passage and this has led some to investigate the risk of rectal injury during posterior mesh kit repair. One series of mesh prolapsed repair kits, with only short-term follow-up, the authors found that they had a 1.1% rectal injury rate [41]. Interestingly, both of the patients were noted to have sustained the rectal injury during the initial dissection and not from the trocar passage. Both patients had the injury repaired primarily and one did eventually have a posterior mesh placed and the other was converted to a more traditional colporrhaphy. Though there is not much data regarding the placement of mesh after rectal injury, we would argue against it. The same study did have 1.6% intra-operative bladder injury rate. Conversely these injuries were secondary to the trocar placement and not dissection.

However, injury to the rectum has been noted in other series of patients treated with mesh kits where rectal injury was not caused by the initial dissection [42]. In this series the rectal injury was found 1 week postoperatively when a rectoscopy, done for refractory dedicatory pain, reveled an arm of the prolapse repair kit mesh traversing the lumen of the rectum. The series had 62 patients with at least part of the surgery including a posterior repair resulting in a 1.6% rectal injury rate.

Patient with pelvic organ prolapsed may elect to undergo treatment by an abdominal approach (open laproscopic with or without robotic assistance). These patients can have a significant amount of posterior defects that the surgeon can attempt to address from the abdominally route. To achieve this, the dissection is carried down toward the perineal body between the vaginal wall and rectum. In one series of 165 women with vaginal vault prolapse undergoing laparoscopic sacrocolpopexy (using a polypropylene mesh) three sigmoid perforations were noted. These were injuries were all noted in women being treated for rectocele, presumably during the posterior dissection. The injuries were all successfully treated by laparoscopy suture repair of the injury that was recognized intra-operatively [43].

Another series of 124 laparoscopic sacrocolpopexy (using multifilament polyethylene terephthalate-polyester) noted two intra-operative rectal injuries (1.6%). There were three bladder injuries (2.4%) noted as well. One of the rectal injuries was immediately recognized and successfully repaired; the procedure proceeded as planed with uneventful follow-up for this patient. There was however one patient that developed a rectovaginal fistula following an occult rectal perforation. This was noted 3 weeks after the surgery and the fistula was debrided and closed with suture. A transitory colostomy was concomitantly performed. This patient unfortunately also developed a lumbosacral spondylodiscitis diagnosed at 4 months, and required prolonged antibiotic therapy before complete resolution [36].

Recognition of a rectal injury, regardless of approach, remains paramount in trying to minimize the morbidity to the patient. Once the injury is realized the surgeon must perform an adequate mobilization of the injured area. The mobilization allows for appropriate exposure so that the injury can be closed in entirety. The mobilization of the rectum away from other tissue is also usually necessary to allow the surgeon to complete the prolapse repair. Lastly this mobilization is critical to allow for a tension free repair.

Next, a two layer closure should be performed. The first layer uses delayed absorbable sutures to close the rectal mucosal defect (usually in a running fashion). The second layer is an imbricated sero-muscular layer using a permanent suture in a Lembert-type fashion. It should also be noted that during the dissection required to mobilize the injured bowel, it is often possible to identify additional tissue (fat, fascia) that can be used to cover the two layered closure.

The final factor in ensuring the best possible outcome from an intra-operative repair of a rectal injury is given patient appropriate postoperative instructions. Ensuring that the patient is having soft bowel movement is paramount. Also patients should avoid anything per rectum for approximately 6 weeks. Fecal diversion is usually not necessary.

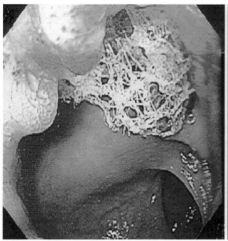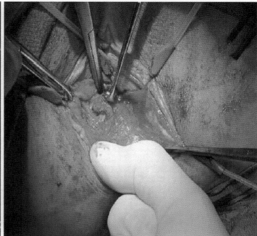

Fig. 4.3 Posterior mesh complication. (**a**) View during a sigmoidoscopy of an eroded (or misplaced) mesh visualized in the lumen of the rectal wall. (**b**) An intra-operative photo of the mesh removal via a transvaginal approach. The surgeons finger is placed in the rectum to aid in the removal of the mesh. Reproduced from Hurtado et al. [44]

Postoperative Identification and Management

One of the concerns about the use of mesh for vaginal prolapse repairs is late complications with mesh extrusion or erosion. This problem can occur in the vaginal lumen, which is much more likely to be discovered on routine pelvic examinations during follow-up. Mesh can also erode into the rectal lumen, which may not be routinely visualized or palpated during a postoperative speculum examination of the vagina. A digital rectal examine should thus be considered part of the postoperative physical exam (especially if a posterior repair was preformed). It requires a high index of suspicion to diagnose problems such as mesh extrusion into the rectum. There are case reports and prolapsed repair series that describe a small, but real, number of women that develop mesh extrusions erosions or misplacements into the rectum recognized postoperatively [44, 45]. Women may present with rectal bleeding, change in bowel habits, worsening dyspareunia several months after posterior prolapsed repair with mesh. Physical examination may be all that is needed to confirm suspicion of a mesh complication but more involved testing with a rigid sigmoidoscope may also be necessary. Figure 4.3 shows an exam-

ple mesh seen by and endoscope in the rectal wall. Borrowing from the trauma literature on penetrating rectal injuries, we know that rigid sigmoidoscopy is much more sensitive than digital rectal exam for uncovering rectal injury. This is a different population with a different mechanism of injury, however if suspicion is high that a rectal injury occurred (or developed) digital rectal exam alone may not be adequate [46].

Cases of rectal vaginal fistula have also been reported with the use of mesh to augment a posterior colporrhaphy and posterior intravaginal slingplasty (see Fig. 4.4) [47]. Women with rectovaginal fistula may present with foul smelling vaginal discharge, systemic signs of infection, and possibly pelvic/perineal adenopathy. Repairs of these fistulas are more involved than repairs of a straight forward mesh extrusions. These repairs often require local tissue flaps. In more complicated cases diverting colostomy may be considered.

Once discovered, attempts to treat the mesh complication can be done endoscopically. This is usually done by cutting the exposed mesh and allowing the injury to heal by secondary intention. However if this is unsuccessful, not possible, or if a more definitive approach is desired a transvaginal excision of mesh is warranted.

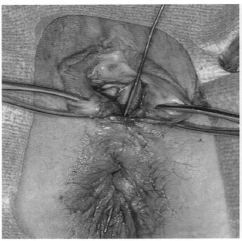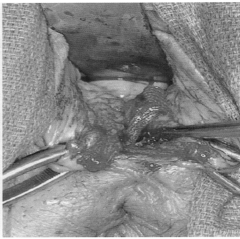

Fig. 4.4 Rectovaginal fistula. (**a**) Rectovaginal fistula demonstrated by a lacrimal duct probe entering the vagina and exiting the anus. (**b**) Posterior intravaginal sling plasty polypropylene mesh protruding though the dissected rectovaginal fistula. Reproduced from Hilger and Cornella [47]

In the event that a transvaginal excision of synthetic mesh is needed the goal is to remove as much (if not all) of the mesh as possible and to repair any violations of the rectum that were discovered or occurred. Based on the extent of the injury and comfort of surgeon these procedures can be done in conjunction with a colorectal surgeon. The authors of this chapter have favored a posterior midline vaginal incision to allow for complete exposure. The vaginal epithelium should then be dissected from the fibromuscularis laterally. The mesh should be identified and in order to facilitate the initial dissection grasping it with an instrument such as an Allis clamp is useful. Ideally the distal edge of the mesh is now identified and freed sharply. At this point the mesh should be dissected off of the rectovaginal septum in a cephalad direction. The use of a finger in the rectum can help the surgeon appreciate the appropriate depth of dissection as well as the area(s) of rectal violation. Further the rectal exam can identify the location of the anal sphincter. Awareness of this location allows us to avoid unnecessary sphincter injury. The mesh should be removed laterally to the pelvic sidewalls to as great an extent as possible. This is often aided by incising the mesh down the middle allowing for dissection above and below the synthetic mesh, freeing it completely.

In many case mesh can become incorporated into the rectal submucosa, or is place through the rectal mucosa and in order to remove it may be necessary to resect a full-thickness portion of the anterior rectal wall. The defect should be closed in at leas two layers in a water tight fashion. A proctoscope or other means of irrigating the rectum (i.e., a catheter) should be used to ensure that the closure is adequate. After the mesh removal and defect repair the rectocele may be present and should be closed without another synthetic material. The vaginal epithelium is then closed.

Other Complications

Mesh extrusion (previously described as erosions) into the vaginal epithelium can also be seen if mesh is used to augment posterior repairs [48]. Dwyer et al. had a 9% overall erosion rate noted with the use of monofilament polypropylene mesh placed in the anterior and posterior compartment found (and one patient who developed a rectovaginal fistula). Posterior vaginal mesh extrusion is handled in much the same way that any mesh extrusion is handled as discussed elsewhere in this book. Observation may be warranted if asymptomatic. Topical local estrogen is another conservative approach, and finally local excision closure of the vaginal epithelium may be necessary.

Lim et al. retrospectively noted a 12.9% incidence of vaginal mesh erosion at 1 year, when a vicryl-prolene mesh was used with posterior colporrhaphy. The authors noted that all of these erosions were dealt with by easily trimming the area, without the need of mesh removal, in the outpatient setting.

References

1. Lowenstein L, Mueller ER. Posterior vaginal prolapse repair. In: Graham Jr SD, Keane TE, editors. Glenn's urologic surgery. New York: Lippincott Williams and Wilkins; 2010. p. 343–9.
2. Hendrix SL, et al. Pelvic organ prolapse in the Women's Health Initiative: gravity and gravidity. Am J Obstet Gynecol. 2002;186(6):1160–6.
3. Richardson AC. The rectovaginal septum revisited: its relationship to rectocele and its importance in rectocele repair. Clin Obstet Gynecol. 1993;36(4):976–83.
4. Kelvin FM, Maglinte DD, Benson JT. Evacuation proctography (defecography): an aid to the investigation of pelvic floor disorders. Obstet Gynecol. 1994;83(2):307–14.
5. Schwandner T, et al. Transvaginal rectal repair: a new treatment option for symptomatic rectocele? Int J Colorectal Dis. 2009;24(12):1429–34.
6. Clemons JL, et al. Risk factors associated with an unsuccessful pessary fitting trial in women with pelvic organ prolapse. Am J Obstet Gynecol. 2004;190(2): 345–50.
7. Goh JTW, Tjandra JJ, Carey MP. How could management of rectoceles be optimized? ANZ J Surg. 2002;72(12):896–901.
8. Wong MTC, et al. Robotic versus laparoscopic rectopexy for complex rectocele: a prospective comparison of short-term outcomes. Dis Colon Rectum. 2011;54(3):342–6.
9. Maher C, et al. Surgical management of pelvic organ prolapse in women. Cochrane Database Syst Rev. 2010;8.
10. Stephenson JJ, et al. Incidence of death and recurring acute coronary syndrome after stopping clopidogrel therapy in a large commercially-insured population in the US. Curr Med Res Opin. 2011;27(6):1079–87.
11. Vasudeva P, et al. Antiplatelet drugs and the perioperative period: what every urologist needs to know. Indian J Urol. 2009;25(3):296–301.
12. Hall R, Mazer CD. Antiplatelet drugs: a review of their pharmacology and management in the perioperative period. Anesth Analg. 2011;112(2):292–318.

13. Touboul C, et al. Major venous hemorrhagic complication during transvaginal cystocele repair using the transobturator approach. Obstet Gynecol. 2008; 111(2):492–5.
14. Wang QY, et al. New concepts in severe presacral hemorrhage during proctectomy. Arch Surg. 1985; 120(9):1013–20.
15. Germanos S, et al. Control of presacral venous bleeding during rectal surgery. Am J Surg. 2010;200(2): e33–5.
16. Ravo B, et al. Complications after stapled hemorrhoidectomy: can they be prevented? Tech Coloproctol. 2002;6(2):83–8.
17. Dodi G, et al. Bleeding, incontinence, pain and constipation after STARR transanal double stapling rectotomy for obstructed defecation. Tech Coloproctol. 2003;7(3):148–53.
18. Harris MA, et al. Stapled transanal rectal resection vs. transvaginal rectocele repair for treatment of obstructive defecation syndrome. Dis Colon Rectum. 2009; 52(4):592–7. doi:10.1007/DCR.0b013e31819edbb1.
19. Phillips C, Hacking N, Monga A. Super-selective angiographic embolisation of a branch of the anterior pudendal artery for the treatment of intractable postoperative bleeding. Int Urogynecol J. 2006;17(3): 299–301.
20. Araco F, et al. Selective embolization of the superior vesical artery for the treatment of a severe retroperitoneal pelvic haemorrhage following Endo-Stitch sacrospinous colpopexy. Int Urogynecol J Pelvic Floor Dysfunct. 2008;19(6):873–5.
21. Rogers RG, et al. A new instrument to measure sexual function in women with urinary incontinence or pelvic organ prolapse. Am J Obstet Gynecol. 2001;184(4): 552–8.
22. Rosen R, et al. The Female Sexual Function Index (FSFI): a multidimensional self-report instrument for the assessment of female sexual function. J Sex Marital Ther. 2000;26(2):191–208.
23. Pancholy AB, Silva WA, Karram MM. Rectocele-anatomic and functional repair. In: Cardoza L, Staskin D, editors. Textbook of female urology and urogynocology. New York: Informa Healthcare; 2010. p. 799–812.
24. Komesu YM, et al. Posterior repair and sexual function. Am J Obstet Gynecol. 2007;197(1):101.e1–6.
25. Abramov Y, et al. Site-specific rectocele repair compared with standard posterior colporrhaphy. Obstet Gynecol. 2005;105(2):314–8.
26. Brandner S, et al. Sexual function after rectocele repair. J Sex Med. 2011;8(2):583–8.
27. Sand PK, et al. Prospective randomized trial of polyglactin 910 mesh to prevent recurrence of cystoceles and rectoceles. Am J Obstet Gynecol. 2001;184(7): 1357–62; discussion 1362–4.
28. Paraiso MFR, et al. Rectocele repair: a randomized trial of three surgical techniques including graft augmentation. Am J Obstet Gynecol. 2006;195(6): 1762–71.

29. Lim Y, et al. A long-term review of posterior colporrhaphy with Vypro 2 mesh. Int Urogynecol J. 2007; 18(9):1053–7.

30. Milani R, et al. Functional and anatomical outcome of anterior and posterior vaginal prolapse repair with prolene mesh. BJOG. 2005;112(1):107–11.

31. Nieminen K, et al. Transanal or vaginal approach to rectocele repair: a prospective, randomized pilot study. Dis Colon Rectum. 2004;47(10):1636–42.

32. Sung VW, et al. Graft use in transvaginal pelvic organ prolapse repair: a systematic review. Obstet Gynecol. 2008;112(5):1131–42.

33. Pancholy AB, Silva WA, Karram MM. Rectocele-anatomic and functional repair. In: Cardoza L, Staskin D, editors. Textbook of female urology and urogynecology. New York: Informa Healthcare; 2001. p. 799–812.

34. Gomelsky A, Penson DF, Dmochowski RR. Pelvic organ prolapse (POP) surgery: the evidence for the repairs. BJU Int. 2011;107(11):1704–19.

35. Gauruder-Burmester A, et al. Follow-up after polypropylene mesh repair of anterior and posterior compartments in patients with recurrent prolapse. Int Urogynecol J Pelvic Floor Dysfunct. 2007;18(9): 1059–64.

36. Sergent F, et al. Mid-term outcome of laparoscopic sacrocolpopexy with anterior and posterior polyester mesh for treatment of genito-urinary prolapse. Eur J Obstet Gynecol Reprod Biol. 2011;156(2):217–22.

37. Claerhout F, et al. Medium-term anatomic and functional results of laparoscopic sacrocolpopexy beyond the learning curve. Eur Urol. 2009;55(6):1459–67.

38. Ghazizadeh S, Nikzad M. Botulinum toxin in the treatment of refractory vaginismus. Obstet Gynecol. 2004;104(5 Pt 1):922–5.

39. Park A, Paraiso MFR. Successful use of botulinum toxin type a in the treatment of refractory postoperative dyspareunia. Obstet Gynecol. 2009;114(2 Pt 2):484–7.

40. Hoffman MS, et al. Injury of the rectum during vaginal surgery. Am J Obstet Gynecol. 1999;181(2):274–7.

41. Abdel-fattah M, Ramsay I, West of Scotland Study. Retrospective multicentre study of the new minimally invasive mesh repair devices for pelvic organ prolapse. BJOG. 2008;115(1):22–30.

42. Altman D, et al. Short-term outcome after transvaginal mesh repair of pelvic organ prolapse. Int Urogynecol J. 2008;19(6):787–93.

43. Granese R, et al. Laparoscopic sacrocolpopexy in the treatment of vaginal vault prolapse: 8 years experience. Eur J Obstet Gynecol Reprod Biol. 2009;146(2): 227–31.

44. Hurtado E, Bailey HR, Reeves K. Rectal erosion of synthetic mesh used in posterior colporrhaphy requiring surgical removal. Int Urogynecol J Pelvic Floor Dysfunct. 2007;18(12):1499–501.

45. Sullivan ES, Longaker CJ, Lee PY. Total pelvic mesh repair: a ten-year experience. Dis Colon Rectum. 2001;44(6):857–63.

46. Hargraves MB, et al. Injury location dictates utility of digital rectal examination and rigid sigmoidoscopy in the evaluation of penetrating rectal trauma. Am Surg. 2009;75(11):1069–72.

47. Hilger W, Cornella J. Rectovaginal fistula after posterior intravaginal slingplasty and polypropylene mesh augmented rectocele repair. Int Urogynecol J Pelvic Floor Dysfunct. 2006;17(1):89–92.

48. Dwyer P, O'Reilly B. Transvaginal repair of anterior and posterior compartment prolapse with atrium polypropylene mesh. BJOG. 2004;111(8):831–6.

Complications of Transvaginal Apical Repairs: Evaluation and Management

5

Kamran P. Sajadi and Sandip P. Vasavada

Introduction

The transvaginal approach to the vaginal apex is commonly performed for pelvic organ prolapse, and offers a minimally invasive alternative to the transabdominal route. Nonetheless, as with any major surgical procedure, there are complications specific to these approaches. Complications common to all procedures, including urinary tract infection, wound infection, venous thrombosis, and neuropraxias, are discussed in Chap. 2. We will focus on major complications related to transvaginal approaches to apical prolapse repair including ureteral or bowel injury, hemorrhage, and peripheral nerve injury.

Ureteral Injury and Obstruction

Ureteral obstruction is a known complication of uterosacral vaginal vault suspension (USVVS), usually related to kinking of the ureter during

K.P. Sajadi, MD
Division of Urology, Oregon Health
and Science University, Portland, OR, USA

S.P. Vasavada, MD (✉)
Center for Female Urology and Reconstructive
Pelvic Surgery, Cleveland Clinic Main Campus,
Mail Code Q10-1, 9500 Euclid Avenue, Cleveland,
OH 44195, USA

Glickman Urological and Kidney Institute,
Cleveland Clinic, Cleveland, OH, USA
e-mail: vasavas@ccf.org

plication of the uterosacral ligament to the vaginal cuff. The distal uterosacral ligament is intimately involved with the cardinal ligament—which contains the uterine vessels—and lies in close proximity to the ureter. Anatomic studies of the ligament demonstrate that the middle and proximal segments may be ideal for use in apical suspension, with the mean±SD distance from the ureter $0.9±0.4$ cm distally, $2.3±0.9$ cm in the middle segment, and $4.1±0.6$ cm proximally (Fig. 5.1) [1]. Obstruction can occur in up to 11% of procedures [2], but the incidence is markedly reduced by performing cystoscopy at the conclusion of the procedure. Indigo carmine is injected intravenously, and cystoscopy is performed to visualize efflux of blue dye from each ureter. If a strong ureteral jet is seen from both sides after the vault suspension has been completed, then ureteral obstruction is unlikely. A study of hysterectomies showed that cystoscopy is cost-effective when the rate of injury is at least 2% [3], and intraoperative as opposed to postoperative diagnosis of ureteral obstruction substantially reduces morbidity [4].

Ureteral Obstruction: Intraoperative Presentation

When there is no efflux from one or both sides, it is important to have a clear plan and algorithm in place for diagnosis and management. First, consider the patient scenario. Reevaluate the patient's history to consider if she has had a prior

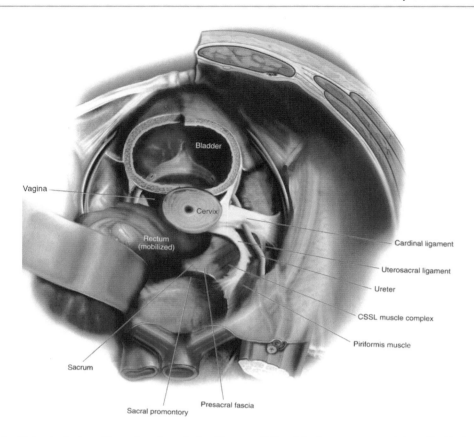

Fig. 5.1 Abdominal view illustrating the relationship between the ureter and the uterosacral ligament. Proceeding cephalad, the uterosacral ligament proceeds medially while the ureter proceeds laterally. Vault suspension to the proximal third therefore has the lowest rate of ureteral obstruction. Illustration from [38]

nephrectomy or ureteral reimplant, in the latter case the ureter may efflux from a different position. If the patient has had any previous abdominal imaging, it can be helpful in identifying the occasional case of a prior nephrectomy or congenital absence of the ipsilateral kidney. In addition, confirm the time of administration of indigo carmine with the anesthesiologist or nurse, as early delivery may mean that all dye has been excreted, or late delivery may mean you have not watched the ureteral orifice long enough. Many different maneuvers have been attempted to promote more rapid excretion of the dye. Most commonly, ensuring adequate hydration by the anesthetist and/or administrating a diuretic such as furosemide may promote more rapid renal

excretion of indigo. Resuming a level position or reverse Trendelenburg to encourage gravitational drainage has also been performed, although these reports are anecdotal.

Once sufficient time has passed to confirm a lack of excretion from one or both sides, there are a few ways to proceed. One option is to cut the more distal (i.e., more lateral) uterosacral plication suture (the uterosacral ligament is closest to the ureter distally) out of the vaginal cuff, and observe if efflux then occurs. With an assistant, it is possible to cut this suture while the cystoscope is still in place. If this suture was the cause, brisk efflux will usually immediately ensue and most pelvic reconstructive surgeons would not attempt to replace the suture in this situation, believing the remaining suspension sutures to be adequate. If efflux does not ensue, remove the remaining sutures on that side, one at a time, proceeding from the most lateral and caudad to the most cranial and medial. It is important to remember, however, that if a concomitant anterior colporrhaphy was performed, that procedure also carries a risk of ureteral obstruction, and it may be prudent to remove those sutures first, because it is easier to repeat an anterior colporrhaphy than an apical suspension.

Occasionally, there will still be a lack of efflux even after removal of all potentially offending sutures. If the patient lacks preoperative upper urinary tract imaging or sufficient historical reason to explain the lack of efflux, a urologic consultation may be prudent. The most common obstacle to performing retrograde ureterography in such cases is that these patients are often not positioned appropriately on the bed or on an appropriate operative table for pelvic fluoroscopy. Therefore, many urologists will attempt blind passage of a wire or ureteral catheter into the ureter to assure patency. If this is done, a flexible tipped, soft hydrophilic wire should be used, and even then there is risk of converting a ureteral kink or obstruction into a ureteral perforation. Making the extra effort to obtain a C-arm and repositioning the patient can significantly improve patient safety. With retrograde ureteropyelography, the urologist can accurately assess the patency of the ureter and make a decision whether or not a stent should be placed. If there is a suspicion of injury and a stent can be passed, it should be left in place for a minimum of 4–6 weeks [4].

Ureteral Obstruction: Postoperative Presentation

Ureteral injury is a potential complication of uterosacral colpopexy even when intraoperative cystoscopy reveals bilateral ureteral efflux. So-called "delayed obstruction" may occur due to excessive scarring between the uterosacral plication and the distal ureter, due to compromise of the ureteral blood supply or perhaps because of inadequate intraoperative examination for efflux. Ureteral obstruction presents in the acute postoperative period with flank pain, nausea and vomiting, and potentially fever. The diagnosis should be confirmed with imaging, and the study of choice in patients with normal renal function is CT Urography (CTU, see Fig. 5.2). The severity of hydronephrosis, site of ureteral obstruction, presence and location of any extravasation, presence or size of a potential urinoma, and the status of the contralateral kidney can all be assessed with a CTU. Once identified, in the acute postoperative period (up to 7 days), cutting the offending colpopexy sutures may be sufficient to relieve the obstruction. It is usually ideal to perform this in the operating room for several reasons. Aside from patient comfort, under anesthesia cystoscopy and retrograde ureteropyelography can be performed at the same time, to confirm patency of the ureter following removal of the suture(s). In addition, given the potential for ureteral edema and the severity of the obstruction, many urologists would choose to place an indwelling ureteral stent after relief of the obstruction. With further delay in presentation or failure to unobstruct in this manner, open abdominal or laparoscopic ureterolysis and reimplant is often necessary, although transvaginal ureterolysis and retrograde stenting has also been reported [5]. In a meta-analysis of USVVS, there was a 1.8% rate of ureteral obstruction, of which 2/3 resolved with suture removal, and the remainder required ureteral reimplantation [6].

Other Apical Suspensions

The sacrospinous ligament is fairly posterior to the path of the ureter, and so sacrospinous ligament fixation (SSLF) is rarely associated with ureteral obstruction. A cohort of women undergoing SSLF found a 3.5% rate of temporary ureteral obstruction [7]. Although 88 of the 200 women studied underwent simultaneous anterior colporrhaphy, all of the ureteral obstructions were right-sided, as were the apical suspensions, implicating the latter. Although no interventions

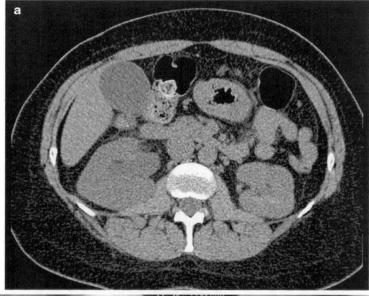

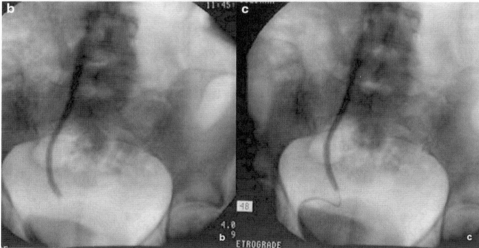

Fig. 5.2 A woman with postoperative suspicion of ureteral injury is found to have right hydronephrosis on a CT (a). Right retrograde ureterography demonstrates medial deviation of the distal ureter, and the distal ureter is not opacified (b). A wire was successfully passed (c), over which a stent was then placed (photograph courtesy of Howard Goldman, MD, Cleveland Clinic, OH)

were required, the study does not explain the presentation or management of these patients. The iliococcygeus suspension has recently gained popularity, with one of the purported benefits being the lack of vital structures in the immediate vicinity of the iliococcygeal fascia. The risk of ureteral injury and obstruction in this procedure is therefore theoretically low, and to our knowledge none have been reported [8].

Hemorrhage

Sacrospinous Ligament Colpopexy or Hysteropexy

Significant hemorrhage is more common with sacrospinous colpopexy or hysteropexy than with other transvaginal apical repairs, largely due

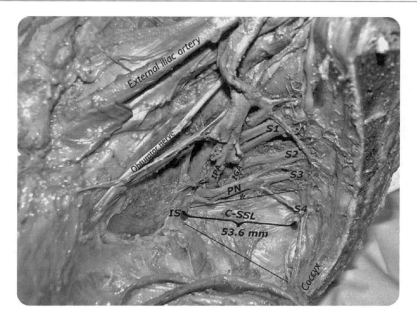

Fig. 5.3 Sagittal cadaveric dissection demonstrating the relationship of the coccygeus-sacrospinous ligament (C-SSL) to the sacral nerve roots and pudendal nerve (PN). Important vascular structures include the internal pudendal artery (IPA) and the more medial inferior gluteal artery (IGA). *Source*: Roshanravan et al. [28]

to the ligament's delicate anatomic location. The sacrospinous ligament, running for about 5 or 6 cm [9] between the ischial spine laterally and the lateral border of the sacrum medially, forms the inferior border of the greater sciatic foramen, through which pass the superior gluteal vessels above the piriformis muscle, and the inferior gluteal and internal pudendal vessels below. The internal pudendal neurovascular bundle runs just inferior and medial to the ischial spine, and therefore suspension sutures should be sufficiently medial and superficial to these structures (Fig. 5.3). Similarly, dissection and suture placement should avoid the cephalad border of the sacrospinous ligament in order to minimize risk to the gluteal vessels and sciatic nerve. Although there is variation in the distance between the ischial spine and pudendal nerve and vessels and the sciatic nerve [10], in general these structures can be avoided by placing suspension sutures in the middle or medial third of the ligament, avoiding the cephalad border of the ligament, and placing sutures through the ligament alone, and not deep through the underlying coccygeus muscle.

Sacrospinous ligament colpopexy or hysteropexy can be performed unilaterally (usually to the right, to avoid the sigmoid colon) or bilaterally, and is approached through either the anterior or posterior vaginal wall. In either case, copious hydrodistension of the vaginal mucosa, especially with epinephrine-containing solutions, can provide not only hemostasis, but also better anatomic delineation of the plane between the vaginal mucosa and muscularis. Meticulous attention to this plane reduces the likelihood of significant bleeding and injury to adjacent viscera (the bladder anteriorly or the rectum posteriorly). SSLF is associated with deviation of vaginal axis posteriorly (and laterally, in the case of unilateral fixation), and therefore increased risk of anterior vaginal wall prolapse recurrence, and many surgeons feel the anterior approach reduces this deviation. In a retrospective cohort study comparing both approaches, there was improved apical and anterior vaginal wall support in the anterior group, and a lower reoperation rate [11]. No randomized controlled studies have compared the two.

We believe the posterior approach offers better control of bleeding because of an increased space in which to place hand-held retractors (Breisky-Navratil) for optimal visualization of the ligament and surrounding structures. With direct visualization, the judicious placement of small surgical clips on bleeding vessels can prevent significant hemorrhage. A comparison of suture placement methods found increased complications with suture placement by palpation as opposed to direct visualization, especially with blood loss and nerve-related complications [12]. Of note, the group criticized the use of a Deschamps needle driver by palpation as opposed to standard needle driver under direct vision, however we use the Deschamps needle driver *under* direct visualization, and feel these differences are due to visualization as opposed to the type of driver.

Bleeding Management

With appropriate judgment, small, slow venous bleeding where the source cannot be directly visualized can be managed by completing the operation, closing, and sufficiently packing the vagina so that pressure can be maintained at least overnight. Alternatively, when significant bleeding occurs, the anesthetist should be notified to monitor hemodynamics, and obtain a blood type and screen or cross-match if not done preoperatively. The extraperitoneal approach of this operation offers the advantage of easy packing with sponges and application of pressure transvaginally to slow the bleeding and allow appropriate time for decision-making and definitive management. After packing the vagina and holding pressure for sufficient time (at least 5 min if bleeding is significant), slowly reexpose the area to assess if the source is visible and amenable to suture or clip application. Arterial bleeding is easier to identify in this situation, but occasionally significant venous ooze makes source identification extremely difficult.

When bleeding is considerable and/or there is question of hemodynamic compromise, then definitive vascular control is necessary. If suspension sutures have been placed or can be placed

quickly, then vault suspension may be completed as rapidly as possible. Attempting to control the bleeding via an open retropubic or abdominal route is invasive, time-consuming, and often unsuccessful, as the expanding retropubic hematoma makes identification of the source, and preservation of important surrounding structures, difficult. Moreover, extensive "surgically significant" collateral circulation exists, and therefore control of the internal iliac artery may be insufficient to stop bleeding [9, 13]. The best definitive management in this case is angiography, either via an interventional radiologist or, if an interventionalist is not readily available, a vascular surgeon. While awaiting the consultation, adequate resuscitation with crystalloid and, once available, packed red cells is prudent. Continue to pack the vagina and apply pressure until arrangements for definitive management have been made.

Occasionally, a patient will present following SSLF with significant postoperative hemorrhage, in which case a similar protocol is usually effective. Again, transvaginal or transabdominal exploration to control bleeding is often difficult and ineffective. Placement of a vaginal packing and attention to hemodynamic monitoring and resuscitation, if necessary, are the next steps while arrangements are made for angiographic control of hemorrhage.

Iliococcygeus Vaginal Vault Suspension

As the iliococcygeus lies distal and anterior to the sacrospinous ligament, and requires less dissection and exposure for placement of suspension sutures, many feel there is less hemorrhage reported with this approach. One comparative study of iliococcygeal vs. sacrospinous fixation found similar rates of hemorrhage and transfusion between the two approaches [14]. Another study of iliococcygeal suspension found a mean estimated blood loss of 358 mL, and 3 of 110 patients had hemorrhage >750 mL [15]. To our knowledge, however, there have been fewer surgical series, anatomical studies, and no randomized controlled trials regarding the iliococcygeal suspension and therefore, much of our knowledge is anecdotal.

Uterosacral Vaginal Vault Suspension

Hemorrhage requiring blood transfusion during USVVS is about 1.3% [6]. Prompt attention to bleeding is necessary because this procedure is intraperitoneal and therefore it can be difficult to control by tamponade alone. In addition, when bleeding is encountered during USVVS, it is important to remember that the most common sources may be the vascular pedicles if a concomitant vaginal hysterectomy was performed. For this reason, leaving suture tags on the pedicles for easy retrieval and examination can be invaluable. Again, the distal uterosacral ligament lies close to the uterine vessels, and therefore targeting suspension sutures towards the middle or proximal uterosacral ligament can minimize bleeding. Minor to moderate bleeding from placement of the uterosacral ligament suture can be controlled by applying tension to the suture until the end of the operation, at which point it can be tied down to stop the bleeding.

Bowel Injury

Sacrospinous Ligament Fixation and Iliococcygeal Suspension

As extraperitoneal operations, the SSLF and iliococcygeal suspension offer the potential advantage of less small bowel and colonic injury. However, the procedures themselves involve perforation into and dissection of the pararectal space and so rectal injury is a known risk that patients should be counseled about preoperatively. Unilateral right-sided SSLF is preferred because this avoids the recto-sigmoid junction, and makes retraction of the rectum easier. Through the posterior approach, copious hydrodissection in the proper plane between the vaginal mucosa and muscularis makes dissection of the vaginal wall off the rectum easier. After

beginning the dissection sharply, with adequate hydrodissection the rectum can usually be bluntly swept off the vagina in patients who have not had previous repairs. Caution is advised when a previous posterior colporrhaphy has been performed, as there is an increased risk of rectal injury in that setting. When there is uncertainty about the plane, keeping a finger behind the vaginal mucosa is helpful on the vaginal aspect, and occasionally a second glove can be worn and a finger placed in the rectum to guide dissection.

After the rectum has been swept off the vagina, when perforating into the pararectal space, the sacrospinous ligament can be exposed by palpating the ischial spine and sweeping the finger medially. When using Breisky-Navratil retractors to expose the ligament, great care is needed in placing these retractors to avoid rectal laceration. First, manual dissection must ensure there is adequate space for the first (thinner) retractor. Second, place the retractor laterally, against the pelvic sidewall, and then rotate it 180° so that it retracts the rectum, rather than inserting it alongside the rectum, which may result in a tear.

Rectal laceration or perforation has been reported in 0.4–4% of SSLF [16–20]. Most rectal injuries occur in the distal anterior rectum upon initial dissection [17, 19]. These injuries are usually small (<2 cm) and can managed with primary closure in 2–3 layers, copious irrigation, and postoperative bowel rest for 2 or 3 days [17]. Many vaginal reconstructive surgeons may repair these injuries themselves, but obtaining a colorectal surgery consult intraoperatively can be helpful for technical and medicolegal reasons. If the injury is readily identifiable, easily accessible, and can be closed in multiple layers in a tension-free manner in a healthy patient without a history of irradiation, then diverting colostomy is usually not necessary.

For sutures that are not placed under direct vision, such as with a suture-capturing device, inadvertent placement of the suture through the rectum can occur. Usually this can be identified intraoperatively with a careful digital rectal examination. If suture is palpable, remove it and replace the suture, and usually there are no sequelae. Identifying rectal placement of suture is essential; however, as there are scattered case reports of significant pararectal infectious complications associated with SSLF [21, 22].

Uterosacral Vaginal Vault Suspension

Despite the intraperitoneal nature of the operation, bowel injury is rare with USVVS, and is reported in less than 1% of cases [6]. Small bowel obstruction (SBO) in particular is very rare, and was first reported in a series in 2006 [23]. Three patients presented with significant nausea and vomiting on postoperative days 1–14 and were found to have possible SBO [23]. After failing conservative management, all subsequently underwent laparoscopy. The source of the obstruction was adhesions in two of the patients, and a prolene suture in the third. One of the patients requiring significant adhesiolysis underwent small bowel resection and enteroenterostomy due to enterotomies during dissection.

Despite the low reported rate of small bowel injury or obstruction, there are several important technical considerations required to keep this rate low. When exposing the uterosacral ligaments, packing of the bowel with tagged, counted laparotomy sponges is usually necessary. The peritoneum should be carefully inspected for abdominal adhesions, the sponges advanced slowly and gently to avoid enterotomies, and gentle retraction on the sponges to minimize trauma. Similarly, these packs should be removed slowly and carefully, and counted, after placing suspension sutures. If performing culdoplasty, care in closing the parietal peritoneum can avoid capturing bowel in the closure.

Evisceration

Small bowel evisceration has been reported following vaginal hysterectomy [24, 25], as well as following transvaginal enterocele and SSLF [26]. Evisceration is a surgical emergency, and although some have had success through a transvaginal route alone, usually a transabdominal route is helpful to assess the viability of the small bowel involved [27].

Neurologic and Pain Complications

Sacrospinous Ligament Fixation

Knowledge and understanding of the nearby anatomy is essential. Suture placement in the middle third of the sacrospinous ligament avoids the region of the pudendal nerve, and staying caudad to the greater sciatic foramen avoids the sciatic nerve [10]. Anatomic studies also reveal, however, that nerves to the coccygeus and levator ani actually pass ventral to the ligament in the middle segment, where sutures are typically placed, and may be encountered during dissection and suture placement [28]. Histologic studies of the ligament itself confirm nerves within the substance of the ligament, especially in the middle segment [29], which explains the potential for pain after this operation. In fact, another cadaveric study found the only nerve-free region of the ligament to be the medial third [30], which is more medial than is often described in the operation.

Buttock or tailbone pain, which may be due to involvement of peripheral nervous branches or to the tension on the ligament, occurs in around 6–14% of patients after SSLF [7, 31, 32]. The majority of cases of postoperative buttock pain resolve spontaneously or with medical management, although in one report 3 of 18 patients with postoperative pain subsequently had chronic pain [32]. Persistent pelvic and perineal pain should raise suspicion of potential pudendal nerve entrapment. History and physical exam will indicate onset of symptoms coincident with surgery, in the sensory distribution of the pudendal nerve. Although removal of the offending suture should not be delayed, a report of a patient who presented 2 years after SSLF noted that they still had complete relief after suture removal even after that length of time from surgery [33].

Uterosacral Vaginal Vault Suspension

The intraperitoneal nature of this operation makes direct visualization of retroperitoneal vasculature and nerves difficult, and therefore a thorough anatomic understanding is necessary. Assessing the position of the ischial spine allows avoidance of the pudendal nerve, which is usually sufficiently far from the uterosacral ligaments [34]. On the other hand, the sacral nerve routes are susceptible during USVVS. A cadaveric study demonstrated that by tenting the uterosacral ligaments distally and ventrally using an Allis clamp before suture placement, the sacral nerve roots can be avoided [34]. Although tension on the ligament is also distributed to the ureter, this effect is seen most dramatically distally, and can be avoided by proximal suture placement [1]. The sacral nerve roots as well as the intrapelvic portion of the sciatic nerve are vulnerable to entrapment during uterosacral suspension, which can explain postoperative pain in some patients [35]. Sensory neuropathies have been reported in 3.8% of patients [36]. Pain tends to present in the acute postoperative period, in the distribution of the S1 through S3 nerve roots, and can be successfully managed by removal of the ipsilateral suspension suture, or with medical management [36, 37].

Summary

Transvaginal apical suspensions can have serious complications, including hemorrhage, visceral injury, and neurologic sequelae. Intimate knowledge of the relevant anatomy can, however, reduce these risks, and the majority of complications can be successfully treated with proper identification and management.

References

1. Buller JL, Thompson JR, Cundiff GW, et al. Uterosacral ligament: description of anatomic relationships to optimize surgical safety. Obstet Gynecol. 2001;97:873–9.
2. Gustilo-Ashby AM, Jelovsek JE, Barber MD, et al. The incidence of ureteral obstruction and the value of intraoperative cystoscopy during vaginal surgery for pelvic organ prolapse. Am J Obstet Gynecol. 2006;194:1478–85.
3. Visco AG, Taber KH, Weidner AC, et al. Cost-effectiveness of universal cystoscopy to identify ureteral injury at hysterectomy. Obstet Gynecol. 2001;97(5 Pt 1):685–92.
4. Kim JH, Moore C, Jones JS, et al. Management of ureteral injuries associated with vaginal surgery for pelvic organ prolapse. Int Urogynecol J Pelvic Floor Dysfunct. 2006;17:531–5.
5. Siddighi S, Yandell PM, Karram MM. Delayed presentation of complete ureteral obstruction deligated transvaginally. Int Urogynecol J Pelvic Floor Dysfunct. 2011;22:251–3.
6. Margulies RU, Rogers MA, Morgan DM. Outcomes of transvaginal uterosacral ligament suspension: systematic review and metaanalysis. Am J Obstet Gynecol. 2010;202:124–34.
7. Lantzsch T, Goepel C, Wolters M, et al. Sacrospinous ligament fixation for vaginal vault prolapse. Arch Gynecol Obstet. 2001;265:21–5.
8. Koyama M, Yoshida S, Koyama S, et al. Surgical reinforcement of support for the vagina in pelvic organ prolapse: concurrent iliococcygeus fascia colpopexy (Inmon technique). Int Urogynecol J Pelvic Floor Dysfunct. 2005;16:197–202.
9. Rane A, Frazer M, Jain A, et al. The sacrospinous ligament: conveniently effective or effectively convenient? J Obstet Gynaecol. 2011;31:366–70.
10. Verdeja AM, Elkins TE, Odoi A, et al. Transvaginal sacrospinous colpopexy: anatomic landmarks to be aware of to minimize complications. Am J Obstet Gynecol. 1995;173:1468–9.
11. Goldberg RP, Tomezsko JE, Winkler HA, et al. Anterior or posterior sacrospinous vaginal vault suspension: long-term anatomic and functional evaluation. Obstet Gynecol. 2001;98:199–204.
12. Pollak J, Takacs P, Medina C. Complications of three sacrospinous ligament fixation techniques. Int J Gynaecol Obstet. 2007;99:18–22.
13. Barksdale PA, Elkins TE, Sanders CK, et al. An anatomic approach to pelvic hemorrhage during sacrospinous ligament fixation of the vaginal vault. Obstet Gynecol. 1998;91:715–8.
14. Maher CF, Murray CJ, Carey MP, et al. Iliococcygeus or sacrospinous fixation for vaginal vault prolapse. Obstet Gynecol. 2001;981:40–4.
15. Meeks GR, Washburne JF, McGehee RP, Wiser WL. Repair of vaginal vault prolapse by suspension of the vagina to iliococcygeus (prespinous) fascia. Am J Obstet Gynecol. 1994;171:1444–52.
16. Hoffman MS, Harris MS, Bouis PJ. Sacrospinous colpopexy in the management of uterovaginal prolapse. J Reprod Med. 1996;41:299–303.
17. Hoffman MS, Lynch C, Lockhart J, Knapp R. Injury of the rectum during vaginal surgery. Am J Obstet Gynecol. 1999;181:274–7.
18. Beer M, Kuhn A. Surgical techniques for vault prolapse: a review of the literature. Eur J Obstet Gynecol Reprod Biol. 2005;119:144–55.

19. Demirci F, Ozdemir I, Somunkiran A, et al. Perioperative complications in abdominal sacrocolpopexy and vaginal sacrospinous ligament fixation procedures. Int Urogynecol J Pelvic Floor Dysfunct. 2007;18:257–61.

20. David-Montefiore E, Barranger E, Dubernard G, et al. Functional results and quality-of-life after bilateral sacrospinous ligament fixation for genital prolapse. Eur J Obstet Gynecol Reprod Biol. 2007;132:209–13.

21. Hibner M, Cornella JL, Magrina JF, Heppel JP. Ischiorectal abscess after sacrospinous ligament suspension. Am J Obstet Gynecol. 2005;193:1740–2.

22. Gafni-Kane A, Goldberg RP, Spitz JS, Sand PK. Extrasphincteric perianal fistulae after sacrospinous fixation for apical prolapse. Obstet Gynecol. 2011; 117:438–40.

23. Ridgeway B, Barber MD, Walters MD, Paraiso MF. Small bowel obstruction after vaginal vault suspension: a series of three cases. Int Urogynecol J Pelvic Floor Dysfunct. 2007;18:1237–41.

24. Moen MD, Desai M, Sulkowski R. Vaginal evisceration managed by transvaginal bowel resection and vaginal repair. Int Urogynecol J Pelvic Floor Dysfunct. 2003;14:218–20.

25. Patravali N, Kulkarni T. Bowel evisceration through the vaginal vault: a delayed complication following hysterectomy. J Obstet Gynaecol. 2007;27:211.

26. Farrell SA, Scotti RJ, Ostergard DR, Bent AE. Massive evisceration: a complication following sacrospinous vaginal vault fixation. Obstet Gynecol. 1991;78:560–2.

27. Rollinson D, Brodman ML, Friedman Jr F, Sperling R. Transvaginal small-bowel evisceration: a case report. Mt Sinai J Med. 1995;62:235–8.

28. Roshanravan SM, Wieslander CK, Schaffer JI, Corton MM. Neurovascular anatomy of the sacrospinous ligament region in female cadavers: implications in sacrospinous ligament fixation. Am J Obstet Gynecol. 2007;197:660.e1–6.

29. Barksdale PA, Gasser RF, Gauthier CM, et al. Intraligamentous nerves as a potential source of pain after sacrospinous ligament fixation of the vaginal apex. Int Urogynecol J Pelvic Floor Dysfunct. 1997;8: 121–5.

30. Lazarou G, Grigorescu BA, Olson TR, et al. Anatomic variations in the pelvic floor nerves adjacent to the sacrospinous ligament: a female cadaver study. Int Urogynecol J Pelvic Floor Dysfunct. 2008;19: 649–54.

31. Meschia M, Bruschi F, Amicarelli F, et al. The sacrospinous vaginal vault suspension: critical analysis of outcomes. Int Urogynecol J Pelvic Floor Dysfunct. 1999;10:155–9.

32. Lovatsis D, Drutz HP. Safety and efficacy of sacrospinous vault suspension. Int Urogynecol J Pelvic Floor Dysfunct. 2002;13:308–13.

33. Alevizon SJ, Finan MA. Sacrospinous colpopexy: management of postoperative pudendal nerve entrapment. Obstet Gynecol. 1996;88:713–5.

34. Siddiqui NY, Mitchell TR, Bentley RC, Weidner AC. Neural entrapment during uterosacral ligament suspension: an anatomic study of female cadavers. Obstet Gynecol. 2010;116:708–13.

35. Schön Ybarra MA, Gutman RE, Rini D, Handa VL. Etiology of post-uterosacral suspension neuropathies. Int Urogynecol J Pelvic Floor Dysfunct. 2009;20: 1067–71.

36. Flynn M, Weidner AC, Amundsen CL. Sensory nerve injury after uterosacral ligament suspension. Am J Obstet Gynecol. 2006;19:1869–72.

37. Lowenstein L, Dooley Y, Kenton K, et al. Neural pain after uterosacral ligament vaginal suspension. Int Urogynecol J Pelvic Floor Dysfunct. 2007;18: 109–10.

38. Vaginal repair of vaginal vault prolapse. In: Baggish, Karram, editors. Atlas of pelvic anatomy and gynecologic surgery. 3rd ed. Elsevier-Saunders; 2011;709.

Complications of Abdominal Sacrocolpopexy

6

Michelle Koski and J. Christian Winters

Introduction

With the aging of our population, pelvic organ prolapse is an increasingly common condition that negatively affects patient quality of life. Vaginal vault prolapse has been reported to occur in as many as 18.2% of all women with prolapse [1], and many would suggest that vaginal vault prolapse is a component of most high-grade anterior compartment descensus. Several repairs exist that reconstitute support to the vaginal vault, and certainly there is no single procedure that is optimal for all patients. Abdominal sacral colpopexy (ASC) offers an effective and durable repair for vaginal vault prolapse [2]. It maximizes functional vaginal length and approximates the normal vaginal axis [3]. ASC should be considered especially in patients with failed prior vaginal repairs, isolated high-grade apical prolapse, and in younger patients with apical prolapse who would like to maintain sexual function [4].

M. Koski
Department of Urology, Medical University
of South Carolina, Charleston, SC 29425, USA

J.C. Winters (✉)
Department of Urology, Louisiana State University,
1542 Tulane Avenue, 5th Floor, Room 547,
New Orleans, LA 70112, USA
e-mail: cwinte@lsuhsc.edu

The procedure may be performed open, laparoscopically, or robotically. In our experience, the key components of the operation though the open or robotic approach include utilization of a permanent, type I macroporous mesh, secure suture fixation of the graft to the sacral promontory and vaginal cuff (Fig. 6.1), complete enterocele reduction and culdoplasty, and the addition of concomitant anti-incontinence procedures as indicated [4]. We affix the vaginal portion of the graft with multiple sutures to distribute the tension evenly over the vaginal apex (Fig. 6.2), and avoid excessive tension between the apex and sacrum (Fig. 6.3). We routinely close the peritoneum over the mesh arm. In this chapter we will address the recognition and management of complications potentially associated with this method of the repair, as well as outline complications that have arisen from other variations.

Intraoperative Complications

In a large meta-review by Nygaard et al. [2], intraoperative complications included hemorrhage or transfusion (0.18–16.9%), cystotomy (0.4–15.8%), enterotomy or proctotomy (0.4–2.5%), and ureteral injury (0.8–1.9%). In patients undergoing the laparoscopic or robotic approach, intraoperative complications associated with pneumoperitoneum and port access may occur which are not unique to colpopexy.

Fig. 6.1 Type 1 macroporous mesh is sutured to the sacral promontory and the vaginal cuff

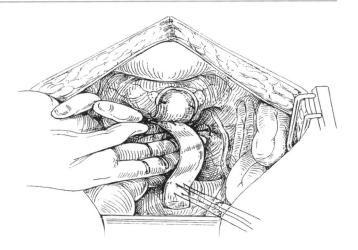

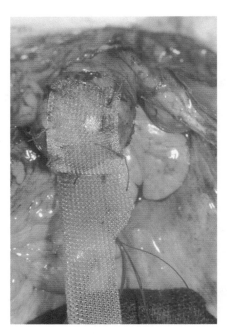

Fig. 6.2 The mesh graft is affixed to the apex of the vagina with multiple sutures for even tension distribution

Hemorrhage

Presacral hemorrhage incurred during the dissection of the sacral promontory is one of the most feared complications of ASC, as well as one of the more commonly reported in the literature [2]. Bleeding from the presacral space may be large volume because the bleeding vessels may retract into the sacrum. Historically, in the 1970s, the

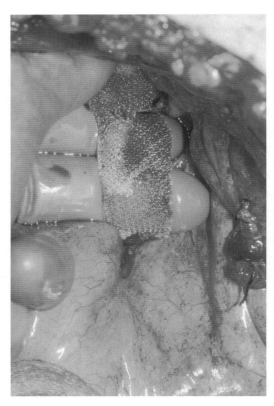

Fig. 6.3 Intraoperative view: graft in final position. A space of two fingerbreadths between the graft and the rectum prevents compression of the rectum under the graft. Incised peritoneum will be closed over graft

operation was described with fixation of the mesh graft to the level of S3–S4 below the sacral promontory in an attempt to create a more natural vaginal axis [5]. After a life-threatening hemor-rhage at this site, Sutton advocated for fixation higher on the sacral promontory at the S1–S2 level [6]. This site allows better visualization of the middle sacral artery and the slight difference in vaginal axis has not resulted in negative out-comes. Careful dissection at the sacral promon-tory should be used to avoid laceration of unseen presacral vessels. Excessive blunt dissection should be avoided to prevent shearing of the pre-sacral veins. Monopolar cautery should be used precisely, and diathermy cautery may be helpful as well. If bleeding occurs in the laparoscopic or robotic approach, increasing the intra-abdominal pressure to 20 cm H_2O may slow the bleeding enough to see the vessel to cauterize. If uncon-trollable bleeding is incurred which is not ame-nable to direct cautery, it may be managed with stainless steel thumbtacks [7], bone wax, or a figure of eight stitch [8].

Cystotomy, Enterotomy, and Ureteral Injury

Injury to the bladder or bowel may occur during dissection or inadvertently. Care should be taken at all points of bladder dissection to maintain a full thickness dissection and avoid cystotomy. Additionally, we try to avoid excessive cautery in the dissection of the bladder from the vagina. If a bladder injury is detected, it should be closed in two layers with absorbable suture and an ade-quately sized urethral catheter should be left for bladder drainage. At this point, it would be at the discretion of the surgeon whether to proceed with mesh attachment to the vaginal apex. Mesh should not be placed adjacent to or in proximity to the cystotomy as it might predispose to erosion of mesh into the bladder or fistula formation [9]. If vesical injury is missed, patients may present with fever, pain secondary to urinoma or urinary ascites.

Enterotomy with any fecal or enteric soilage precludes placement of mesh. The bowel injury

should be repaired and the case concluded. This illustrates the benefit of preoperative bowel prep-aration. If enterotomy is missed, patients with unrecognized bowel injuries often present 1–2 days postoperatively and may lack the typical signs of peritonitis. Patients may present with low grade fever and leucopenia with a left shift. If the injury was incurred in a laparoscopic case, they may have severe pain at one of the trocar sites. The clinician should maintain a high index of suspicion to order a computed tomography (CT) scan in these patients.

The ureters should be identified early on in the case to avoid injury from dissection or entrap-ment or kinking in the culdoplasty sutures. To insure patency of the ureter we perform cystos-copy after the conclusion of the case with admin-istration of indigo carmine or methylene blue to clearly visualize ureteral efflux.

Postoperative Complications

Postoperative complications in a comprehen-sive review included urinary tract infection (2.5–25.9%), wound infection or separation (0.4–19.8%), ileus (1.1–9.3%), deep venous thrombosis or pulmonary embolism (0.4–5.0%), and small bowel obstruction (SBO) (0.6–8.6%), and inci-sional hernia requiring repair (0.4–15%). Additionally, mesh erosion was noted at an over-all rate of 3.4% in the 2,178 patients reviewed in this meta-analysis [2].

Vaginal Mesh Erosion

Key signs and symptoms of vaginal mesh erosion include persistent pain, discharge, and occasion-ally dyspareunia for the woman and/or her part-ner. Suture erosions are typically asymptomatic [10, 11]. A comprehensive review of ASC quoted an overall mesh erosion rate of 3.4% [2], although rates of erosion quoted in the literature vary [10, 12–14]. While mesh erosions after ASC typically occur 4–24 months after surgery [10, 12], they may also present several years later [15]. Because of this, determining an accurate erosion rate in series is complicated by length of follow-up. Additionally, mesh type, surgical technique, and modifiable factors may affect the rate of erosion.

Mesh type appears to affect erosion rates based on comparison of the literature, although there have been no standardized trials comparing different materials. In the Nygaard meta-analysis, polypropylene carried an erosion rate of 0.5% in comparison to 3.1% for polyethylene terephthalate (Mersilene; Johnson & Johnson), 3.4% for polytetrafluoroethylene (Gore-Tex; W.L. Fore, Flagstaff, AZ), 5.0% for polyethylene (Phillips Sumika, Polypropylene Co., Houston, TX) and 5.5% for Teflon (E.I. DuPont de Nemours and Co.) [2]. No conclusions were made in this review regarding whether certain mesh types predispose to erosion because in this setting they could not control for other variables (method of graft placement, concurrent hysterectomy, etc.). However, certainly, particular mesh materials are more at risk for erosion. Govier et al. found a 23.8% graft complication rate (mesh erosion or infection) in a retrospective review of 21 patients who underwent ASC using a silicone coated polyethylene preformed graft [13]. A subanalysis of the Colpopexy and Urinary Reduction Efforts (CARE) study found a nearly fourfold increased risk of mesh erosion if Gore-Tex mesh was used compared to non-Gore-Tex mesh, which reached statistical significance and altered their use of Gore-Tex mesh [14].

Biologic materials are not without complication. Allograft fascia lata has been described as a biologic alternative to mesh. This material precludes the risk of mesh erosion. However, reports of failures associated with attenuation or absence of the fascia lata graft in reoperation [16, 17], presumably secondary to autolysis, have led to decreased use of this material. A retrospective cohort study comparing polypropylene mesh to Pelvicol (CR Bard, Murray Hill, NJ) and autologous fascia found a higher rate of failures as well as erosions and other graft-related complications in the Pelvicol group (although it should be noted that Pelvicol was used more frequently in patients

undergoing concomitant hysterectomy) [18]. Similar findings of high rates of graft-related complications and unacceptable failure rates were found with porcine grafts [19].

A modifiable risk factor for erosion after ASC identified by the CARE trial analysis was tobacco use [14]. In their group of 322 patients, smoking was associated with a fivefold increased risk of erosion. A retrospective study of 499 patients undergoing ASC found a nonsignificant trend of smokers requiring more than one surgery for effective treatment of vaginal mesh erosion [20]. The dominant theory is that microvascular vasospasm with associated hypoxia may lead to poor wound healing and vaginal mesh erosion in smokers [15].

Approach and technique affect mesh erosion rates. If graft or suture is introduced through the vagina in sacral colpoperineopexy, erosion rates are increased. In a retrospective review of 273 patients, there was no statistically significant difference in mesh erosion rates for patients undergoing ASC (3.2%) or purely abdominal sacral colpoperineopexy (4.5%). In patients undergoing sacral colpoperineopexy with vaginal introduction of mesh or sutures, the erosion rates increased to 16% (vaginal placement of sutures) and 40% (vaginal mesh), which maintained statistical significance on multivariate analysis. These patients exhibited a shorter time to mesh erosion as well, with median time to erosion 15.6 months for ASC, 12.4 months for abdominal sacral colpoperineopexy, 9.0 months in the suture group ($P<0.005$), and 4.1 months in the vaginal mesh group ($P<0.0001$) [21].

The role of concomitant hysterectomy in mesh erosion after ASC has been debated. In the CARE subanalysis [15], concurrent abdominal hysterectomy was performed in 26% of the patients, who incurred a 14% risk of erosion as compared to 4% in women who had undergone prior hysterectomy. This represented a fivefold increased risk of erosion. Culligan et al. found a statistically significant increase in erosion rates in patients undergoing concomitant hysterectomy in a retrospective review of 245 patients (27.3% erosion in those undergoing hysterectomy, 1.3% erosion without hysterectomy) [22]. A retrospective review of 313 patients found a statistically significant fivefold risk of mesh erosion in women on estrogen with concomitant hysterectomy [23]. Of note, they found no significant difference in erosion rates in those undergoing concurrent hysterectomy in the non estrogen group, or in the overall group as well. This data implies that either estrogen or hysterectomy may increase erosion rates. In our experience, it seems hysterectomy would be the most likely risk factor. In contrast, in a retrospective review of 124 patients undergoing ASC (60 with hysterectomy and 64 without), Brizzolara et al. found a low overall mesh erosion rate of 0.8% and no significant difference in mesh erosions in the hysterectomy group [12]. They attributed their success to two-layer closure of the cuff, careful handling of tissues and use of antibiotic irrigation [12]. Based on these findings, if a small vaginal laceration is encountered during colpopexy, we close the laceration in two layers as described in the previous study. In reviewing outcomes of colpopexy following hysterectomy, the significance of the CARE subanalysis, as opposed to retrospective reviews, is that it was prospectively designed to capture complications, including mesh and suture erosions, at regular study intervals in the first 2 years.

In cases of mesh erosion after combined hysterectomy and ASC, the erosion site is usually at the cuff. This may be secondary to potential vaginal bacterial contamination of the mesh from the opened vagina during hysterectomy. Alternatively, poor healing may occur at the cuff secondary to a devascularizing effect of cuff closure combined with mesh vaginal attachment sutures [15]. Some authors advocate supra-cervical hysterectomy as an alternative to total hysterectomy at the time of ASC [13]. Currently, the practice of concomitant hysterectomy and ASC remains controversial.

In cases of erosion of Type I mesh (Dacron, Marlex, Prolene), treatment with antibiotics and trimming and covering of the mesh is sufficient [11]. Because of the macroporous nature of the mesh, it is expected that macrophages will pass, making complete removal of the graft unnecessary. Additionally, eroded Type III mesh (combinations of multifilament and macroporous components: Teflon, Mersilene) may be treated

with partial removal and reclosure of vaginal flaps [11]. However, infected Type II mesh (microporous material: Gore-Tex) must almost always be removed completely, as its microporous nature creates a bacterial sanctuary where access to antibiotics and the immune response is reduced [11, 15].

Conservative therapy with observation and topical estrogen may be initially attempted in small mesh erosions of type I or III mesh (<1 cm). Local excision of mesh is utilized as first line therapy as well, or in cases of failed conservative therapy. In a series of vaginal erosions of Ethibond (Ethicon, Somerville, NJ) suture and Marlex and Mersilene mesh, patients presented at an average of 14 months postoperatively (range 4–24). All patients were initially treated with vaginal estrogen and 8 weeks of pelvic rest. Two patients with suture erosions resolved with this regimen, but all five patients with mesh erosion required surgical intervention and were successfully treated with vaginal mesh excision and flap advancement [10]. In another series, local surgical excision of exposed mesh carried a reported efficacy rate of 50% [20]. If the upper portion of the mesh is infected, it must be removed [15]. In the CARE subanalysis, 6% of patients experienced mesh/suture erosion. Most of the women with mesh erosion (13/17) underwent at least one surgery for partial or total mesh removal. Two patients completely resolved, 6 had persistent problems, and 5 were lost to follow-up [15]. Of the four women who elected observation, none experienced resolution [15].

Well-circumscribed areas of mesh extrusion may be approached vaginally. We excise only the exposed area with an additional margin of 1–2 cm; not all of the mesh needs to be excised. Surgical exposure of apical mesh extrusions in the postsacrocolpopexy patient is more challenging than in distal vaginal extrusions. When the apex is well supported, it may be difficult to pull the apex into the forefront of the surgical field. We use a Lone Star retractor (Cooper Surgical, Trumbull, CT) with sharp hooks placed proximal to the mesh to expose as well as possible. Hydrodissection may be utilized around the area of the extrusion. We grasp the edge of the vaginal

Fig. 6.4 Cystoscopic view of mesh erosion into the bladder

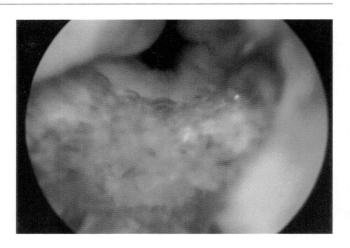

margin and dissect laterally between the vaginal margin and the mesh with Metzenbaum scissors to create vaginal flaps that extend about 2 cm circumferentially. If the edge of the mesh is available, we grasp that edge and begin our dissection underneath the mesh. If an edge is not accessible, we incise the mesh and isolate each resultant edge in an Allis clamp. Oftentimes, the mesh will peel off the underlying tissue with a combination of blunt and sharp dissection. We keep the scissor tips pointing toward the mesh. Once the mesh has been separated back to the edges of the initial dissection we inspect the quality of the edges of our vaginal margins. If there is any question about the quality of the tissue, we will excise or debride the edges. Finally, we reapproximate the vaginal flaps with absorbable suture in a tension-free closure with no mesh under the suture line. Other authors have advocated a partial colpocleisis type approach [20]. If the initial extrusion is extensive or if prior vaginal approaches have failed, an abdominal approach may be attempted. Abdominal excisions are associated with higher blood loss, longer hospitalization, and additional morbidity [20].

In all cases, the approach to extrusions is vaginal unless there is other intra-abdominal pathology warranting correction. In an abdominal approach, extensive scarring and adhesions will be encountered. A full bowel preparation is recommended and vaginal localization can be assisted with the use of an EEA sizer and or a Lucite vaginal stent. Partial removal of offending

mesh is acceptable unless gross infection is present. The vaginal defect should be repaired in two layers using absorbable sutures. In cases of poor tissue quality, a biologic interposition over the vaginal cuff or omentum may be utilized to assist in cuff healing.

Erosion of Mesh into Bladder or Bowel

Patients with mesh erosion into the bladder after ASC may present with hematuria, irritative voiding symptoms, recurrent urinary tract infections, or chronic bladder stones. Diagnosis of this problem hinges on a high index of suspicion and a low threshold to perform cystoscopy. Maintaining a full thickness of the bladder without cystotomy during dissection, or alternatively, minimizing bladder mobilization may help in avoiding this complication.

Patsner reported a case of erosion of polypropylene mesh and Prolene suture into the bladder base presenting 4 months after ASC who was treated with open excision after two failed cystoscopic attempts [24]. Yamamoto et al. report a vesicovaginal fistula after abdominal hysterectomy and ASC which occurred adjacent to the edge of the mesh and required abdominal repair [9]. In our experience, we have not had a mesh or suture erosion into the bladder secondary to ASC, but we have acquired a skill set from dealing with vesical mesh erosions from other causes (Fig. 6.4). Depending on the site of erosion and the amount

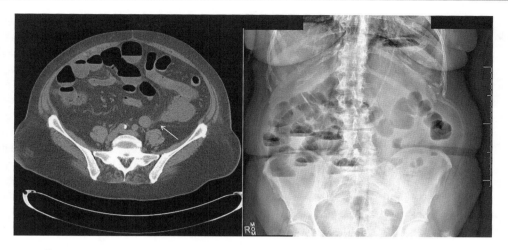

Fig. 6.5 Radiographic images of a patient with partial small bowel obstruction after abdominal sacral colpopexy. The CT scan shows distended loops of bowel with a transition point marked with an *arrow*

of mesh, a cystoscopic approach may be attempted. If this fails or is precluded by position or mesh volume, an open cystorrhaphy may be necessary. If the mesh is near the ureteral orifice, the surgeon should consider a retrograde pyelogram or a ureteral stent to delineate the ureter. In a retrospective review of intravesical mesh management cases (from various causes), Frenkl et al. concluded that, in their experience, sutures were managed most successfully with endoscopic techniques, where mesh was best managed with cystorrhaphy [25].

There have been only three reported incidences of mesh erosion into the bowel. In a rare report of mesh erosion into the sigmoid colon 8 years after ASC, the patient was noted to have stool in her vagina and was ultimately treated with sigmoid colon resection with a low colorectal reanastamosis and omental J-flap placement [26]. Kenton et al. described a Gore-Tex graft erosion into the rectum with spontaneous passage of the graft 7 years post-ASC without fistula formation [27]. Hopkins and Rooney describe a small bowel fistula secondary to adhesion of a loop of terminal ileum to an exposed mesh that had been "minimally retroperitonealized" [28]. Based on this, they advocate retroperitonealization of the mesh as a way to prevent adhesion of bowel. Most early descriptions of sacrocolpopexy describe closing the peritoneum over the graft. Other authors question the utility of this step. In a

small study of 35 women, 3 had postoperative bowel obstructions, all resulting from intestine trapped under the mesh, despite careful retroperitonealization [29]. Due to the low incidence of bowel mesh erosions, it is unlikely that this question will be addressed in a standardized fashion. In order to prevent these complications, we would advise meticulous placement of the mesh with careful attention to ensure an adequate space between the mesh and the sigmoid colon. We routinely close the peritoneum over the mesh.

Ileus and Small Bowel Obstruction

The reported incidence of postoperative ileus is a median 3.6% (range 1.1–9.3%) of patients and reoperation for SBO is a median 1.1% (range 0.6–8.6%) after ASC in meta-analysis [2]. This review was comprised mostly of retrospective reports. The findings from a subanalysis of the CARE trial supported these findings in the framework of a large prospective trial [30]. Of their 322 patients, 5.9% had postoperative gastrointestinal conditions resulting in reoperation, prolonged hospitalization, or readmission. Four patients (1.2%) required reoperation and all were found to have small bowel entrapment in, or adhesion to, the abdominal wall incision (Fig. 6.5). Overall, the rate of SBO was 1.9–2.5% and the rate of ileus was 2.2–2.8%. Age was found to have a significant association with ileus [30]. Prior abdominal surgery was not significantly associated, but the study was not sufficiently powered to rule this out. Of note, 18% of their patients experienced nausea, vomiting and bloating postoperatively and they make note that 20–30% of patients may experience these symptoms after general anesthesia for any surgery [31].

Recurrence

Recurrent vaginal vault prolapse after ASC with permanent mesh is rare. The success rate, when defined as lack of apical prolapse postoperatively, ranges from 78 to 100% [2]. Baessler et al. proposed that rare cases of symptomatic apical recurrence are usually secondary to detachment of the mesh from the vagina and that separation of the mesh from the sacrum is much less common [11]. If the mesh is still secured to the sacrum, they describe attaching a new mesh to it, which is then sutured to the vagina. They warn against removal of the original mesh due to the high risk of hazard to the ureter and bowel in a potentially difficult dissection. Addison et al. reiterate this in their series of recurrences, all resulting from disruption of the mesh from the vaginal apex (one of these cases secondary to a dissection of an enterocele beneath the mesh, causing disruption) [32]. They advocate performing a meticulous culdoplasty with permanent sutures and attachment of the mesh to the vaginal vault with multiple permanent sutures placed through the entire thickness of the vagina over a broad area as methods to help prevent recurrence [32].

Unmasking of Occult Stress Incontinence

We routinely assess for occult SUI preoperatively with either urodynamics or cough stress test with the prolapse reduced. Rates of urodynamic SUI with prolapse reduction have been reported ranging from 25 to 100% in symptomatically continent women using various methods of reduction [33]. Patients undergoing ASC are at significant

risk for developing bothersome stress urinary incontinence, even in the absence of preoperative symptoms. This was well illustrated in the CARE study [34]. In a prospective, controlled trial of 322 previously stress-continent women, 23.8% who underwent Burch colposuspension at the time of ASC showed postoperative SUI compared to 44.1% who underwent ASC alone. Those in the ASC alone group were also more likely to report bothersome SUI symptoms as compared to the Burch group (24.5% vs. 6.1%) [34]. Women who demonstrated preoperative SUI with prolapse reduction were more likely to report postoperative SUI, regardless of concurrent colposuspension (controls 58% vs. 38% ($P=0.04$) and Burch 32% vs. 21% ($P=0.19$)) [33]. In this study, the majority of women who did not leak with prolapse reduction did not leak after prolapse surgery (60%). In addition, women who did have a Burch procedure still experienced an approximately 30% rate of recurrent SUI. Based on these findings, we use urodynamics to counsel our patients and identify who might best benefit from concurrent anti-incontinence procedures, but we also inform our patients that a negative test does not preclude postoperative incontinence. We prefer midurethral sling concurrently in patients undergoing ASC with symptomatic or occult SUI detected on screening. If women have significant obstructive symptoms on urodynamics with the prolapse reduced, we will perform ASC without sling. If a woman has no occult SUI or symptoms of SUI, patients choose whether or not to undergo concomitant sling. Our bias is to not place a sling at that time. If patients develop SUI after ASC alone, a midurethral sling can be placed at a later date with minimal difficulty.

Osteomyelitis

Osteomyelitis after ASC is rare, and is generally heralded by persistent new low back pain. Weidner et al. described two cases of lumbosacral osteomyelitis after ASC, both treated successfully and definitively with prolonged parenteral antibiotic therapy guided by aspirated cultures and neither requiring mesh removal [35].

One patient presented with unremitting severe low back pain 5 years after ASC, and the second patient presented 2 months postoperatively. Both sacral fixations were performed with Ticron (Davis and Geck, Wayne, NJ) suture. Both were diagnosed on MRI, which is the most sensitive method for detecting osteomyelitis and defining the extent of the infection. Plain films and bone scan may be diagnostic, but are less sensitive than MRI. The authors suggest maintaining a higher level of suspicion for osteomyelitis in patients with a history of degenerative disc disease [35], as patients with degenerative disc disease are predisposed to infection due to disruption of the vertebral endplate and neovascularization of disc spaces, which allows bacteria into a normally avascular space [36]. In the rheumatologic literature, Cailleux et al. reported on five cases of sacral osteomyelitis after ASC (of a retrospective review of 45 patients with sacral osteomyelitis) [37]. Initial symptoms occurred at an average of 38 days postoperatively. In three of the patients, the same bacterial species was identified in urine cultures 1–4 days postoperatively as in the biopsy of the infected bone.

Since these initial series, there have been more reports, usually in the form of case report. Nosseir et al. reported a case secondary to titanium tacks that resolved with parenteral antibiotics [38]. Muffly et al. reported a case of osteomyelitis and infected mesh with a sinus tract after robotic hysterectomy and ASC which required discectomy, sacral debridement, and mesh removal [39]. Another case of sacral osteomyelitis with concomitant mesh erosion and sinus formation required mesh removal and tract resection [40]. Taylor et al. described a case that presented with vaginal erosion of mesh and osteomyelitis with progressive neurologic symptoms requiring a decompressive laminectomy [41].

We advocate empiric routine preoperative IV antibiotics and meticulous surgical technique with mesh and other permanent implants. Patients with degenerative disc disease may be at increased risk of osteomyelitis and should be treated with care as well as a higher index of suspicion postoperatively. MRI should be used to rule out osteomyelitis in the carefully selected patient, and if possible, CT-guided aspiration and culture should be performed to guide antibiotic therapy. Isolated osteomyelitis may respond to prolonged antibiotics alone. In cases that fail antibiotics or in patients with mesh erosion, infection, or sinus tracts, surgery may be required. The urologist should maintain a low threshold to consult infectious disease, orthopedics, and/or neurosurgery as indicated by the patient's presentation.

Conclusion

Sacrocolpopexy is a well-established standard of care for the surgical correction of vaginal vault prolapse. It has become minimally invasive with the robotic and laparoscopic approach. In many ways it is now a more comparable alternative to vaginal apical repair operations. Complications occur at a low incidence [2]. For the vast majority of patients, this procedure provides a gratifying outcome which is durable and anatomic. A thorough knowledge of anatomy, graft biology, and potential complications is optimal in order to assure this procedure may be performed as safely and efficiently as possible.

References

1. Winters JC, Cespedes RD, Vanlangendonck R. Abdominal sacral colpopexy and abdominal enterocele repair in the management of vaginal vault prolapse. Urology. 2000;56:55–63.
2. Nygaard IE, McCreery R, Brubaker L, et al. Abdominal sacrocolpopexy: a comprehensive review. Obstet Gynecol. 2004;104:805–23.
3. Given FT. Vaginal length and sexual function after colpopexy for complete uterovaginal eversion. Am J Obstet Gynecol. 1993;169:284–7.
4. Winters JC, Delacroix Jr S. Abdominal Sacral Colpopexy. In: Graham SD, Keane TE, editors. Glenn's urologic surgery. 7th ed. Philadelphia: Lippincott Williams & Wilkins; 2010. p. 349–54.
5. Birnbaum SJ. Rational therapy for the prolapsed vagina. Am J Obstet Gynecol. 1973;115:411–9.
6. Sutton GP, Addison WA, Livengood III CH, et al. Life-threatening hemorrhage complicating sacral colpopexy. Am J Obstet Gynecol. 1981;140:836–7.
7. Timmons MC, Kohler MF, Addison WA. Thumbtack use for control of presacral bleeding with description of an instrument for thumbtack application. Obstet Gynecol. 1991;78:313–5.

8. Lane FE. Modified technique of sacral colpopexy. Am J Obstet Gynecol. 1982;142:933.

9. Yamamoto Y, Nishimura K, Ueda N, et al. Vesicovaginal fistula caused by abdominal hysterectomy and sacrocolpopexy with polypropylene mesh (Gynemesh): a case report. Hinyokika Kiyo. 2010;56:517–20.

10. Kohli N, Walsh PM, Roat TW, et al. Mesh erosion after abdominal sacrocolpopexy. Obstet Gynecol. 1998;92:999–1004.

11. Baessler K, Leron E, Stanton SL. Sacrohysteropexy and sacrocolpopexy. In: Stanton SL, Zimmern P, editors. Female pelvic reconstructive surgery. New York: Springer; 2002. p. 189–90.

12. Brizzolara S, Pillai-Allen A. Risk of mesh erosion with sacral colpopexy and concurrent hysterectomy. Obstet Gynecol. 2003;102:306–10.

13. Govier FE, Kobashi KC, Kozlowski PM, et al. High complication rate identified in sacrocolpopexy patients attributed to silicone mesh. Urology. 2005;65:1099–103.

14. Cundiff GW, Varner E, Visco AG, et al. Risk factors for mesh/suture erosion following sacrocolpopexy. Am J Obstet Gynecol. 2008;199:688.e1–5.

15. Bensinger G, Lind L, Lesser M, et al. Abdominal sacral suspensions: analysis of complications using permanent mesh. Am J Obstet Gynecol. 2005;193:2094–8.

16. Fitzgerald MP, Mollenhauer J, Bitterman P, Brubaker L. Functional failure of fascia lata allografts. Am J Obstet Gynecol. 1999;181:1339–46.

17. Fitzgerald MP, Edwards SR, Fenner D. Medium-term followup on use of freeze-dried, irradiated donor fascia for sacrocolpopexy and sling procedures. Int Urogyn J. 2004;15:238–42.

18. Quiroz LH, Gutman RE, Shippey S, et al. Abdominal sacrocolpopexy: anatomic outcomes and complications with pelvicol, autologous, and synthetic graft materials. Am J Obstet Gynecol. 2008;198:557.e1–5.

19. Claerhout F, De Ridder D, Van Beckevoort D, et al. Sacrocolpopexy using xenogenic acellular collagen in patients at increased risk for graft-related complications. Neurourol Urodyn. 2010;29(4):563–7.

20. Quiroz LH, Gutman RE, Fagan MJ, et al. Partial colpocleisis for the treatment of sacrocolpopexy mesh erosions. Int Urogynecol J Pelvic Floor Dysfunct. 2008;19:261–6.

21. Visco AG, Weidner AC, Barber MD, et al. Vaginal mesh erosion after abdominal sacral colpopexy. Am J Obstet Gynecol. 2001;184:297–302.

22. Culligan PJ, Murphy M, Blackwell L, et al. Long-term success of abdominal sacral colpopexy using synthetic mesh. Am J Obstet Gynecol. 2002;187:1473–82.

23. Wu JM, Wells EC, Hundley AF, et al. Mesh erosion in abdominal sacral colpopexy with and without concomitant hysterectomy. A J Obstet Gynecol. 2006;194:1418–22.

24. Patsner B. Mesh erosion into the bladder after abdominal sacral colpopexy. Obstet Gynecol. 2000;95:1029.

25. Frenkl TL, Rackely RR, Vasavada SP, et al. Management of iatrogenic foreign bodies of the bladder and urethra following pelvic floor surgery. Neurourol Urodyn. 2008;27:491–5.

26. Rose S, Bunten CE, Geisler JP, et al. Polypropylene mesh erosion into the bowel and vagina after abdominal sacral colpopexy. J Pelvic Med Surg. 2006;12:45–7.

27. Kenton KS, Woods MP, Brubaker L. Uncomplicated erosion of polytetraflouroethylene grafts into the rectum. Am J Obstet Gynecol. 2002;187:233–4.

28. Hopkins MP, Rooney C. Entero-mesh vaginal fistula secondary to abdominal sacrocolpopexy. Obstet Gynecol. 2004;103:1035–6.

29. Pilsgaard K, Mouritsen L. Follow-up after repair of vaginal vault prolapse with abdominal colposacropexy. Acta Obstet Gynecol Scand. 1999;78:66–70.

30. Whitehead WE, Bradley CS, Brown MB, et al. Gastrointestinal complications following abdominal sacrocolpopexy for advanced pelvic organ prolapse. Am J Obstet Gynecol. 2007;197:78.e1–7.

31. Watcha MF, White PF. Postoperative nausea and vomiting. Its etiology, treatment, and prevention. Anesthesiology. 1992;77:162–84.

32. Addison WA, Timmons MC, Wall LL, et al. Failed abdominal sacral colpopexy: observations and recommendations. Obstet Gynecol. 1989;74:480–3.

33. Visco AG, Brubaker L, Nygaard I, et al. The role of preoperative urodynamic testing in stress-continent women undergoing sacral colpopexy: the Colpopexy and Urinary Reduction Efforts (CARE) randomized surgical trial. Int Urogynecol J Pelvic Floor Dysfunct. 2008;19:607–14.

34. Brubaker L, Cundiff GW, Fine P, et al. Abdominal sacrocolpopexy with Burch colposuspension to reduce urinary stress incontinence. New Engl J Med. 2006;354:1557–66.

35. Weidner AC, Cundiff GW, Harris RL, et al. Sacral osteomyelitis: an unusual complication of abdominal sacral colpopexy. Obstet Gynecol. 1997;90:689–91.

36. Cranney A, Feibel R, Toye BW, et al. Osteomyelitis subsequent to abdominal-vaginal sacropexy. J Rheumatol. 1994;21:1769–70.

37. Cailleux N, Daragon A, Laine F, et al. Spondylodiscites infetieuses après cure de prolapses genital: A propos de 5 cas. J Gynecol Obstet Biol Reprod. 1991;20:1074–8.

38. Nosseir SB, Kim YH, Lind LR, et al. Sacral osteomyelitis after robotically assisted laparoscopic sacral colpopexy. Obstet Gynecol. 2010;116:513–5.

39. Muffly TM, Diwadkar GB, Paraiso MF. Lumbosacral osteomyelitis after robot-assisted total laparoscopic hysterectomy and sacral colpopexy. Int Urogynecol J Pelvic Floor Dysfunct. 2010;21:1569–71.

40. Hart SR, Weiser EB. Abdominal sacral colpopexy mesh erosion resulting in a sinus tract formation and sacral abscess. Obstet Gynecol. 2004;103:1037–40.

41. Taylor GB, Moore RD, Miklos JR. Osteomyelitis secondary to sacral colpopexy mesh erosion requiring laminectomy. Obstet Gynecol. 2006;107:475–7.

Colpocleisis: Current Practice and Complications

Lior Lowenstein and Shay Erisson

Introduction

The term colpocleisis is derived from the ancient Greek term "kolpos," which refers to a fold in the Greek tunic and "cleisis," which stands for occlusion or closure. Colpocleisis is the obliterative alternative to reconstructive surgery, offered to women with stage II–IV Pelvic Organ Prolapse (POP) who are at high risk to surgery and no longer wish to preserve coital function per vagina.

Over the last decades the popularity of colpocleisis has declined from as high as 17,200 procedures in 1992 to around 900 procedures in 1997 [1]. Nevertheless, colpocleisis has an important role in the management of POP, especially with the aging of the population and the loss of coital function is offset by the positive impact in the daily activities.

Terminology

Colpocleisis is normally employed for treatment of posthysterectomy vaginal vault prolapse or advanced uterovaginal prolapse. Total colpocleisis usually refers to the removal of most or all of the vaginal epithelium from within the hymenal ring posteriorly to within 0.5–2.0 cm of the external urethral meatus, anteriorly [2, 3].

During complete colpocleisis, the epithelial and lamina proprial layers are removed down to the fibromuscular layer. The operation attaches the anterior fibromuscular layer to the posterior fibromuscular layer, effectively closing the vaginal tube and replacing it back into the abdominal cavity. A partial colpocleisis refers for the most part to Le-Forte [4] and its modifications [5], i.e., removing two areas of vaginal mucosa anteriorly and posteriorly and subsequently creating a series of imbrication sutures to create a tissue platform. By preservation of the lateral vaginal epithelium one potentially permits drainage of serosanguinous fluid postoperatively as well as any postmenopausal bleeding remote from surgery [6]. Other terms used to describe these procedures include total or partial colpectomy, vaginal extirpation, complete procidentia, and total or subtotal vaginectomy [7].

Indications

There is no standardized guideline to choose colpocleisis over reconstructive surgery. While it is generally accepted that it may be utilized in Stage II–IV POP, the surgeon must consider the best surgical option in terms of duration of surgery, blood loss, recovery time, immediate and delayed postoperative complications, risk of foreign

L. Lowenstein (✉) • S. Erisson
Urogynecology Service, Department of Obstetrics and Gynecology, Technion-Israel Institute of Technology, Rambam Health Care Campus, Halya 8, Haifa 31096, Israel
e-mail: lowensteinmd@gmail.com

H.B. Goldman (ed.), *Complications of Female Incontinence and Pelvic Reconstructive Surgery*, Current Clinical Urology, DOI 10.1007/978-1-61779-924-2_7, © Springer Science+Business Media, LLC 2013 body, and comorbidities affecting surgical risk. Satisfaction and compatibility with the patient's expectations are increasingly important factors that come into play; thus, the patient's desire for future vaginal intercourse, postoperative expectations, body-image, and fear of prolapse recurrence are inherent to choice of procedure [8].

In general terms, the impetus to perform colpocleisis should follow the rationale that prolonged reconstructive surgery or general anesthesia is contraindicated for women with recurrent POP following previous surgical attempts to repair POP. The real question remaining is the desire to retain the potential for sexual intercourse per vagina. In a study that surveyed older adults on their sexuality and health, researchers found that the prevalence of sexual activity among women aged 57–64, 65–74, 75–85 years of age were 62%, 40%, and 17%, respectively [9]. However, these prevalence rates are overestimating sexual activity per vagina. Furthermore, the odds ratio for being sexually active among those who reported their health to be "poor" or "fair" as compared to "very good" or "excellent" was 0.36 for women. Put together with the epidemiologic data that those who reach the age of 85 years can expect to live on average about 7 more years [10], the frail segment of this population are good candidates for colpocleisis.

Preoperative Considerations and Evaluation

Typically, obliterative procedures are less invasive, require shorter operative times and have less surgical risks than traditional vaginal reconstructive procedures [11].

Assessing the elderly patient with urogenital prolapse requires a holistic approach, taking into account the operational anatomic plane, desired functional pelvic floor endpoints, concomitant urinary incontinence evaluation, and choice of complementary procedures. In addition, the patient's physiology and potential perioperative complications need to be accounted and planned for in advance.

Considerations

Anatomic evaluation
Urinary symptoms
General comorbidity risk stratification
Choice of anesthesia

Anatomic Evaluation

Maximum extent of the prolapse should be assessed in the standing position unless the patient cannot support her own weight, in which case the prolapse assessment may be carried out with the patient supine or seated in a birthing chair. In both situations the surgeon performs a digital vaginal examination while the woman strains to push the vaginal bulge out. Prolapse should be measured in the anterior, posterior, and apical dimensions of the vaginal walls and recorded in the POP quantification system format [12].

Urinary Evaluation

Older women with advanced prolapse are at increased risk for urinary retention, which may be complicated by hydronephrosis and/or ureteral obstruction [13]. A study conducted by Fitzgerald et al. in 2002 showed that 89% of women with elevated postvoid residual volumes (>100 mL) will experience resolution of the urinary retention after their prolapse is surgically corrected [14]. All patients should undergo determination of postvoid residual volume by either straight catheter or bladder scanner. Urine dipstick analysis or urine analysis needs be performed to evaluate for urine infection and hematuria.

Historically, urinary incontinence (UI) occurs postoperatively in up to 27% of patients, representing the strongest deterrent against colpocleisis [15]. De novo stress incontinence is attributed to anatomic distortion with distal vaginal dissection and downward traction on the urethra; as a consequence, contemporary techniques avoid distal dissection and often utilize high perineorrhaphy. The other mechanism by which UI occurs postoperatively is due to unmasking of existent, occult stress urinary incontinence (SUI) due to "un-kinking" of the bladder neck with prolapse reduction. In this setting, selected patients undergo incontinence procedures to complement the obliterative procedure, with the risk of postoperative urinary retention considered against the morbidity of postoperative stress incontinence [16–19].

Assessment of SUI in symptomatic women should include a cough stress test with the bladder filled to a standardized volume such as 300 mL, in a standing or supine position. A negative stress test should be repeated with the prolapse reduced. Cystometry is also warranted should the patient report symptoms of urinary retention or mixed incontinence. The role of complex urodynamics is debatable. Urodynamics has not been shown to be sensitive in differentiating severe prolapse from detrusor overactivity as a cause of poor bladder emptying. Of interest, a literature review by Roovers and Oelke [20] posits that there is little evidence suggesting that preoperative urodynamic investigation improves the outcome of treatment.

General Risk Stratification

Increasing age is associated with increased rates of complications and mortality especially in those beyond age 80, where mortality with urogynecologic surgery is 2.8 out of 1,000 [11].

However, in women 80 years and older, fewer complications occur with obliterative surgery than with reconstructive surgery (17.0% vs. 24.7%, $P < 0.01$), making it an attractive surgical approach [21]. Still, preoperative risk stratification and minimization of postoperative complications are prudent and should be addressed through preventive measures and lab investigations.

It is noteworthy that cardiac output after age 60 is more dependent on diastolic filling and stroke volume. Furthermore, it responds poorly to sympathetic stimuli and has to compensate for a reduced secretion of water and sodium loads due to declining renal mass and filtration ability. Thus, perioperative fluid management is

paramount [22] and antihypertensives should be given the day of surgery and restarted immediately after surgery. ADL (activities of daily living) status is another important parameter. Poor functional status is predictive of pulmonary complications and should prompt a rigorous assessment and postoperative preparedness with incentive spirometry.

Other factors that need to be taken into account are baseline dementia which increases the risk of acute postoperative delirium and nutritional status which influences recovery time and the durability of the repair.

Recommended preoperative laboratories and testing in the older woman (>65 years) include hematocrit, blood urea nitrogen, glucose, creatinine, and electrocardiogram.

Choice of Anesthesia

No benefit has been demonstrated favoring one type of anesthesia in the older patient undergoing surgery. General, regional, or local anesthesia technique should be tailored to the patient's needs and desires and anesthesiologist and surgeon preference and training [23].

Obliterative Surgery Techniques: Le-Forte/Partial Colpocleisis, Complete Colpocleisis, Perineorrhaphy, Levator Myorrhaphy, Hysterectomy

In our institute we perform the colpocleisis according to Le Fort technique.

In case of uterovaginal prolapse, a cervical dilation and uterine curettage are performed to ensure there is no intrauterine pathology, and we begin the colpocleisis by marking rectangles on the anterior and posterior vaginal walls with a sterile marker; this facilitates maintaining orientation throughout the procedure. We begin with the posterior vaginal wall dissection to minimize obscuring the surgical field by blood. The vaginal epithelium is incised and removed from the underlying muscularis using Metzenbaum scissors with the surgeon's nondominant finger underlying the epithelium for guidance and traction. The anterior vaginal wall flap of mucosa is removed in a similar fashion. Rectangular strips of vaginal mucosa of approximately equal size are removed from the anterior and posterior surfaces of the protruding vagina leaving a canal of approximately 3 cm on each side. Care is taken not to remove vaginal mucosa from the area beneath the urethra. Dissecting and placing sutures near the bladder neck places downward traction on the posterior urethra and may increase the risk postoperative SUI. In the case of vaginal vault prolapse, we still perform a partial colpocleisis and remove two rectangles of vaginal epithelium, leaving a small patch of mucosa at the apex marked to maintain orientation during the surgery. Once the mucosa is stripped off the underlying fascia, attention is paid to achieve hemostasis before the vaginal canal and the uterus are closed. The muscularis layers from the anterior and posterior vagina are brought together with imbricating interrupted 2-0 polyglactin 910 sutures (Vicryl®, Ethicon, Johnson and Johnson). With each row of imbricating sutures, an interrupted suture is placed on the lateral edge of the mucosa to approximate the anterior and posterior vaginal epithelium together to form a lateral tunnel. All women undergo cystoscopy to ensure that there is no cystotomy and that bilateral urine efflux from the ureteral offices is seen. To facilitate the visualization of ureteral efflux, we give 5 mL indigo carmine intravenously. Intravenous furosemide may be given if after 10–15 min no efflux is seen from either ureteral orifice.

Perineorrhaphy is done at the end of the procedure to reduce the size of the genital hiatus, Two Allis clamps are placed superiorly on the genital hiatus to demarcate where we ultimately want the inferior border of the introitus after the perineorrhaphy. After the perineorrhaphy, the genital hiatus should allow passage of one finger. A diamond-shaped flap of epithelium is marked and removed. The perineal body is reconstructed greatly reducing the size of the genital hiatus using a series of interrupted 2-0 polyglactin 910 sutures (Vicryl®, Ethicon, Johnson and Johnson). The skin is then closed with a running subcuticular suture of Vicryl 3-0 (Vicryl®, Ethicon, Johnson and Johnson).

Outcomes

There is no level I or II evidence concerning the efficacy of colpocleisis and published data is comprised primarily of case-series. Only a few case-series defined their outcomes in standardized terms of anatomy, function, and satisfaction. Nonetheless, both partial and complete colpocleisis emerge as highly effective and safe procedures for advanced POP with anatomic success rates ranging between 90 and 100%, symptomatic recurrence between 0 and 10% and satisfaction between 86 and 100% [24].

Perioperative Complications

Perioperative complications have been reported to occur in 0.2–26% of general gynecologic procedures [25]. In 2004, Giannice et al. found that to be an underestimate when observing women >70 undergoing gynecologic oncology surgery; according to their series, the perioperative complication rate is 38% [26]. In regards to the urogynecologic population, Lambrou et al. found the complication rate to be as high as 46%, regardless of age [25]. A report from the Cleveland Clinic on 267 patients >75 who underwent urogynecologic surgery between the years 1999 and 2003, noted a perioperative complication rate of 25.8% [27], most likely reflecting a "healthier" cohort of patients.

Data on perioperative complications with colpocleisis are scant and case-series-based. At best we could supply a scale and narrative to such complications and generalize individual case-series for the benefit of preoperative risk stratification and recommended adjunct surgical measures.

As generally practiced, we categorize colpocleisis-associated complications as intra and postoperative as well as major and minor in significance.

Complications of Colpocleisis

Intra-operative complications are rare with colpocleisis (Table 7.1). Numbers range from null [28] to a case of intra-operative ureteral occlusion

Table 7.1 Summarizes the risks and advocates appropriate interventions

Issue	Background	Clinical recommendation
Deep venous thrombosis/thromboembolic events	Older patients have 20–40% risk of deep venousthrombosis because of advanced age (60 years) and length of surgery	Perioperative use of sequential pneumatic compression devices and selective use of heparin prophylaxis, early ambulation
Cardiovascular	Perioperative myocardial infarction associated with 50% mortality rate	Perioperative-blocker use in the high- and moderate-risk patient
Pulmonary	Increased perioperative morbidity and mortality rates with development of pneumonia	Pulmonary toilet with deep cough, incentive spirometry, early ambulation
Neuropathies	Neurologic injuries caused by nerve compression and ischemia as a result of patient positioning	Careful patient positioning with attention to peroneal, femoral, ulnar, and sciatic nerves with padd stir-ups, avoid hyperflexion of extension of the lower extremities
Hypothermia	Decreased immunologic response, prolonged wound healing, increased perioperative cardiac events	Intra-operative forced warm air blanket use, warmed intravenous fluids
Infectious disease	Clean contaminated procedures: mixed flora of the vagina	Perioperative dose of first-generation cephalosporin
Pharmacology	Decreased pharmacologic metabolic rates in older patients. Risk of oversedation and delirium	Avoidance of polypharmacy, sedatives, and anticholinergic medications
Delirium	Abrupt change in cognition of conscious-ness, postsurgical prevalence estimate 37%, at risk for long-term cognitive deficiencies and increased mortality, underdiagnosis	Avoid merperidine and anticholinergic agents including the promethazine, minimize hospital stay, allow a companion to stay at bedside, maintain circadian pattern
Urinary tract infection	Pelvic floor surgery postoperative rates up to 44%	Screen is new-onset bladder or voiding symptoms

in Von Pechmann's series [29] and 5.2% in Kevin's et al. review of all urogynecologic surgeries [27].

Major postoperative complications occur in about 4% [30], among which and most common overall is blood transfusion, reaching 22% in Von Pechman's series [5].

Minor surgical complications, such as UTI, vaginal hematoma, cystotomy, fever, and thrombophlebitis, occur in approximately 15%. Consistent across studies is a 5% adverse event rate of cardiac, thromboembolic, pulmonary, and cerebrovascular morbidity. Infrequent complications include pyometra [31] and vaginal evisceration [32].

Mortality is approximately 1 in 400 cases [8] and through 2008, only three deaths were reported, one of which is multiorgan failure and may have been related to the procedure [4, 15]. In comparison, Cleveland Clinic's series 6 weeks

mortality rate of 0.07% is just short of three times higher [27].

Complications in Cases with Concomitant Hysterectomy

Notably, concomitant hysterectomy done to avoid infrequent complications, such as pyometra, was not found to be more successful [21] and is currently not advocated unless uterine extirpation is medically justified. However, since colpocleisis alone denies access to the uterine cavity it mandates preoperative assessment of the endometrial lining for pathology as well as for possible postmenopausal bleeding. Importantly, concomitant hysterectomy is likely to increase adverse events due to an operative time increase from 90 to 120 min on average and up to 52 min longer [5], and a blood loss increase from 150 to 250 mL on average [11].

Postoperative Persistent or De Novo Stress Urinary Incontinence: Current Opinion

The postoperative report of urinary incontinence after colpectomy is common [33–35], and as discussed previously, is a grievance that should be avoided. Fitzgerald et al. reported up to 27% de novo SUI in previously continent women as well as persistence of SUI in 28% of preoperatively symptomatic women [10].

Preoperative assessment of such patients is critical and challenging. Encouragingly, the long-term dilemma of employing prophylactic tension-free vaginal tape (TVT) in patients undergoing prolapse repair, including colpocleisis, is currently reviewed in the Outcomes Following Vaginal Prolapse Repair and Mid Urethral Sling (OPUS), randomized controlled trial run by the Pelvic Floor Disorders Network [36]. A hint at what their findings may be with regards to persistence of symptoms can be found in a recent study by Abbasy et al. in 2009 where mid-urethral slings were employed concomitantly with colpocleisis in women suffering from stage II–IV prolapse. In this cohort of 38 patients, 31 of which suffered from SUI symptoms, only four had persistent SUI postoperatively (~13%) and there only was one case of de novo SUI.

It should be noted that the spectrum of urinary incontinence extends beyond SUI to urge incontinence, mixed incontinence, etc. It is beyond the scope of this text to delve into the intricacies of these different entities; however, in a recent study by Fitzgerald it was found that urge incontinence after colpocleisis decreased from 41 to 15%, 1 year after surgery.

Perioperative Management

Aside from careful preoperative assessment using ASA/CCI scoring and selecting the appropriate type of anesthesia, the following measures should be employed to decrease perioperative morbidity—this recommendation is based on our own experience.

Prior to incision—patients should receive a single dose of broad spectrum antibiotics.

Inpatient supervision—is recommended for at least 24 h; however, some healthy and active patients can be discharged the day of surgery. Follow up in the clinic is usually in 2 weeks time.

Cardiovascular/pulmonary risk management—patients with high cardiovascular risk should be prescribed alpha blockers and incentive spirometry.

Thromboembolism Prophylaxis

- *Moderate-risk patients* with early ambulation prospects should use sequential compression devices.
- *High risk patients* should be given low molecular weight heparin 1 day postoperatively when bleeding risk subsides.

Surgical pain: In the immediate postoperative period, pain can be managed with IV ketorolac and oral acetaminophen as well as hydrocodone as needed. Ibuprofen is routinely used after the first 24 h.

Surgical site pain can be managed via Ice-Packs and in situ bupivicaine around the perineorrhaphy wound.

Diet: A regular diet is started immediately after surgery.

Foley catheter removal: Before removal is carried out a voiding trial should be performed. If voiding is inadequate the Foley should be replaced. (*Once Foley is removed, a course of antibiotics Colmay be given as UTI prophylaxis.)

References

1. Boyles S, Weber A, Meyn L. Procedures for pelvic organ prolapse in the United States, 1979–1997. Am J Obstet Gynecol. 2003;188(1):108–15.
2. Thompson HG, Murphy Jr CJ, Picot H. Hysterocolpectomy for the treatment of uterine procidentia. Am J Obstet Gynecol. 1961;82:748–51.
3. Rubovits W, Litt S. Colpocleisis in the treatment of uterine and vaginal prolapse. Am J Obstet Gynecol. 1935;29:222–30.

4. Wyatt J. Le Fort's operation for prolapse, with an account of eight cases. J Obstet Gynaecol Br Emp J. 1912;22:266–9.
5. Ubachs JM, van Sante TJ, Schellekens LA. Partial colpocleisis by a modification of LeFort's operation. Obstet Gynecol. 1973;42:415–20.
6. FitzGerald MP, Richter HE, Siddique S, Thompson P, Zyczynski H, Weber A, for the Pelvic Floor Disorders Network. Colpocleisis: a review. Int Urogyn J. 2006; 17:261–71.
7. Bradbury WC. Subtotal vaginectomy. Am J Obstet Gynecol. 1963;86:663–71.
8. Abbasy M, Kenton K. Obliterative procedures for pelvic organ prolapse. Clin Obstet Gynecol. 2010;53(1):86–98.
9. Elkadry EA, Kenton KS, FitzGerald MP, et al. Patient-selected goals: a new perspective on surgical outcome. Am J Obstet Gynecol. 2003;189:1551–7.
10. Federal Interagency Forum on Aging-Related Statistics. Older Americans 2008: key indicators of well-being. Federal interagency forum on aging-related statistics. Washington, DC: U.S. Government printing office; 2008.
11. Sung VW, Weitzen S, Sokol ER, et al. Effect of patient age on increasing morbidity and mortality following urogynecologic surgery. Am J Obstet Gynecol. 2006;194:1411–7.
12. Bump RC, Mattiasson A, Bo K, et al. The standardization of terminology of female pelvic organ prolapse and pelvic floor dysfunction. Am J Obstet Gynecol. 1996;175:10–7.
13. Beverly CM, Walters MD, Weber AM, et al. Prevalence of hydronephrosis in patients undergoing surgery for pelvic organ prolapse. Obstet Gynecol. 1997;90: 37–41.
14. Fitzgerald MP, Kulkarni N, Fenner D. Postoperative resolution of urinary retention in patients with advanced pelvic organ prolapse. Am J Obstet Gynecol. 2000;183:1361–3.
15. Fitzgerald MP. Colpocleisis and urinary incontinence. Am J Obstet Gynecol. 2003;189:1241–4.
16. Fitzgerald MP, Richter HE, Bradley CS, et al. Pelvic support, pelvic symptoms, and patient satisfaction after colpocleisis. Int Urogynecol J Pelvic Floor Dysfunct. 2008;19:1603–9.
17. Van Huisseling JCM. A modification of Labhardt's high perineoplasty for treatment of pelvic organ prolapse in the very old. Int Urogynecol J Pelvic Floor Dysfunct. 2009;20:185–91.
18. Murphy M, Sternschuss G, Haff R, et al. Quality of life and surgical satisfaction after vaginal reconstructive vs. obliterative surgery for the treatment of advanced pelvic organ prolapse. Am J Obstet Gynecol. 2008;198:573.e1–7
19. Agarwala N, Hasiak N, Shade M. Graft interposition colpocleisis, perineorrhaphy, and tension-free sling for pelvic organ prolapse and stress urinary incontinence in elderly patients. J Minim Invasive Gynecol. 2007;14(6):740–5.
20. Roovers JWR, Oelke M. Clinical relevance of urodynamic investigation tests prior to surgical correction of genital prolapse: a literature review. Int Urogynecol J. 2007;18:455–60.
21. Hoffman MS, et al. Vaginectomy with pelvic herniorrhaphy for prolapse. Am J Obstet Gynecol. 2003; 189:364–71.
22. Katz PR, Grossberg GT, Potter JF, et al. Geriatric syllabus for the specialists. New York: American Geriatrics Society; 2002.
23. Segal JL, Owens G, Silva WA, et al. A randomized trial of local anesthesia with intravenous sedation vs general anesthesia for the vaginal correction of pelvic organ prolapse. Int Urogynecol J Pelvic Floor Dysfunct. 2007;18:807–82.
24. Wheeler TL, Gerten KA, Garris J. Obliterative vaginal surgery for pelvic organ prolapse. Obstet Gynecol Clin North Am. 2009;36:637–58.
25. Lambrou NC, Buller JL, Thompson JR, Cundiff GW, Chou B, Montz FJ. Prevalence of perioperative complications among women undergoing reconstructive pelvic surgery. Am J Obstet Gynecol. 2000;183:1355–8.
26. Giannice R, Foti E, Poerio A, Marana E, Mancuso S, Scambia G. Perioperative morbidity and mortality in elderly gynecological oncological patients (O70 years) by the American Society of Anesthesiologists physical status classes. Ann Surg Oncol. 2004;11:219–25.
27. Stepp KJ, Barber MD, Yoo E-H, Whiteside JL, Paraiso MF, Walters MD. Incidence of perioperative complications of urogynecologic surgery in elderly women. Am J Obstet Gynecol. 2005;192(5):1630–6. doi:10.1016/j.ajog.2004.11.026.
28. Latthe PM, Karri K, Arunkalaivanan AS. Colpocleisis revisited. Obstet Gynaecol. 2008;10:133–8. doi:10.1576/toag.10.3.133.27414.
29. Von Pechmann WS, et al. Total colpocleisis with high levator plication for the treatment of advanced pelvic organ prolapse. Am J Obstet Gynecol. 2003;189:121–6.
30. FitzGerald MP, Richter HE, Siddique S, Thompson P, Zyczynski H, Weber A, for the Pelvic Floor Disorders Network. Colpocleisis: a review. Int Urogyn J. 2006;17:261–7.
31. Roth TM. Pyometra and recurrent prolapse after Le Fort colpocleisis. Int Urogynecol J Pelvic Floor Dysfunct. 2007;18:687–8.
32. Moore RD, Miklos JR. Repair of a vaginal evisceration following colpocleisis utilizing an allogenic dermal graft. Int Urogynecol J Pelvic Floor Dysfunct. 2001;12:215–7. doi:10.1007/PL00004035, doi:10.1007/s00192-006-0201-z.
33. Falk H, Kaufman S. Partial colpocleisis: the Le Fort procedure (analysis of 100 cases). Obstet Gynecol. 1955;5:617.
34. Hanson GE, Keettel WC. The Neugebauer Le Fort operation (a review of 288 colpocleisis). Obstet Gynecol. 1969;34:352–7.
35. Pratt JH, Baker RK. Urinary incontinence following the Le Fort operation: report of a case. Obstet Gynecol. 1960;16:722–3.
36. Wei J, Nygaard I, Richter H, et al. Outcomes following vaginal prolapse repair and mid urethral sling (OPUS) trial—design and methods. Clin Trials. 2009;6:162–71.

Transvaginal Mesh Complications

Farzeen Firoozi and Howard B. Goldman

Introduction

The lifetime risk of requiring pelvic surgery for vaginal prolapse or incontinence for a woman in the United States is 11%, with a risk for reoperation of 29% [1]. Traditional vaginal repairs for prolapse using only the patient's native tissues have had reported rates of recurrence ranging from 10 to 50% depending on the compartment repaired [2]. In the last 10 years, there have been advancements in pelvic floor reconstructive surgery to create repairs that are reproducible with improved subjective and objective outcomes.

Initial attempts were made to augment transvaginal repairs using biologic grafts or absorbable synthetic mesh. In terms of anterior vaginal wall augmented repairs, Meschia et al. compared outcomes of anterior colporrhaphy with and without a porcine dermis onlay graft (Pelvicol™ [Bard

Medical, Covington, GA]). The objective failure rate at 1 year, determined by pelvic exam, was 20% in the anterior colporrhaphy group vs. 7% in the porcine dermis onlay group [3]. In 2005, Gandhi et al. reported their experience with the use of solvent dehydrated cadaveric fascia lata (Tutoplast® [RTI Biologics, Inc., Alachua, FL]) in augmenting anterior vaginal wall repairs. Outcomes of anterior colporrhaphy with or without the cadaveric fascia lata were compared. The authors reported no difference in the objective and subjective outcomes between the two groups at 13 months follow up [4] in addition, Weber et al. failed to show any difference in cure rates between Vicryl mesh repairs vs. traditional anterior repairs [5].

The first trial to compare mesh vs. nonmesh repairs in the management of posterior wall vaginal prolapse was published by Sand et al. in 2001. In this study, absorbable Vicryl mesh was used for the augmented repair arm. The authors found virtually no difference in rectocele recurrence rates between the two groups [6]. In 2006, Paraiso et al. compared posterior colporrhaphy, site-specific repair and site-specific repair with porcine small intestine submucosal onlay graft for rectocele repair. From an objective standpoint, there was a higher recurrence rate of rectocele in the graft onlay group vs. the posterior colporrhaphy group. When comparing all three groups, there was no difference in subjective report of prolapse symptoms [7]. As a result of these types of studies, the use of biologic grafts or absorbable synthetic mesh had been largely abandoned

F. Firoozi, MD (✉)
Center for Pelvic Health and Reconstructive Surgery,
The Arthur Smith Institute for Urology,
Hofstra North Shore-LIJ School of Medicine,
233 7th Street, Suite 203, Garden City, NY 11530, USA
e-mail: farzeenfiroozi@aol.com

H.B. Goldman, MD
Center for Female Pelvic Medicine and Reconstructive
Surgery, Glickman Urologic and Kidney Institute,
The Cleveland Clinic, Cleveland, OH, USA

Lerner College of Medicine, Case Western
Reserve University, Cleveland, OH, USA

H.B. Goldman (ed.), *Complications of Female Incontinence and Pelvic Reconstructive Surgery*,
Current Clinical Urology, DOI 10.1007/978-1-61779-924-2_8, © Springer Science+Business Media, LLC 2013

as an alternative for augmenting traditional vaginal repairs of anterior and posterior compartment prolapse.

In terms of apical prolapse, the gold standard has been the abdominal sacrocolpopexy utilizing mesh attached to the vaginal wall. Success rates for managing apical prolapse repairs using mesh via an abdominal route range between 85 and 100% [2]. The safety of this approach has been well established in numerous studies reported over the last several decades [8].

The use of transvaginal mesh was initially adopted on a large scale after the introduction of synthetic slings for the treatment of urinary incontinence [9]. The safety of synthetic mesh slings has been well established over the last 15 years. The use of synthetic mesh slings for urinary incontinence has shown significant efficacy, durability, and safety, and led the way for innovation towards transvaginal mesh prolapse repairs. This was an intuitive step on the progression of improved transvaginal repairs, especially since biologic and absorbable synthetic mesh trials in the past had failed to demonstrate superiority to traditional repairs. The newly designed synthetic mesh kit procedures were first approved by the Food and Drug Administration (FDA) in 2003. Since their introduction over 8 years ago, a multitude of mesh kit procedures have become available on the commercial market. Although each is designed slightly differently the common goal has been to establish a new transvaginal repair that would prove safe, with improved efficacy and durability when compared to traditional repairs.

Hiltunen et al. reported a significant difference in anterior wall recurrence rates between their traditional repairs vs. their nonabsorbable mesh augmented repairs—38.7% and 6.7%, respectively [10]. Nguyen and Burchette found in their randomized controlled trial that the traditional repair arm had a recurrence rate of 45%, vs. 13% in the nonabsorbable mesh augmentation group [11]. In 2011, a randomized controlled trial of transvaginal mesh kit repair vs. traditional colporrhaphy for anterior vaginal wall prolapse was published in the New England Journal of Medicine by Altman et al. The overall rate of objective success, based on pelvic organ prolapse quantification (POP-Q) stages, was significantly higher in the mesh group (60%) compared to the traditional colporrhaphy group (35%) [12]. The purported benefit in most of these studies was the objective superiority of repairs involving nonabsorbable mesh augmentation. In addition, many of these studies showed trends towards improvements in subjective outcomes in those with mesh but these findings were not significant at the time points evaluated.

The use of synthetic mesh in transvaginal prolapse repairs has not been without controversy. At the heart of the controversy lies the concern by its opponents, that complications related to mesh use outweigh the benefit of augmenting repairs with synthetic mesh. The main issues at hand are the risks of pain, dyspareunia, and mesh extrusion or perforation requiring corrective surgery. Adding significant legitimacy to this side of the debate was the initial white paper published by the FDA in 2008 regarding the use of transvaginal mesh for both incontinence and prolapse surgery. The overall tone of the report was in keeping with the main concern of the detractors of mesh use, namely the risk for intra- and postoperative complications. The recommendations included the proper counseling of patients as to the potential risks of mesh use in incontinence and prolapse surgery. A recent update in July 2011 further expressed the concern for use of synthetic mesh for prolapse surgery, but very clearly separated the use of mesh for urinary incontinence— somewhat of an acknowledgement to the arguments made by many experts that the safety of synthetic mesh slings had been well established over almost 2 decades of study.

There are two general theories that explain the occurrence of mesh complications. The first is that synthetic mesh implanted in the vagina is simply prone to causing pain, extrusion, or perforation. The other is that it is generally problems with appropriate surgical technique that accounts for many mesh complications [13]. We will discuss this portion of the debate in our next section. Regardless, while the use of synthetic mesh has shown some utility in augmenting traditional transvaginal repairs of prolapse a very real aspect of these repairs are the potential intra- and postoperative complications related to the use of mesh. In this chapter, we will review techniques for avoiding complications, recognizing technical issues intra-operatively, and managing complications postoperatively.

Avoiding Complications of Transvaginal Mesh Repairs

Preoperative Considerations

Preoperative preparation of patients for transvaginal mesh repairs begins with optimization of vaginal tissue. We recommend the initiation of vaginal estrogen supplementation 4–6 weeks preoperatively to improve perioperative tissue quality. There are currently many options on the market including Premarin cream, Estrace cream, Vagifem, and E-string. The continued use of local hormone replacement postoperatively is recommended to maintain tissue quality and to facilitate tissue healing.

Certain patient populations with impaired wound healing or damaged vaginal skin may be at greater risk for mesh extrusion. Patients who have had pelvic radiotherapy, those on steroids and possibly smokers are examples of these types of patients. Very careful consideration of risk profiles and an acknowledgement of increased rates of extrusion should be undertaken before surgery is performed in this population.

Intra-operative Considerations

A cornerstone of transvaginal mesh repair is developing the proper plane of dissection. Probably the best way to accomplish this is with copious hydrodissection of the vaginal wall to aid in the actual sharp and blunt dissection that follows. The vaginal wall incision is made through the viscerofascial layer to the potential space (filled with a gelatinous fluid after hydrodissection) between the fascial layer (either pubocervical or prerectal) and the underlying viscera. This plane is much deeper than the typical superficial plane external to the viscerofascial layer used for a traditional repair. If the superficial plane is

inadvertently utilized for mesh placement vaginal wall necrosis and ulceration or extrusion may ensue. In addition to vaginal wall extrusion, the risk for vaginal/pelvic pain and dyspareunia are increased by dissection and mesh placement in too superficial a plane.

Once dissection is completed hemostasis is of utmost importance. Initial postoperative pain following transvaginal mesh repairs can be secondary to perioperative bleeding. This is typically in the form of a hematoma, which can exert pressure on the vaginal tissues eliciting pain. In addition to pain, hematomas can also delay healing and promote wound separation. Wound separation in the setting of mesh use may result in extrusion of the synthetic material. For these reasons, it is paramount that adequate hemostasis is achieved at the completion of the case and a tight vaginal pack is typically placed overnight as well.

Dissection should be adequate to allow the mesh to lay flat over the defect both side to side and proximal to distal. When a trocar-based system is used one must take care to make the lateral dissection wide enough to allow the arms to be spread as they pass through that area to avoid bunching of the mesh. Bunching and buckling of the mesh can predispose to pain and extrusion.

Similar to placement of synthetic mesh slings, the mesh placed during transvaginal repair is meant to be placed without tension. The main reason for this surgical tenet is the avoidance of postoperative vaginal/pelvic pain. Whether a trocar or trocarless kit is used, there should be no tension after completion of mesh placement. This can be done by loosening the arms if a trochar-based system is used, and making a releasing incision in the body of the mesh if necessary. Again, the goal is placement of a tension-free system.

Prior to closure, the practice of vaginal wall trimming (common to traditional repairs) needs to be avoided in transvaginal mesh repairs. Only excoriated areas should be removed and only in a very judicious fashion. The reasoning behind minimization of vaginal wall trimming relates to the competency of the wound. A wound under tension has the increased risk of developing a possible separation or compromised coverage of the underlying mesh predisposing to extrusion of the synthetic graft.

Postoperative Considerations

A Foley catheter and vaginal packing are typically left indwelling at the completion of the case. The vaginal packing serves to tamponade the vagina and reduce the risk of postoperatively bleeding and can be removed within 24 h after surgery.

Intra-operative Complications

With correct dissection, bleeding involving the vaginal wall or the tissue remaining deep to this dissection plane should be minimal during transvaginal mesh repairs. If bleeding does occur on either the vaginal wall or plane of mesh placement, hemostasis can typically be achieved with electrocautery. If bleeding persists, absorbable suture placed in figure of eight interrupted fashion can be used as a further means of hemostasis. Bleeding can also occur with passage of external trocars or internal trocars with both anterior and posterior approaches. The first maneuver should be direct compression at the site of bleeding. If bleeding persists, optimal exposure of the site of bleeding is paramount. Typically, the source of bleeding is an aberrant vessel which cannot be managed with compression alone. Once further dissection is performed and exposure of the bleeding vessel is achieved, judicious placement of small clips may be performed to halt further bleeding. Some surgeons use hemostatic agents such as Floseal if there is venous oozing in a deep area where it is difficult to see. If significant bleeding cannot be controlled packing followed by embolization must be considered.

Another potential intra-operative complication of transvaginal mesh repair is injury to other pelvic organs including the bladder or rectum. If bladder injury occurs, multilayer closure of the cystotomy should be performed with absorbable suture. A Foley catheter should be left indwelling for approximately 10 days prior to cystogram for

confirmation of bladder healing. If a rectal injury is encountered, consultation with surgery is recommended. The ultimate decision of primary repair of rectal injury vs. repair with diversion is at the discretion of the consultant surgeon. With either bladder or rectal injury, placement of mesh at the same setting is discouraged. The main concern for mesh placement would be a risk for mesh perforation of the organ given compromised tissue healing and infection after an injury.

Evaluation of Mesh Complications

History

There are a litany of complaints that patients can present with after transvaginal mesh repair. In this chapter we will concentrate on patients who present with mesh extrusions and perforations. In 2010, the ICS and IUGA created a classification system to help promote a universal language that could be used by all pelvic floor surgeons in order to aid with reporting of mesh complications. The new classification system uses three components to describe complications related to the use of prosthesis/grafts, which include the category (C), time (T) and site (S). The C includes the anatomical site which the graft/prosthesis complication involves and identifies degree of exposure. More severe complications would involve increasing migration/protrusion into surrounding anatomical structures, opening into surrounding organs, and systemic compromise. The T for the complication is when it is clinically diagnosed. There are three time periods used: intra-operative to 48 h, 48 h to 6 months, and over 6 months. The S selection of this division incorporates the current sites where the graft/prosthesis complications have been noted.

The first step in taking a history from a patient involves documenting the presenting complaint, which can include dyspareunia, prolonged vaginal discharge, severe incontinence, rectal discharge, recurrent prolapse, urinary tract infection, defecatory dysfunction, and thigh drainage or infection. Vaginal and pelvic pain are also presenting complaints, which are covered in another chapter.

A complete review of systems should be performed, specifically those symptoms which have occurred since the time of surgery. If the original case was performed by another surgeon, the preoperative records, operative reports, and any other hospital reports should be reviewed. Any intraoperative issues such as bleeding or injury to pelvic organs or problems that occurred postoperatively such as prolonged bladder catheterization, blood transfusion, or need for reoperation should be closely reviewed. These issues tend to signify a complicated postoperative course, which may relate to the complication at hand. Finally, a detailed history of any events that followed surgery is useful in any future medical or surgical management of mesh complications. Good documentation of one's findings is critical as these cases may end up under medicolegal review.

Physical Exam

The focused physical exam involves a complete genitourinary exam which includes a thorough pelvic exam with a speculum with internal or external light source. Before the speculum exam, careful initial palpation can be performed to elicit any areas of pain. These areas can be associated with folded over mesh, contracted mesh, or taut arms of the mesh if present. Care should be taken to evaluate each vaginal compartment in mapping out all areas of pain. Often it is easier to palpate extruded mesh than to see it and thus a very careful palpation of the entire vaginal surface should be performed.

In terms of the speculum pelvic exam, systematic evaluation of the entire vagina should be carried out. Any areas of mesh extrusion should be documented. If a patient complains of pain over the mesh—the specific sites of pain should be mapped out. Other important findings such as fistulae should be evaluated closely. Other urologic testing such as cystoscopy to rule our mesh perforation, cystogram or methylene blue test to confirm presence of fistula, and urodynamics for bladder dysfunction may also be performed based on presenting symptoms. Those patients who present with rectal bleeding or discharge should be evaluated with proctoscopy.

Management of Mesh Complications

Mesh Extrusion

Complications from transvaginal mesh repairs may present days to years after initial surgery. Vaginal mesh extrusion typically occurs as a result of wound separation, infection or vaginal atrophy. Typically, mesh extrusion noted in the immediate postoperative period, usually within 6 weeks, is a result of wound separation. If the wound does not appear infected, additional attempt at wound closure may be offered under local anesthesia with or without sedation. If the wound appears infected, a short course of antibiotics may rectify the issue, with close observation to ensure closure of the wound. Vaginal estrogens should be applied during this time. If the infection persists, then excision of the exposed area is recommended.

Vaginal mesh extrusion noted more than 6 weeks after surgery may be due to technical error, local infection, vaginal atrophy, or wound separation secondary to hematoma. Initial conservative therapy with local estrogen may be offered in order to avoid reoperation. If conservative therapy fails, partial or complete mesh excision should be pursued. Typically only the areas of mesh that are involved in an extrusion need to be excised—much of the uninvolved mesh can usually be safely left behind. Some very small extrusions can be excised under local anesthesia in the office by just cutting the exposed portion and allowing the vaginal skin to heal over the area. Many patients with point tenderness can be treated in a similar fashion with just those areas causing tenderness excised. In such cases one must carefully map out the areas of pain preoperatively as there will be no extruded mesh to guide you at the time of operation.

Surgical Technique for Excision of Mesh Extrusion

Under either intravenous sedation or general anesthesia, the patient is placed in the dorsal lithotomy position and the vagina and lower abdomen are prepped and draped in standard fashion. One percent lidocaine with 1:200,000 epinephrine is used to infiltrate under the vaginal skin around the site of the extrusion. Bilateral vaginal flaps are created extending at least 2 cm lateral to the visible mesh. One cm of skin immediately around the mesh is usually discarded. The mesh is then incised in the midline and dissected off of the bladder or rectum in either direction at least 1–2 cm lateral to where the skin will be closed. Once the lateral extent of the mesh is dissected, the mesh is excised. The vaginal wall is then closed in a single layer with absorbable suture. A vaginal packing is placed and removed later in the recovery room.

Mesh Perforation

Once mesh perforation of the bladder or rectum has been diagnosed, mapping of the areas of perforation must be documented. Mesh perforation of the bladder is typically seen at the bladder base or lateral bladder walls where mesh arms can sometimes be found (Fig. 8.1). If the mesh has been in the bladder for an extended period of time, calcification of the synthetic material may occur. We have described the purely transvaginal excision of bladder and rectal mesh perforation

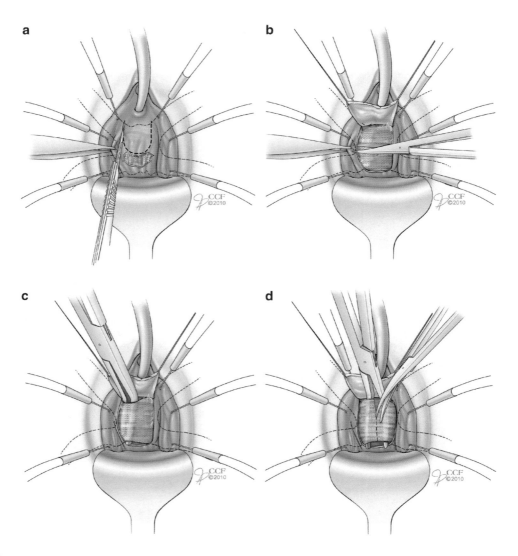

Fig. 8.1 (**a–h**) Excision of transvaginal mesh

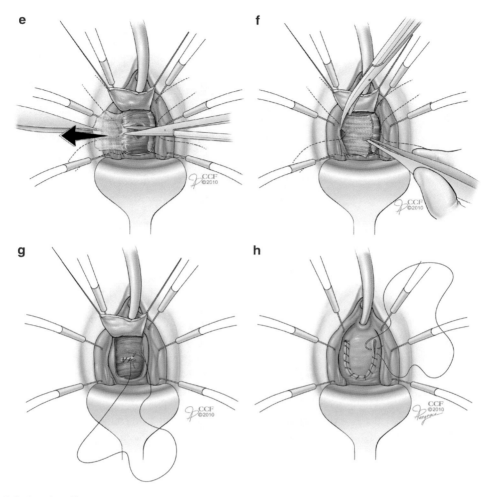

Fig. 8.1 (continued)

as safe and efficacious [14] and feel that often the easiest way to remove the mesh is via the same route it was placed.

Surgical Technique for Excision of Mesh Perforation of the Bladder

Under general anesthesia, the patient is placed in the dorsal lithotomy position and the vagina and abdomen are prepped and draped in standard fashion. Retrograde pyelograms are performed to rule out ureteral involvement (if there is ureteral involvement, a JJ stent is placed retrograde or a percutaneous nephroureteral stent is left indwelling to maintain continuity of the urinary tract during reconstruction). If no ureteral involvement is noted, temporary bilateral open-ended ureteral stents are inserted. 1% lidocaine with 1:200,000 epinephrine mixture is infiltrated under the vaginal skin and an inverted U-shaped incision is made. The vaginal wall is dissected to create an inverted U-flap, which serves as the final layer of closure for the repair (in cases where there is a vesico-vaginal fistula [VVF] closer to the vaginal apex a true (noninverted) U-flap is created with the bottom of the U at the VVF site) (Fig. 8.1a). Dissection of the vaginal skin is performed laterally from the U-flap towards the pelvic sidewall (Fig. 8.1b). When only a small area of mesh has eroded into the bladder the remainder may be found relatively superficially under the

Picture 1 Mesh perforation
into rectum

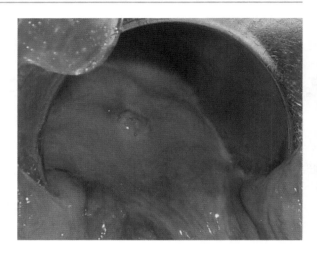

vaginal wall. If a substantial amount of mesh has eroded into the bladder the mesh may not be as easy to find and the detrusor muscle may need to be incised vertically in the area of the mesh (which can be determined with cystoscopic guidance) until one comes across it. A right angle clamp can be used to mobilize the mesh off the bladder in the midline (Fig. 8.1c). An incision is made in the midline of the mesh after which the lumen of the bladder is visible (Fig. 8.1d). Any remaining overlying tissues (superficial to the mesh) are bluntly and sharply dissected. By grasping on the midline (incised edge) of the mesh and pulling laterally, the bladder wall underneath the mesh is carefully peeled off using both sharp and blunt dissection. If there is a fistula present, it can be seen in its entirety at this point (Fig. 8.1e). The mesh is incised as far laterally as feasible and removed (Fig. 8.1f). The ureteral catheters can be both palpated and visualized. The mucosal layer is reapproximated using 3-0 absorbable suture taking care to stay medial to the ureteral catheters. The detrusor layer is then closed in two layers using 2-0 vicryl suture (Fig. 8.1g). The anterior vaginal wall is closed with 2-0 vicryl suture (Fig. 8.1h). Although not mandatory, the open-ended ureteral stents can be replaced with JJ ureteral stents to prevent any potential ureteral obstruction from inflammation and edema involving the bladder. A vaginal packing is placed and an 18 French Foley catheter is left per urethra.

Another option for removal of mesh perforation of the bladder would be a transabdominal approach. A Pfannenstiel incision is made in the lower abdomen. The incision is carried down to the level of the rectus fascia using electrocautery. The rectus fascia is incised transversely and the space of Retzius is entered. The bladder is filled via the indwelling Foley catheter to aid in identification. The bladder is then bivalved with a vertical incision using electrocautery. The mesh can now be visualized. The incision is carried down to the mesh. Bladder flaps are now created lateral to the body of the mesh. The mesh is then excised. The vaginal wall is closed using 2-0 absorbable suture. If possible a portion of omentum should be mobilized and placed as an interposition graft between the vagina and bladder. The bladder is then closed in two layers with 2-0 absorbable suture. A vaginal packing is placed and an 18 French Foley catheter is left per urethra.

We prefer the transvaginal approach and find it to be less morbid for the patient.

Surgical Technique for Excision of Mesh Perforation of the Rectum

Under general endotracheal anesthesia, the patient is placed in the jackknife position, the perineum and buttocks are prepped and the rectum is cleaned with betadine irrigation. A Hill Ferguson retractor is placed to aid in visualization (Picture 1). Mucosal flaps are developed around the exposed mesh. The mesh is then dissected off of the underlying rectal wall and excised. The mucosal flaps are closed with vicryl suture.

Palpable Tender Mesh Arm in Fornix of Vagina

Occasionally, a patient will note pain near the fornix and one can palpate a tense arm of mesh at that spot. In such cases, division of the mesh arm may ameliorate the patient's symptoms. Under IV sedation and local or general anesthesia palpate the arm of interest, inject some lidocaine with epinephrine in the vaginal wall overlying it, incise through the vaginal skin at that site, identify and dissect out the mesh arm and then cut it and close the vaginal skin.

Conclusion

The use of synthetic mesh for the management of pelvic organ prolapse has been debated for the past few years. At the heart of the controversy lies the concern that complications related to mesh use outweigh any benefit of augmenting repairs with mesh. Although studies have shown objective benefit to mesh augmentation of transvaginal repairs, particularly in the anterior compartment, there is still concern about potential complications [12, 15]. On the other hand many believe that the issue is not mesh itself but to a large degree the surgical techniques in use by many [13]. While all would agree that complications can occur there are published case series in the literature of transvaginal mesh repairs performed in the hands of experts with very low complication rates. Furthermore, most complications after transvaginal mesh repairs have been shown to be manageable with resolution of most presenting complaints [16]. The authors have extensive experience in the management of mesh complications secondary to the use of commercially available kits and in our experience, these complications are generally able to be successfully managed transvaginally with minimal morbidity [17].

References

1. Olsen AL, Smith VJ, Bergstrom JO, et al. Epidemiology of surgically managed pelvic organ prolapse and urinary incontinence. Obstet Gynecol. 1997;89:501–6.
2. Maher C, Feiner B, Baessler K, et al. Surgical management of pelvic organ prolapse in women. Cochrane Database Syst Rev. 2010;(4):CD004014.
3. Meschia M, Pifarotti P, Bernasconi F, et al. Porcine skin collagen implants to prevent anterior vaginal wall prolapse recurrence: a multicenter, randomized study. J Urol. 2007;177:192–5.
4. Gandhi S, Goldberg RP, Kwon C, et al. A prospective randomized trial using solvent dehydrated fascia lata for the prevention of recurrent anterior vaginal wall prolapse. Am J Obstet Gynecol. 2005;192:1649–54.
5. Weber AM, Walters MD, Piedmonte MR, et al. Anterior colporrhaphy: a randomized trial of three surgical techniques. Am J Obstet Gynecol. 2001;185:1299–304; discussion 1304–6.
6. Sand PK, Koduri S, Lobel RW, et al. Prospective randomized trial of polyglactin 910 mesh to prevent recurrence of cystoceles and rectoceles. Am J Obstet Gynecol. 2001;184:1357–62; discussion 1362–4.
7. Paraiso MF, Barber MD, Muir TW, et al. Rectocele repair: a randomized trial of three surgical techniques including graft augmentation. Am J Obstet Gynecol. 2006;195:1762–71.
8. Maher CF, Feiner B, DeCuyper EM, et al. Laparoscopic sacral colpopexy versus total vaginal mesh for vaginal vault prolapse: a randomized trial. Am J Obstet Gynecol. 2011;204:360.e1–7.
9. Ulmsten U, Petros P. Intravaginal slingplasty (IVS): an ambulatory surgical procedure for treatment of female urinary incontinence. Scand J Urol Nephrol. 1995;29:75–82.
10. Hiltunen R, Nieminen K, Takala T, et al. Low-weight polypropylene mesh for anterior vaginal wall prolapse: a randomized controlled trial. Obstet Gynecol. 2007;110:455–62.
11. Nguyen JN, Burchette RJ. Outcome after anterior vaginal prolapse repair: a randomized controlled trial. Obstet Gynecol. 2008;111:891–8.
12. Altman D, Vayrynen T, Engh ME, et al. Anterior colporrhaphy versus transvaginal mesh for pelvic-organ prolapse. N Engl J Med. 2011;364:1826–36.
13. Goldman HB, Fitzgerald MP. Transvaginal mesh for cystocele repair. J Urol. 2010;183:430–2.
14. Firoozi F, Goldman HB. Transvaginal excision of mesh erosion involving the bladder after mesh placement using a prolapse kit: a novel technique. Urology. 2010;75:203–6.
15. Sanses TV, Shahryarinejad A, Molden S, et al. Anatomic outcomes of vaginal mesh procedure (Prolift) compared with uterosacral ligament suspension and abdominal sacrocolpopexy for pelvic organ

prolapse: a Fellows' Pelvic Research Network study. Am J Obstet Gynecol. 2009;201 519.e1–8.

16. Ridgeway B, Walters MD, Paraiso MF, et al. Early experience with mesh excision for adverse outcomes after transvaginal mesh placement using prolapse kits. Am J Obstet Gynecol. 2008;199:703.e1–7.

17. Firoozi F, Ingber MS, Moore CK, et al. Purely transvaginal/perineal management of complications from commercial prolapse kits using a new prostheses/grafts complication classification system. J Urol, 2012;187(5):1674–9.

Pain Complications of Mesh Surgery

9

Lisa Rogo-Gupta and Shlomo Raz

Introduction

Pelvic reconstructive surgery offers many treatments for pelvic organ prolapse. Surgical solutions include vaginal, laparoscopic, and abdominal approaches with native vaginal tissue, fascia autografts and allografts, xenografts, and synthetic absorbable and nonabsorbable mesh. Augmentation of traditional vaginal prolapse techniques using nonabsorbable synthetic mesh demonstrated low morbidity and high anatomic success when initially described. This seemingly reassuring data resulted in the rapid and widespread adoption of such techniques by Gynecologists and Urologists worldwide. Innumerable manufactured products ("kits") for single or multiple compartment prolapse repair are available to pelvic surgeons. Mesh kits have many commonly known advantages such as tension-free placement design, simple technique that is easily repeated with minimal training, and short operative time and disadvantages including price, retraction, adherence, and the potential long-term effect of vaginal atrophy on the health of the mesh implant.

There is no international consensus regarding standard practice of mesh in vaginal surgery. The continuous modifications and rapid introduction of new products make long-term evaluation of any single product challenging. Multiple organizations have cited the insufficient evidence to support mesh in vaginal surgery [1, 2]. The American College of Obstetricians and Gynecologists (ACOG) modified their prior recommendations considering mesh experimental; stating patients considered for vaginal mesh should be informed of the potential complications and lack of long-term data [3]. The Society of Gynecologic Surgeons (SGS) highlighted the lack of reliable evidence to support recommendations regarding the use of mesh for posterior compartment prolapse and stated the risks may outweigh the benefits [4]. Similarly, the Society of Obstetricians and Gynaecologists of Canada (SOGC) stated that the transvaginal mesh devices using trocar placement for prolapse repair should be considered novel techniques and patients should be counseled regarding potential serious adverse sequelae [5]. The Cochrane Collaboration highlighted the insufficient evidence to support the use of mesh repair of posterior compartment prolapse in their recent review [6]. Despite cautionary advice, the enthusiasm surrounding synthetic mesh has continued to increase.

Complications of pelvic reconstruction are generally mild and self-limited (Table 9.1). Pain is a common complication of mesh surgery; however its presentation and clinical implications vary greatly. Pain may initially present in the immediate or delayed postoperative period, varying in quality from mild dyspareunia to severe

L. Rogo-Gupta • S. Raz (✉)
Division of Pelvic Medicine and Reconstructive Surgery, Department of Urology, University of California Los Angeles, 200 Medical Plaza, Suite #140, Los Angeles, CA 90095, USA
e-mail: sraz@mednet.ucla.edu

H.B. Goldman (ed.), *Complications of Female Incontinence and Pelvic Reconstructive Surgery*,
Current Clinical Urology, DOI 10.1007/978-1-61779-924-2_9, © Springer Science+Business Media, LLC 2013

Table 9.1 Dindo classification

Grade	Definition
I	Deviation from the normal postoperative course, requiring therapies such as antiemetics, antipyretics, analgesics, diuretics, electrolytes, and physiotherapy
II	Additional pharmacological treatments, blood transfusion, or total parenteral nutrition
III	Requiring surgical, endoscopic, or radiological intervention
IIIa	Intervention not under general anesthesia
IIIb	Intervention under general anesthesia
IV	Life-threatening complication requiring ICU management
IVa	Single organ dysfunction, including dialysis
IVb	Multiorgan dysfunction
V	Death of a patient

Adapted from Dindo et al. [42]

debilitating pain rendering the patient unable to sit or walk. Physicians offer medical and surgical options including trigger-point injections, pelvic floor physiotherapy, epidural injections, mesh incisions and excisions, topical and oral medications. Although most patients who undergo mesh placement do not suffer from pain, a number of patients experience a chronic, debilitating pain that is not responsive to these management strategies. Many patients may never experience resolution of pain.

In this chapter we will review the general categories of mesh complications, focusing primarily on pain. Improved understanding of pain after mesh placement is essential to our ability to treat these patients. Evaluation of patients with pain after mesh surgery should take into consideration all contributing factors including mesh properties, surgical methods, and host responses. In this chapter, we will (1) describe the multifactorial etiology of pain after mesh placement; (2) correlate patient symptoms with the anatomy of mesh placement; (3) provide recommendations for evaluation and treatment; (4) suggest strategies to prevent these complications.

Pelvic Reconstructive Surgery

Epidemiology

Pelvic floor reconstruction has gained much interest from the medical field and general population in recent years. From the medical

perspective, with a record number of women simultaneously approaching menopause, the healthcare system must anticipate and prepare for the increasing demands on geriatric healthcare. From the population perspective, rising healthcare costs and financial strains in the setting of healthcare reform have left many wondering if they will be able to afford the healthcare they will inevitably require.

According to United States population projections, over 81 million women will be over age 45 by the year 2030, increasing to over 95 million by 2050. After 2030, these women will comprise approximately 23% of the total population [7]. Women have an 11% lifetime risk of undergoing surgical management for pelvic organ prolapse and traditional repair techniques carry a 30% failure risk. This combination of increasing number of patients with prolapse and significant numbers requiring one or more surgeries will result a flood of patients seeking care from pelvic surgeons. The anticipation of this sudden increase in care needs adds additional pressure on the field to develop new techniques with higher long-term success rates.

Risk factors for pelvic organ prolapse have been identified but no preventative care treatment plan is currently in place in the United States. Risk factors include age, parity, obesity, menopause, genetic predisposition, and chronic illnesses that increase pelvic strain. The majority of patients appear to suffer from chronic increased intra-abdominal pressure (i.e., obesity, asthma/cough, constipation) combined with tissue damage from childbearing. The symptoms of mild prolapse often remain manageable until the hormonal, neurological, and muscular strains of the perimenopausal period combine resulting in a weak and dysfunctional pelvic floor. The combined urologic, gynecologic, and gastroenterological symptom profile brings these patients to medical attention. The challenge of pelvic surgery is not only to recreate pelvic support, but also to rehabilitate lifelong behavioral patterns that have ultimately cumulated in the dysfunction.

Pelvic organ prolapse repair is recommended for symptomatic patients. The treatment of asymptomatic patients is debated amongst experts. Treatment is generally recommended for patients with subjective complaints causing them to seek medical attention or objective findings that require medical intervention. Commonly reported symptoms include vaginal bulge, obstruction of urination or defecation, and dyspareunia. Further discussion with patients may uncover unrecognized symptoms of prolapse including splinting, pelvic pain, and inadequate emptying. Objective findings in patients with prolapse include hydronephrosis, ulceration of prolapsed organs, urinary retention, abnormal pressure-flow urodynamics, or cystoscopic findings of urinary obstruction. Lack of sexual satisfaction is also an indication for prolapse repair, and improvement in sexual function has been demonstrated following pelvic reconstructive surgery [8, 9].

The current definition of pelvic organ prolapse contributes to the discrepancy in subjective symptoms and objective findings. Perfect pelvic organ support is defined as POP-Q stage 0; however, 75% of asymptomatic women have greater than stage 1 prolapse on physical examination. This suggests that 75% of asymptomatic women should be classified as having prolapse. The discrepancy also exists in the evaluation of patients following pelvic organ prolapse repair. Satisfactory surgical outcome is often defined as the pelvic organs higher than 1 cm proximal to the hymen, despite the observation that 40% of women do not meet these criteria, many of whom are satisfied with their surgical outcome.

Materials

Pelvic reconstruction offers a variety of techniques using various combinations of autologous, biologic, and synthetic materials. All areas of prolapse have been addressed in the evolution of pelvic reconstruction including urethral support for stress incontinence, vaginal wall for anterior and posterior wall prolapse, and uterus or vaginal cuff in apical prolapse (Table 9.2).

Autologous vaginal tissue is well tolerated when used in vaginal reconstruction but carries a higher failure rate. When autologous vaginal tissue is utilized in reconstruction for prolapse, the reconstruction carries ~30% risk of recurrence requiring additional surgery. Autologous abdominal wall or fascia lata grafts have improved durability when compared to vaginal grafts. This true human fascia is durable and its use in reconstruction significantly improved long-term anatomic outcome with only 10% failure risk [10, 11]. Pain at the site of graft harvest can be considerable. Additional complications include prolonged immobility due to pain at the harvest site and unfavorable cosmetic outcome. Autologous fascia grafts are also limited by size. Harvest of larger grafts increases the risk of pain, worsens cosmesis, and weakens the harvest site. Therefore, despite the durability of autologous fascia, it is not routinely utilized for repair of pelvic reconstruction.

The use of biological grafts eliminates the pain of autologous harvest. Biological grafts include cadaveric fascia lata and abdominal fascia, and xenografts of dermis or intestine. Biologic grafts are not permanent. Material loss over time has been demonstrated and is due to multiple factors including the intrinsic donor tissue quality, structural changes due postharvest processing, radiation, graft rejection, and reabsorption without remodeling of surrounding tissues.

Synthetic mesh is a part of a surgical evolution attempting to maintain durability of repair while minimizing pain of autologous tissue harvesting. Initially introduced to repair uterine prolapse, synthetic mesh has become the preferred method for repairing pelvic organ prolapse [12]. Synthetic grafts are intended to facilitate minimally invasive

Table 9.2 Materials in pelvic reconstruction

Compartment	Synthetic	Organic
Anterior (urethra)		
Bone-anchored	InFast (AMS)	
Retropubic	SPARC (AMS)	BioArc[a] (AMS)
	Align, Uretex (Bard)	Pelvicol, PelviLace[a] (Bard)
	Advantage, Lynx (Boston Scientific)	Stratasis TF[a] (Cook)
	T-Sling (Caldera)	
	I-STOP (CL Medical)	
	Supris (Coloplast)	
	TVT, TVT-Abbrevo, TVT-Exact (Gynecare)	
	Sabre (Mentor)	
Infrapubic	Ophira (Promedon)	
	INfast Ultra (AMS)	
Obturator fascia	Adjust (Bard)	
	Miniarc (AMS)	
	TVT-Secur (Gynecare/Ethicon)	
Transobturator	Monarc (AMS)	BioArc-TO[a] (AMS)
	Align-TO, Uretex-TO (Bard)	Pelvicol-TO, PelviLace-TO[a] (Bard)
	Obtryx, Solyx, Uratape (Boston Scientific)	
	T-Sling (Caldera)	
	TVT-O (Gynecare/Ethicon)	
	I-STOP (CL Medical)	
	Aris, Ob-tape (Mentor-Porges)	
Anterior (bladder)		
Armed	Perigee (AMS)	Avaulta Plus, PelviSoft[a] (Bard)
	Avaulta, Avaulta Solo, Pelvitex (Bard)	
	Gynemesh-PS, Prolift, Prolift-M (Gynecare)	
Nonarmed	Elevate (AMS)	
	Gynemesh, Prosima (Gynecare)	
Apical (vault, uterus)		
Armed	Avaulta, Avaulta Solo (Bard)	Avaulta Plus[a] (Bard)
	Prolift, Prolift-M (Gynecare)	
	IVS Tunneler (Tyco)	
Nonarmed	Elevate (AMS)	
	Prosima (Gynecare)	
Posterior (rectum)		
Armed	Apogee (AMS)	Avaulta Plus, PelviSoft[a] (Bard)
	Avaulta, Avaulta Solo, Pelvitex (Bard)	
	Prolift, Prolift-M (Gynecare)	
Nonarmed	Prosima (Gynecare)	
Any compartment	Prolene Soft (Ethicon)	Repliform[b] (Boston Scientific)
		Dermal Allograft[b] (Bard)

[a]Porcine
[b]Human dermis

pelvic organ prolapse repairs using tension-free placement techniques. They provide broad vaginal coverage without the need to trim or suture to the graft directly. Synthetic grafts, like biological grafts, eliminate the risk of painful autologous harvesting but have been associated with prolonged postoperative pain. Mesh is available for prolapse of the anterior, apical, and posterior compartments. Anterior compartment mesh repairs include both trocar-guided and trocarless (also known as single incision) products for repair of urethral hypermobility and bladder prolapse.

Table 9.3 Mesh classification

Type	Pore size	Material	Product	Fiber type

I	Macroporous	Polypropylene	Free
			  Prolene (Ethicon)
			  Marlex (Bard)
			Kit
			  Apogee, Perigee (AMS)
			  Avaulta (Bard)
			  Prolift (Gynecare)
				Monofilament

II	Microporous	Polytetrafluoroethylene (PTFE)	Gore-Tex (Gore)	Multifilament
III	Macro/micro	Polyethylene Polypropylene/polyglactin 910 Polyglactin 910 Polyethylene terephthalate	Mersilene (Ethicon) Vypro (Ethicon) Vicryl (Ethicon)	Multifilament
IV	Submicro	Silicone		Monofilament

Macroporous >75 μm, microporous <75 μm

Table 9.4 Reaction to mesh

Stage	Onset (weeks postoperative)	Reaction	Implication
I	0–2	Inflammation, capillary proliferation, granular tissue formation, giant cell appearance	Critical process for tissue stability, strength
II	0–2	Granular tissue stabilization, lymphocyte appearance	
III	2–4	Inflammation resolves, capillary reduction	Mesh retracts 20–30% during scar formation
IV	4–6	Dense fibrous tissue formation, giant cell presence	

Trocar-guided mesh for the anterior compartment contains four arms, all of which traverse the adductor muscles (two superiorly and two inferiorly). Trocarless mesh for the anterior compartment is fixated intravaginally in two points in the obturator fascia, without penetration of the adductor muscles, and two points in the sacrospinous ligament.

Multiple mesh materials have been used in vaginal reconstruction and some are associated with infection, graft rejection, and pain. Mesh classification systems are utilized in clinical and research settings to describe different mesh materials (Table 9.3). Mesh is categorized by properties that influence the incidence of complications including material, pore size, and fiber type. The first widely used synthetic sling material for urethral prolapse was Mersilene as described in 1962 by Williams and Te Linde [13]. Subsequent published reports of painful erosions and infections

of Mersilene stimulated the development of a Silicone sling introduced in 1985 which demonstrated similar complications [14, 15]. Polypropylene was introduced in 1996 and has so far demonstrated the lowest complication rates of all available slings [16]. Pore size is thought to contribute to infection and pain as it relates to the immune system's ability to effectively combat bacterial infection. Mesh surface area has also been implicated in many complications [17], as increased size may increase bacterial contamination, inflammatory response, and release of more noxious degradation products.

Mesh placed in vaginal surgery is not inert [18] (Table 9.4). The active process of tissue incorporation and mesh degradation begins immediately following insertion. This process is responsible for the routine postoperative pain and discomfort that occurs during the first 3 months following insertion. During the immediate post-operative period, inflammation is followed by the formation of granular tissue. This granular tissue foundation is critical to strength and stability as it is converted into dense fibrous tissue beginning 4–6 weeks following insertion, peaking at approximately 6–12 weeks. Tissue incorporation occurs concurrently with mesh shrinkage. Ultrasound data consistently demonstrates 30–60% decrease in mesh size at 4–12 weeks compared to size at insertion [19]. The concurrent processes of tissue in growth and mesh shrinkage may cause significant pain, particularly in patients who undergo trocar-guided mesh placement. Adherence of the mesh arms in the lateral pelvic wall is a point against which tension increases during the processes of tissue in growth and mesh shrinkage.

Complications of Mesh in Pelvic Reconstructive Surgery

Evaluation of long-term complications after mesh placement is challenging. Multiple trials noted vaginal mesh exposure during postoperative examinations. These patients were treated with a variety of topical medications and office procedures. The early presentation of vaginal mesh exposure resulted in halting of many trials designed to study the outcomes of synthetic mesh grafts. The overall morbidity of this complication is relatively low and does not significantly impact patient's quality of life following mesh placement [20]. Research halted in the early postoperative period due to exposure fails to describe the more severe pain that continues past the immediate postoperative period. Complication evaluation is also hindered by the rapid introduction of novel mesh techniques as complications are identified [21]. For example, the currently available techniques for synthetic mesh placement include armed grafts, nonarmed grafts, absorbable and nonabsorbable sutures, staples, plastic tines, or pressure compression. Given the complexity of pain syndromes as discussed in this chapter, both patients and physicians would

benefit from the publication of long-term follow-up data on mesh complications.

Multiple tools exist to monitor the outcomes of mesh placement in reconstructive surgery. In addition to the publication of surgeon experience, organized data collection services monitor complications and publish their findings for public viewing. The Manufacturer and User Facility Device Experience (MAUDE) is a U.S. Food and Drug Administration (FDA) database of voluntarily reported adverse events involving medical devices [22]. Using this data the FDA released a Public Health Notification (PHN) [23] warning physicians and patients on the risks of mesh in vaginal surgery. International data is also being collected, as synthetic mesh use in pelvic reconstruction is not limited to the United States [24].

Perioperative Considerations

Imprecise mesh placement may predispose to complications and vaginal pain. Mesh placed in the vaginal epithelium may cause necrosis and ulceration. Necrotic vaginal tissue will ultimately present as pain, vaginal ulceration, vaginal bleeding, mesh exposure, or dyspareunia. Patients who undergo concomitant vaginal procedures are at risk for this complication due to the extensive dissection of the surrounding vaginal tissues. Similarly, suture line integrity is essential to decreasing the risk of painful complications of vaginal mesh surgery. Wound disruption due to poor suture selection, improper suture placement, or excessive tensioning may result in bleeding under the vaginal wall, infection, and mesh exposure. Synthetic delayed absorbable sutures are most commonly used for closure of vaginal incisions following mesh placement [25]. Polyglactin 910 (Vicryl: Ethicon, Somerville, NJ) and Polyglycolic acid (Dexon: Sherwood/Davis & Geck, St. Louis, MO) are commonly used because they maintain good tensile strength during the initial stages of vaginal healing with minimal inflammatory response.

Perioperative bleeding may contribute directly or indirectly to pain following mesh placement.

Hematoma formation may cause pressure to surrounding tissues and discomfort perioperatively making position change and prolonged sitting uncomfortable. Hematomas may also create sinus tracts, delay healing, and cause wound separation. Vaginal packing is most commonly used to provide local compression and decrease perioperative bleeding immediately postoperatively.

Infection contributes to prolonged pain after mesh placement. Bacterial contamination has been documented during vaginal surgery despite standard infection prevention techniques [26]. Precautions to decrease infection with mesh placement have been described and include preoperative chlorhexidine washes, hair removal, intraoperative administration of intravenous antibiotics, solutions of antibiotics or betadine, sheaths to protect mesh from contamination at insertion, and postoperative oral antibiotics [27]. Mesh contamination in vaginal surgery is similar to contamination after surgical placement of foreign material in other surgical literature [28]. Contamination may result in the formation of biofilms surrounding the mesh which produce a low-grade infection that may not present symptomatically until months following mesh insertion. Symptoms of chronic, low-grade infections caused by biofilms include fatigue, fevers, chills, and constant fluid drainage. These infections may progress to cause pain, visible cellulitis, wound separation, purulent discharge, abscess, or pelvic organ infection including genitourinary, gastrointestinal, or musculoskeletal.

Host tissue characteristics influence the pattern of pain after mesh placement. Neovascularization speed may influence the rate of mesh incorporation and shrinkage. Connective tissue metabolism may influence the rate of degradation and chemical breakdown. Hormonal status has been implicated as a contributing factor to mesh complications; however clinical studies have been inconsistent. In vitro estrogen-deprivation of vaginal and periurethral tissues decreased tissue integrity, which contributes to increase risk of vaginal bleeding, poor wound healing, and susceptibility to infection. Rarely, patients may experience an abnormal foreign body response resulting in a chronic inflammatory process [29].

Etiology of Mesh Pain

Routine postoperative pain is self-limited. The duration of postoperative pain is variable, typically present during the initial stages of healing and shrinkage as mentioned earlier in this chapter. Most often the pain is dull, constant, exacerbated by activity, and relieved with rest or oral pain medications. Increases in intra-abdominal pressure during voiding, defecation, lifting, or intercourse may also exacerbate pain. Treatment for routine postoperative pain should be directed towards relieving the exacerbating factors. Options include local (rest, ice, warm soaks, topical medications) and systemic (oral pain control, stool softeners).

A group of patients will experience an abnormal pain pattern, either pain persisting beyond the routine postoperative period or absence of immediate postoperative pain and appearing weeks after surgery. Initial evaluation of these patients includes a detailed physical examination and relevant diagnostic and imaging studies (detailed later in this chapter). The goal of this evaluation is to identify common complications whose treatment, medical or surgical, may improve or resolve the pain entirely. Mesh removal will successfully improve or resolve pain. Examples of pain complications that are identifiable on initial evaluation include mesh visualization (perforation, erosion, extrusion) and fluid collections (hematoma, abscess). Studies to diagnose these complications include cystoscopy, CT, and magnetic resonance imaging (MRI).

Chronic mesh pain syndrome (CMPS) refers to a complex condition that develops in a small number of patients with pain following mesh reconstruction (Table 9.5). CMPS is characterized by the development of chronic pain symptoms following mesh insertion persisting past the routine postoperative period [30]. This description is consistent with literature describing the onset of other chronic pain syndromes, such as chronic pelvic pain syndrome (CPPS), following multiple initial causative events. Patients with CMPS are identified using the following criteria. First, pain must initiate following mesh placement. A careful history and chart review should be used for confirmation. Second, pain must

Table 9.5 Chronic mesh pain syndrome (CMPS)

Characteristics	Definition
Initiated by mesh	Pain only present following mesh placement
Chronic	Pain past the postoperative period (>90 days)
Refractory	Pain refractory to treatment of identifiable, potentially reversible causes of pain
Disproportion	Pain out of proportion to physical examination findings
Regional symptoms	Presence of ≥1 of the following symptoms, due to neuronal sensitization and cross-talk
Visceral hyperalgesia	Enhanced pain sensitivity in the same and nearby organs
Allodynia	Pain due to stimuli that do not normally provoke pain
Hyperalgesia	Increased response to painful stimuli
Diffuse location	Poorly delineated margins due to relative paucity of nerve endings in viscera
Systemic symptoms	Presence of ≥1 of the following symptoms
Allergic/immunologic	Rash, hypersensitivity, inflammation, fevers
Referred hyperalgesia	Tenderness at remote superficial sites

persist past the routine postoperative period. Pain lasting more than 3 months postoperatively should be considered abnormal. Third, pain must be refractory to medical and surgical treatment of other complications. Patients who present with pain after mesh placement should undergo the recommended examination and testing. Complications should be treated. Patients whose pain persists despite these treatments should be considered for the diagnosis of CMPS. Notably, treatment with mesh removal does not resolve pain. Fourth, pain intensity is considerably greater than routine pain and is not relieved by routine therapies. Pain is out of proportion to physical examination findings. Lastly, regional and systemic symptoms develop as a result of neuronal sensitization, cross-talk, and pain centralization.

Different from self-limiting postoperative pain, CMPS is a pathologic condition caused by the transformation of local vaginal pain into a multiorgan systemic process. Pain should be treated as an ongoing pathologic process instead of a variation of routine postoperative pain. Treatment is challenging given the cascade of events that is not entirely reversible by mesh removal. Risk factors are unknown. A combination of mesh material, surgical technique, and host factors are likely contributors. Multiple case reports and case series have been published to increase awareness of this condition [31].

CMPS is the result of abnormal neuronal activation (Fig. 9.1a). Following the initial event (mesh placement), neuronal up regulation results in simultaneous sensitization of pain pathways in the spinal cord and central nervous system (CNS), along with pelvic organ cross-talk. These abnormal neuronal activation pathways, when continuously stimulated, result in the formation of abnormal somatic-visceral responses. As a result of this pathway, routine postoperative pain driven by pain input is converted to a process whose focus of neural activity is located in the CNS. The long-term peripheral and central release of neurotrophic factors stimulates these sensory pathways resulting in permanent sensory changes, a process referred to as sensitization. Patients who have undergone sensitization often suffer from referred hyperalgesia, visceral hyperalgesia, allodynia, hyperalgesia, and disproportion.

Innervation of Mesh Pain

Pain signals from the pelvic organs travel with somatic nerves, sympathetic and parasympathetic fibers (Fig. 9.1b). Organs located intraperitoneal (ureter, uterus, ovaries, bladder) send pain and temperature signals via the sympathetic nervous system. Preganglionic sympathetic fibers originate at the spinal cord levels T9–L1, exit through the ventral spinal roots, pass through the sympathetic trunks, and synapse at the inferior mesenteric ganglion. Postganglionic fibers

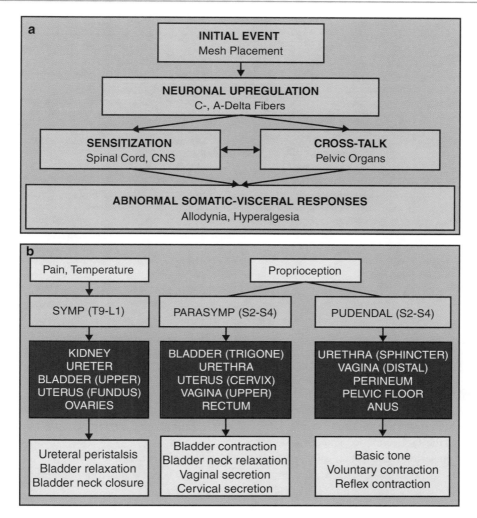

Fig. 9.1 (a) Development of abnormal pain responses. Abnormal neuronal activation is a key component of chronic mesh pain syndrome. (b) Pelvic innervation. Pain signals from the pelvic organs travel with somatic nerves, sympathetic and parasympathetic fibers

then travel through the superior hypogastric plexus and inferior hypogastric (pelvic) plexus prior to synapsing on the pelvic organs to increase peristalsis, inhibit bladder detrusor contraction, increase bladder neck contractility, and control vasoconstriction.

Parasympathetic pelvic nerves (S2–S4) provide proprioception from the rectum, bladder trigone, urethra, cervix, and upper vagina. These afferent fibers travel through the parasympathetic pelvic splanchnic nerves to the sacral plexus, sensory ganglia, and the ventral spinal cord at

level S2–S4. Preganglionic sympathetic fibers originate at the spinal cord level S2–S4, exit through the ventral spinal roots, travel through the sacral plexus, and travel as long pelvic splanchnic nerves until synapsing in the pelvic ganglia. Short postganglionic fibers promote bladder contraction, bladder neck relaxation, and vaginal secretions.

The pudendal, ilioinguinal, and femorocutaneous nerves are often involved in chronic mesh pain. The pudendal nerve (S2–S4) senses proprioception and pain from the distal vagina, urethra,

Table 9.6 Anatomy of mesh pain

Mesh		Etiology of pain			
Location	Organ	Nerve	Muscle	Bone	Viscera
Retropubic	Urethra	Ilioinguinal	Anterior rectus	Pubic symphysis	Urethra Bladder Vagina
Transobturator	Urethra Bladder	Femorocutaneous Posterior cutaneous Pudendal Perineal Inferior anal Obturator	Adductor longus Adductor brevis Adductor magnus Gracilis Obturator externus Obturator internus	Pubic symphysis Ischial rami Ischial spines	Urethra Bladder Vagina
Sacral	Vault Uterus	Sacral roots Lumbosacral plexus Pelvic plexus	Piriformis Obturator internus	Ischial spines Sacrum	Vagina Uterus Rectum
Sacrospinous	Bladder Vault Uterus Rectum	Pudendal Sciatic	Gluteus maximus Levator ani	Ischial spines Ischial tuberosities	Bladder Vagina Uterus Rectum

pelvic floor, and perineum. Efferent fibers provide motor function to the pelvic floor, vagina, perineum, and urethral and anal sphincters. The pudendal nerve courses in close proximity to pelvic organs and can be injured in pelvic reconstructive surgery. The pudendal nerve travels posterior to the sacrospinous ligament and enters the pelvis posterior to the ischial spine, providing innervation to perineal structures including the bulbospongiosus, ischiocavernosus, clitoris, anal canal (including external anal sphincter and puborectalis muscles), and urethral sphincter. The ilioinguinal nerve (L1) may be damaged after passage of trocars through the suprapubic area. The ilioinguinal nerve arises at level T12 and provides sensation to the suprapubic and upper, outer portions of the perineum. Patients who undergo mesh with retropubic trocar entry sites who present with pain should be evaluated for ilioinguinal nerve involvement. The posterior femorocutaneous nerve (S1–S3) originates from dorsal divisions of S1–S2 and ventral divisions of S2–S3 as part of the sacral plexus. The nerve enters the pelvis through the greater sciatic foramen below the piriformis muscle. Branches of the posterior femorocutaneous nerve provide sensation from the posterior thigh, perineum lateral to the labia, and lateral genitalia.

Anatomy of Mesh Pain

A thorough understanding of pelvic anatomy is essential to evaluating complex mesh pain. The identification of mesh pain should trigger evaluation for other related complications (Table 9.6).

Musculoskeletal

Mesh may become incorporated into surrounding muscle. Trauma to the muscle can be directly to muscle fibers or indirectly via traction, local hematoma, and secondary fibrosis causing restriction and pain in movement. Direct muscle injury is less common and more difficult to diagnose. Clinical presentation of mesh pain of the pelvic or extremity muscles includes isolated spasm, pain with position change, or activity-related fatigue relieved by rest. Pain is typically intermittent and activity-related. Pelvic organ muscle involvement may present as dyspareunia or dysfunction of urination or defecation. Mesh placed superficially in the vaginal muscularis instead of the adventitia may cause pain with any manipulation of the vaginal canal and intercourse may be intolerable as a result.

Muscular pain following retropubic mesh placement is primarily a result of trauma to the anterior rectus muscle. Trauma may be direct or

Fig. 9.2 (**a**) Hip adductors. The pectineus, adductor longus, gracilis, and adductor magnus may be involved in mesh pain. Nerves in close proximity are also included. (**b**) Lumbosacral plexus. The lumbosacral nerve, sciatic nerve, and pudendal nerve are particularly vulnerable during apical compartment suspension

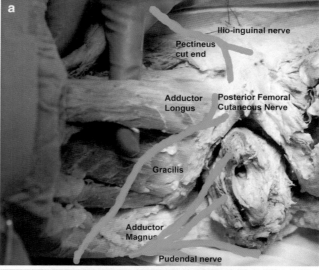

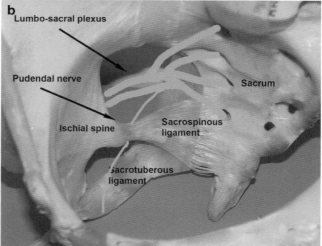

indirect as described above. The pain is typically positional and relieved with rest.

Muscular injury after transobturator trocar-guided mesh placement may cause severe pain with walking or joint movement. Obturator muscle involvement presents as pain with abduction, lateral thigh rotation, and walking. The hip adductors are also at considerable risk during placement of a transobturator mesh. The adductor longus, adductor brevis, adductor magnus, gracilis, and obturator externus muscles all originate along the inferior pubic and ischial rami in close proximity to mesh placement (Fig. 9.2a). These muscles are responsible for hip flexion, thigh adduction, medial and lateral rotation. Innervation is provided by the obturator nerve (L2–L4) and sciatic nerve (L4–S3). Pain is exacerbated by movement of the hip and thigh and relieved with rest. The levator ani muscles may also be affected causing pelvic pain, dyspareunia, or pain with prolonged standing.

Pain may occur following apical prolapse repair by multiple techniques. Mesh fixated to the sacrospinous ligament may damage the surrounding musculature. Involvement of the coccygeus muscle overlying the sacrospinous ligament or the piriformis muscle may be a considerable source of pain. Pain from the levator muscle may occur if placement is inferior to the sacrospinous ligament causing pelvic or gluteal pain radiating to the distal pelvis and vagina. Distal vaginal vault suspensions utilizing the ileococcygeus muscle, or high levator myorrhaphy, may also experience movement-induced gluteal area pain. The piriformis muscle along the anterior sacrum may cause pain after apical compartment repair. Innervation is provided by the piriformis nerve (L5–S2) and functions to laterally rotate the thigh.

Patients who undergo posterior compartment mesh repair with trocar-guided lateral mesh arms may experience pain in the levator muscles or gluteus maximus. Gluteus maximus innervation is provided by the inferior gluteal nerve (S1). Patients may present with pain exacerbated by sitting, external hip rotation and hip extension, Injury to the external anal sphincter muscles may cause pain or defecatory dysfunction including constipation or incontinence of flatus or stool.

Mesh may be anchored to the bony pelvis intentionally or as a result of fibrous adherence following placement. Bone-related mesh pain may be dull or sharp, constant or intermittent. Bone pain after retropubic sling is caused by trocar passage along the posterior aspect of the superior pubic rami posterior to the obturator grove. Trocar passage during placement of a transobturator mesh is in close proximity to the inferior pubic rami. Anterior vaginal wall mesh placed with trocar guidance travels along the lateral inferior aspect of the ischial rami until emerging medially into the vaginal canal just posterior to the descending rami. Physicians are recommended to avoid the superior pubic rami that are in close proximity to the obturator artery and nerve.

Sacral involvement should be suspected in patients with bone pain following sacrocolpopexy. Ischial spines and ischial tuberosities may be damaged during vaginal approaches to posterior compartment repair. Placement of posterior mesh arms in close proximity to these prominences may cause pain by direct trauma or mesh fixation.

Patients who have abnormal pain caused by posterior mesh arms report difficulty with prolonged sitting.

Periosteum can be damaged during trocar passage or irritated by infected or adherent mesh causing persistent pain. Mild periosteal inflammation is mild and self-limited and does not require evaluation. Severe localized pubic pain suggestive of osteitis or osteomyelitis requires a diagnostic bone scan. Pain may radiate to nearby muscles.

Visceral

Visceral pain may be caused by trocar placement, mesh penetration, or organ obstruction. Mesh penetration pain is typically dull, constant, and exacerbated by usage of the related organ from muscular inflammation. The affected organ may be in pain with any movement including peristalsis, contraction, filling, or emptying. Pelvic organ prolapse (recurrent or new) may also cause pain or obstruction after mesh placement.

Mesh may penetrate the urethral or bladder after vaginal reconstruction. Hematuria, recurrent infections, and urethral pain that extends past the routine postoperative period is suspicious for mesh penetration and should be evaluated. Detrusor overactivity may be caused by mesh penetration, improper location, or excessive lateral adherence. Urinary obstruction from improper placement may also present as pain. Urinary obstruction following transobturator sling typically requires the patient to lean forward while voiding.

Vaginal mesh complications may present with or without exposure. Palpable mesh cords or bands in the lateral fornices below the vaginal epithelium may present with vaginal pain or be identified incidentally on examination. Mesh folding, shrinkage, and excess tensioning all contribute to formation of mesh cords. Pain with intercourse is also a common complaint following mesh reconstruction.

Mesh penetration into the uterus/cervix may occur following apical prolapse repair. Symptoms include abnormal bleeding, cramping, infections, or pain.

Mesh penetration into bowel or anal sphincter may present as bleeding, infection, obstruction, or incontinence. Patients who report rectal bleeding postoperatively should be evaluated for mesh perforation. Symptoms including fever, erythema, persistent fullness, or malodorous drainage may reflect an ongoing infectious process. Constant rectal pain, fecal urgency or incontinence, and pain relieved by defecation are signs of rectal obstruction.

Lymphovascular

Perioperative bleeding, recognized or unrecognized, may result in hematoma formation. Up to 25% of patients undergoing retropubic slings have postoperative hematomas visible on MRI [32]. Branches of the obturator vessels may be injured by trocar passage over the superior pubic rami close to the obturator foramen. Trocar passage in the lateral vagina may cause bleeding in branches of the pudendal artery. Hemorrhage from damage to the uterine or internal iliac vessels has also been described.

Chronic inflammatory states following mesh placement can cause an increase in lymphatic fluid production resulting in a chronic increase in drainage. Patients with preexisting poor pelvic venous drainage may also be at risk for pain.

Neurological

Intraoperative nerve damage presents immediately following the procedure. Sharp pain in a specific nerve distribution presenting in the immediate postoperative period suggests intraoperative nerve damage and should be treated. Nerve injury at the time of retropubic mesh placement is rare but has been reported [33]. The most common injury is damage to branches of the ilioinguinal nerve (L1) following lateral skin perforation. Less commonly, incorrect trocar use during retropubic mesh placement may also affect the obturator nerve.

Nerve pain that presents in the postoperative period and persists into the delayed postoperative period should be considered an example of mesh pain and trigger evaluation for other etiologies as well. This includes nerve entrapment and the pelvic organ cross-talk or sensitization.

Transobturator mesh placement may damage branches of the femorocutaneous, posterior cutaneous, pudendal, perineal, inferior anal, or obturator nerve. The obturator internus nerve (L5–S1) innervates the obturator internus muscle that is intentially traversed by trocar-guided mesh products. The anterior, lateral, and posterior femoral cutaneous nerves (L2–S3) provide sensation to the inner aspect of the thigh and lateral perineum where transobturator trocars typically exit the skin. If trocar placement is in close proximity to the labia majora, labial branches of the pudendal nerve may also be involved. The pudendal nerve branches that may be damaged by anterior compartment mesh procedures include the dorsal clitoral nerve (clitoris), posterior labial nerves (posterior labia), and perineal nerves (midperineum). Posterior mesh procedures are more likely to damage posterior pudendal nerve branches such as the inferior anal nerves (perineal body, anus).

Sacrospinous mesh fixation for reconstruction of the apical or posterior compartments may damage multiple pelvic nerves. The lumbosacral nerve plexus on the piriformis muscle, sciatic nerve superolateral to the sacrospinous ligament, and pudendal nerve as it passes posterior to the ischial spines are particularly vulnerable during apical compartment suspension (Fig. 9.2b). Patients with these injuries typically present with buttock or posterior leg pain, loss of sensation, or motor function. Sacrocolpopexy by any approach can cause damage to the presacral nerves at the sacral promontory.

Posterior compartment repair may cause injury to the lumbosacral plexus, sciatic nerve, or pudendal nerve. These nerves are at risk during both trocar-guided and nontrocar-guided mesh procedures. Trocars pathways typically begin at the perineum through the ischial fossa and the levator muscles to the perirectal space.

Evaluation of Patients with Mesh Pain

History

Evaluation of patients with pain after mesh placement begins with a detailed history to identify de novo pain that is discrete from routine postoperative pain as described above. Mesh pain persists past the immediate postoperative period, is activity-related, intense out of proportion to objective findings, and demonstrates characteristics of CPPS. Whether the etiology of mesh pain is irreversible nerve damage or a progressive pathological pain response remains unclear.

Pain is clearly documented at each visit. The essential details include exacerbating and relieving factors, quality, radiation, severity, and time course. Activities that exacerbate pain are noted; including prolonged sitting or hip flexion, to identify involved musculoskeletal components. Symptoms of obstructive urination, defecation, or dyspareunia suggest misplacement. These findings are often associated with retraction of the vaginal epithelium. Prolonged vaginal, bladder, or rectal bleeding suggests ulceration, infection, or organ penetration. Timing of pain onset in relation to tissue incorporation, mesh breakdown and shrinkage should be considered.

Mesh visualization should be documented using standard nomenclature. A mesh complication categorization scheme has been developed and published by the International Continence Society and the International Urogynecologic Association, and is intended to facilitate communications amongst physicians [34] (Table 9.7). General approach to mesh visualization should take into consideration the time of presentation, symptom severity, and associated symptoms.

Perform a complete review of systems to identify de novo systemic symptoms. Allergic or immune reactions to mesh components may present immediately or in the delayed postoperative period. New diagnoses of systemic illness following mesh placement should alert the physician to consider mesh as a contributing factor. Special notice should be taken when new autoimmune, inflammatory, or allergic illnesses do not respond to traditional management. If available, compare the patients' symptoms to the initial review of systems performed prior to mesh placement. Identify concurrent pelvic complaints of pressure, pain, dyspareunia, and pelvic organ prolapse above the introitus. Patients with these symptoms may have preexisting pain syndromes such as chronic pelvic pain, painful bladder syndrome, interstitial cystitis, fibromyalgia, vulvodynia, dysmenorrhea, and chronic constipation.

Table 9.7 Mesh terminology

Terminology	Definition
Contraction	Reduction in size
Prominence	Parts project beyond a surface
Penetration	Entering
Separation	Physically disconnected
Exposure	Displaying or making accessible
Extrusion	Passage gradually out of a body tissue
Perforation	Abnormal opening into a hollow organ
Dehiscence	Bursting open along natural or sutured lines

Adapted from Haylen et al. [34]

These diagnoses imply a significant component of pelvic floor dysfunction and myofascial pain. Patients with these diagnoses are poor candidates for mesh prolapse repair. Insertion of vaginal mesh with fixation to the pelvic floor will only exacerbate the preexisting condition [35].

Obtain and review Operative Reports and prior History and Physical Examination forms for patients with pain. Complications or intraoperative challenges such as bleeding, prolonged operative time, and intraoperative consultations should be identified. The performance of concomitant procedures and use of other mesh products should also be noted. For example, it is important to obtain information on concomitant procedures with special attention to any discrepancy between planned and performed procedures. Length of antibiotic therapy, prolonged catheter management, blood transfusions, and ICU care are signs of a complicated surgical course.

Minor surgical complications may contribute to mesh pain. Minor complications are generally considered to include hematoma formation, vaginal or urinary infection, or urinary retention. Detailed conversation with the patient regarding the perioperative events may also provide additional information regarding surgical complications.

Obtain detailed information on medical and surgical treatments for pain after mesh placement. Discuss the patient's impression of improvement following these treatments. For example, patients with pain due to mesh attachment to the levator plate may find relief with anti-inflammatory agents or rest. This pain would be exacerbated by stimulating therapies such as pelvic floor physiotherapy.

Physical Examination

Physical examination is essential to identify the cause of pain. Begin by palpating the path of mesh, tines (if applicable), and location of trocar placement. Identify areas that recreate the patient's pain when palpated. Perform a careful vaginal examination for signs of mesh exposure or erosion. Evaluate the urethra and bladder after mesh for anterior and apical prolapse. Valuable information can be obtained by minimally invasive evaluation methods including postvoid residual for urinary obstruction, bladder filling using indigo carmine for perforation or fistula, cystourethroscopy for perforation, obstruction or misplacement, urodynamics for voiding and storage dysfunction, and voiding cystourethrogram for all indications. Patients who have undergone apical and posterior compartment repairs and present with defecatory dysfunction may require digital rectal examination, sigmoidoscopy, and evaluation of defecatory function using dynamic MRI, or defecography. Patients with de novo rectal bleeding should be evaluated for rectal perforation with sigmoidoscopy.

Ultrasound may provide additional objective information regarding mesh location. Mesh location, direction, size, extrusion, penetration, and folding may be identified by ultrasound. This information may be particularly valuable when Operative Reports are unavailable or when patients have undergone prior mesh incisions or partial excisions (Fig. 9.3a, b).

Complete pelvic imaging may reveal contributing factors for pain. MRI may reveal relevant pathology such as fluid collections, abscesses, prolapse, bone anchors, disc herniation, pelvic masses, and visceral obstruction. However, if intracavitary coils are used, adequate visualization of mesh will not be achieved. Bone scans can also be used to identify signs osteitis or osteomyelitis.

Treatment

Patients presenting with asymptomatic or minimally symptomatic vaginal mesh exposure may present days or years after placement. Mesh visualization identified in the immediate postoperative period is most commonly a direct result of vaginal epithelium separation, or incision dehiscence. Additional attempts at surgical closure may be offered. If the process appears infectious, the mesh may be salvaged with courses of clindamycin or metronidazole. Infections that fail medication management require excision of the prominent mesh portions or total excision to prevent recurrence.

When mesh is visualized in the delayed postoperative period (>6 weeks), this exposure may be due to weakened vaginal epithelium, local infection, chronic inflammation, complications of vaginal healing or mesh shrinkage, or improper placement. Mesh extrusion is typically a result many factors, including but not limited to chronic infection, improper placement, and vaginal atrophy. Vaginal atrophy may be conservatively treated with local or transdermal estrogen. Patients with mesh extrusion who fail medical management should be evaluated for surgical excision of mesh partially or in its entirety. Patients with multiple risk factors for mesh extrusion are more likely to require complete excision given the risk of recurrent extrusion following partial excision.

Mesh incision and partial excision are only recommended for patients with organ obstruction in the absence of pain or infection. Infection is not limited to exposed mesh segments alone. Removing exposed mesh portions in the presence of active infection is followed by recurrent exposure frustrating both patient and physician. Additional surgical attempts at mesh removal become increasingly technically challenging due to mesh retraction and tissue incorporation of remaining portions.

Surgeons treating patients with mesh pain caused by mesh, fixation materials, abscess, or hematoma should be prepared to remove all mesh portions. Partial excision may improve, but is unlikely to completely resolve, mesh pain.

Fig. 9.3 (a) 3D ultrasound image for mesh evaluation. Seventy year old G3P3 with lower abdominal pain, urinary retention for 2 years following retropubic sling (TVT). Ultrasound reveals sling in normal position. (b) 2D ultrasound image for mesh evaluation. Forty-six-year-old G2P2 with pelvic pain, urinary incontinence, dyspareunia for 1 year following transobturator sling (unknown type). Ultrasound reveals sling with displacement of unilateral arm

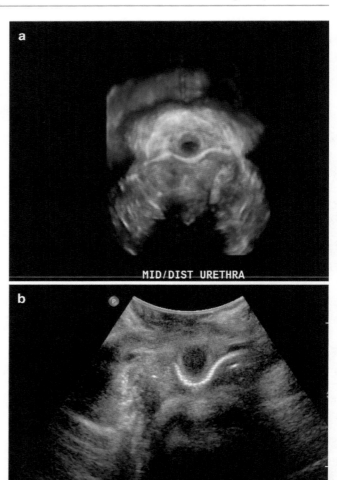

Patients with complex mesh pain as described in this chapter receive the maximum benefit from early complete mesh removal to decrease the risk of pain somatization and centralization. Published series note an 88% improvement following mesh removal in patients with severe mesh pain [36].

Technical difficulty of surgical mesh removal is determined by mesh type and location. Armed mesh through the transobturator membrane requires a technically challenging removal. To successfully remove armed mesh segments in their entirety, the obturator membrane must be perforated and dissection carried out laterally. Additional incisions in the lateral thighs may be required to adequately free the arms from the surrounding soft tissues. We suggest preoperatively marking the lateral puncture sites to facilitate intraoperative dissection. If the lateral incisions cannot be identified by patient symptoms or scarring, gentle traction on the medial portion of the mesh arms may be used as a guide. The mesh should be followed from skin incision to the intersection of the adductor muscles and dissected free in a circumferential fashion.

Muscle fibers often must be dissected when mesh has become incorporated into the surrounding fibers. Large defects in the vaginal wall may occur with mesh removal and surgeons ought to be prepared to utilize rotational vaginal flaps, labial flaps, or skip flaps for reconstruction. Following complete healing and resolution of other symptoms such as pain, infection, bleeding, urinary or defecatory dysfunction, evaluation for additional surgery for persistent incontinence or prolapse can begin if clinically indicated.

The decision to proceed with mesh removal for refractory pain should not be avoided due to fear of recurrent incontinence or prolapse. Literature has demonstrated recurrent prolapse following mesh removal may not require immediate surgical correction. Patients who undergo incision of urethral slings are continent in 60% of cases in many large series [37]. Following mesh removal for other compartment prolapse, recurrence is highest for the anterior compartment, which carries a 19% risk of recurrent bladder prolapse. This is consistent with published opinion that fibrotic tissue from mesh placement and its removal is at least as durable as traditional colporrhaphy alone.

Consultations by other physicians may be warranted for patients presenting with illnesses involving other organ systems. However, evaluation and management of the mesh complication must continue. During initial pain evaluation and treatment planning, patients with uncontrolled pain may require Pain Management assistance to select an appropriate medication regimen. The onset of additional symptoms may warrant consultation by Gastroenterology, Rheumatology or Allergy/Immunology. Consultants may provide useful information regarding patient illnesses, however for all illnesses or pain de novo following mesh placement, the authors recommend strong consideration of mesh removal to obtain the best potential to improve patient quality of life.

Despite thorough evaluation and treatment, mesh pain may persist. The centralization of pain may not be completely reversible if sensitization and cross-talk have already created significant abnormal somatic-visceral responses.

Prevention

Intraoperative and perioperative considerations may minimize the risk of mesh complications. Preoperatively, caution should be taken when offering mesh placement at the time of concomitant vaginal procedures to avoid extensive vaginal dissection and increased infection risk. Intraoperative hemostasis and infection prevention are essential. Vaginal packing should be used postoperatively for additional hemostasis and infection prevention.

Litigation is an important concern for physicians inserting vaginal mesh [38]. In addition to adequate preoperative counseling, physicians ought to document discussion with patients regarding the FDA warning on vaginal mesh, and the risks, benefits and alternatives to vaginal mesh reconstruction. Education of both patients and physicians for early signs and symptoms of mesh complications will improve patient selection, outcome, and overall satisfaction.

Conclusion

In conclusion, evaluation and treatment of patients with pain after mesh placement is more complex than previously described. The majority of patients presenting with pain after mesh placement experience a self-limited, routine postoperative pain. However, an unknown number of these patients develop complex mesh pain with symptoms similar to those of CPPS. As an increasing number of patients undergo repair of pelvic organ prolapse with synthetic mesh, physicians must be prepared for the presentation of more complex, multiorgan system complications that may require partial or complete mesh removal. Some patients may never have complete resolution of pain despite mesh removal. The origin of complex mesh pain is unknown. Patients with mesh complications present with a myriad of subjective and objective findings that may be suggestive of a physical reaction to mesh, technical placement complications, or mesh rejection over time.

Management of patients with mesh pain should focus on both physical and emotional recovery. The impact of pain after mesh placement is often underappreciated. Patients must be encouraged to seek support and rehabilitation services in extreme cases. When additional operative interventions are warranted, patients should have appropriate expectations regarding their recovery and be informed of the risk of recurrent pelvic organ prolapse.

Evaluation of the current approach to vaginal reconstruction is warranted. The goal of reconstructive surgery is to provide successful outcomes and to improve quality of life. In searching for improved anatomic outcomes we have adopted synthetic mesh, but at what cost? In a field where treatment success is difficult to quantify [39] and subjective outcomes do not correlate with anatomic outcomes [40, 41], which should prevail? For this reason, these authors share the opinion that successful objective outcome is insufficient reason to continue mesh prolapse repairs in the absence of adequate demonstration of comparably successful subjective outcome.

References

1. Savary D, Fatton B, Velemir L, Amblard J, Jacquetin B. What about transvaginal mesh repair of pelvic organ prolapse? Review of the literature since the HAS (French Health Authorities) report. J Gynecol Obstet Biol Reprod. 2009;38:11–41.
2. Morrisroe S, Lee U, Raz S. The use of mesh in vaginal prolapse repair: do the benefits justify the risks? Curr Opin Urol. 2010;2:275–9.
3. ACOG Practice. Bulletin Number 85, September 2007 (replaces practice bulletin number 79, February 2007). Clinical management guidelines for obstetrician-gynecologists. Am J Obstet Gynecol. 2007;110:707–29.
4. Murphy M. Society of Gynecologic Surgeons systematic review: clinical practice guidelines on vaginal graft use from the society of gynecologic surgeons. Obstet Gynecol. 2008;112:1123–30.
5. Walter J. Transvaginal mesh procedures for pelvic organ prolapse: Society of Obstetricians and Gynaecologists of Canada technical update. J Obstet Gynaecol Can. 2011;33:168–74.
6. Maher C, Feiner B, Baessler K, Adams EJ, Hagen S, Glazener CM. Surgical management of pelvic organ prolapse in women. Cochrane Database Syst Rev. 2007;3:CD004014.
7. United States Census Bureau, 2004. U.S. interim projections by age, sex, race, and hispanic origin. http://

www.census.gov/ipc/www/usinterimproj. Accessed 1 Jan 2011.
8. Nieminen K, Hiltunen R, Heiskanen E, Takala T, Niemi K, Merikari M, et al. Symptom resolution and sexual function after anterior vaginal wall repair with and without polypropylene mesh. Int Urogynecol J Pelvic Floor Dysfunct. 2008;19:1611–6.
9. Kuhn A, Burkhard F, Eggemann C, Mueller MD. Sexual function after suburethral sling removal for dyspareunia. Surg Endosc. 2009;23:765–8.
10. Beck RP, Grove D, Arnusch D, Harvey J. Recurrent urinary stress incontinence treated by fascia lata sling procedure. Am J Obstet Gynecol. 1974;120:613–21.
11. Beck RP, McCormick S, Nordstrom L. The fascia lata sling procedure for treating recurrent genuine stress incontinence. Obstet Gynecol. 1988;72:699–703.
12. Huguier J, Scali P. Posterior suspension of the genital axis on the lumbosacral disk in the treatment of uterine prolapsed. Presse Med. 1958;66:781–4.
13. Williams TJ, Te Linde RW. The sling operation for urinary incontinence using Mersilene ribbon. Obstet Gynecol. 1962;19:241–5.
14. Stanton SL, Brindley GS, Holmes DM. Silastic sling for urethral sphincter incompetence in women. Br J Obstet Gynaecol. 1985;92:747.
15. Duckett JRA, Constantine F. Complications of silicone sling insertion for stress urinary incontinence. J Urol. 2000;163(6):1835–7.
16. Rodriguez LV, Raz S. Prospective analysis of patients treated with distal urethral polypropylene slings for symptoms of stress urinary incontinence: 5-year outcomes. J Urol. 2003;170:849–51.
17. Ostergard DR. Polypropylene vaginal mesh grafts in gynecology. Obstet Gynecol. 2010;116:962–6.
18. Clavé A, Yahi H, Hammou JC, Montanari S, Gounon P, Clavé H. Polypropylene as a reinforcement in pelvic surgery is not inert: comparative analysis of 100 explants. Int Urogencol J Pelvic Floor Dysfunct. 2010;21:261–70.
19. Garcia-Urena MA, Vega Ruiz V, Diaz Godoy A, Baez Perea JM, Marin Gomez LM, Carnero Hernandez FJ, et al. Differences in polypropylene shrinkage depending on mesh position in an experimental study. Am J Surg. 2007;193:538–42.
20. Niro J, Phillipe AC, Jaffeux P, Ambiard J, Velemir L, Savary D, et al. Postoperative pain after transvaginal repair of pelvic organ prolapse with or without mesh. Gynecol Obstet Fertil. 2010;38:648–52.
21. Moore RD, Davila GW. Vaginal mesh kits for prolapse 2010: update in technology and techniques to minimize complications. Female Patient. 2010;35:33–7.
22. The Manufacturer and User Facility Device Experience (MAUDE). http://www.accessdata.fda.gov/scripts/cdrh/cfdocs/cfmaude/search.cfm. Accessed 1 Jan 2011.
23. The United States Food and Drug Administration Medical Device Alerts and Notices on Surgical Mesh. http://www.fda.gov/MedicalDevices/Safety/AlertsandNotices/ucm142636.htm. Accessed 1 Jan 2011.

24. National Institute for Health and Clinical Excellence. Surgical repair of vaginal wall prolapse using mesh 2008. http://guidance.nice.org.uk/IPG267. Accessed 1 Feb 2011.

25. Greenberg JA, Clark RM. Advances in suture material for obstetric and gynecologic surgery. Rev Obstet Gynecol. 2009;2:146–58.

26. Culligan P, Heit M, Blackwell L, Murphy M, Graham CA, Snyder J. Bacterial colony counts during vaginal surgery. Infect Dis Obstet Gynecol. 2003;11:161–5.

27. Darouiche RO, Wall Jr MJ, Itani KM, Otterson MF, Webb AL, Carrick MM, et al. Chlorhexidine-alcohol versus povidone-iodine for surgical site antisepsis. N Engl J Med. 2010;362:18–26.

28. Gristina AG. Biomaterial-centered infection: microbial adherence versus tissue integration. Science. 1987;237:1588–95.

29. Junge K, Bunnebosel M, von Trotha K, Rosch R, Klinge U, Neuman UP, Jansen PL. Mesh biocompatibility effects of cellular inflammation and tissue remodeling. Langenbecks Arch Surg. 2012;397: 255–70.

30. Delavierre D, Rigaud J, Sibert L, Labat JJ. Definitions, classifications and terminology of chronic pelvic and perineal pain. Prog Urol. 2010;20:853–64.

31. Lin LL, Haessler AL, Ho M, Betson LH, Alinsod RM, Bhatia NN. Dyspareunia and chronic pelvic pain after polypropylene mesh augmentation for transvaginal repair of anterior vaginal wall prolapse. Int Urogynecol J Pelvic Floor Dysfunct. 2007;18:675–8.

32. Giri SK, Wallis F, Drumm J, Saunders JA, Flood HD. A magnetic resonance imaging-based study of retropubic haematoma after sling procedures: preliminary findings. BJU Int. 2005;96(7):1067–71.

33. Fisher HW, Lotze PM. Nerve injury locations during retropubic sling procedures. Int Urogynecol J Pelvic Floor Dysfunct. 2011;22:439–41.

34. Haylen BT, Freeman RM, Swift SE, Cosson M, Davila GW, Deprest J, et al. An International Urogynecological Association (IUGA)/International Continence Society (ICS) joint terminology and classification of the complications related directly to the insertion of prosthesis (meshes, implants, tapes) & grafts in female pelvic floor surgery. Int Urogynecol J Pelvic Floor Dysfunct. 2011;22:3–15.

35. Butrick CW, Sanford D, Hou Q, Mahnken JD. Chronic pelvic pain syndromes: clinical, urodynamic, and urothelial observations. Int Urogynecol J Pelvic Floor Dysfunct. 2009;20:1047–53.

36. Feiner B, Maher C. Vaginal mesh contraction: definition, clinical presentation, and management. Obstet Gynecol. 2010;115:325–30.

37. Marcus-Brown N, von Theobald P. Mesh removal following transvaginal mesh placement: a case series of 104 operations. Int Urogynecol J. 2010;21:423–30.

38. Mucowski SJ, Jumalov C, Phelps JY. Use of vaginal mesh in the face of recent FDA warnings and litigation. Am J Obstet Gynecol. 2010;203:103.e1–4.

39. Barber MD, Brubaker L, Nygaard I, Wheeler II TL, Schaffer J, Chen Z, et al. Defining success after surgery for pelvic organ prolapse. Obstet Gynecol. 2009;114:600–9.

40. Nieminen K, Hiltunen R, Takal T, Heiskanen E, Merikari M, Niemi K, et al. Outcomes after anterior vaginal wall repair with mesh: a randomized, controlled trial with a 3 year follow-up. Am J Obstet Gynecol. 2010;203:235.e1–8.

41. Withagen MI, Milani AL, den Boon J, Vervest HA, Vierhout ME. Trocar-guided mesh compared with conventional vaginal repair in recurrent prolapse. A randomized controlled trial. Obstet Gynecol. 2011;117:242–50.

42. Dindo D, Demartines N, Clavien PA. Classification of surgical complications. Ann Surg. 2004;244:931–7.

Retropubic Bladder Neck Suspensions

10

Elizabeth R. Mueller

Introduction

Open abdominal retropubic procedures for urinary incontinence were widely performed in the United States starting in the 1950s till the turn of the century when the use of transvaginal synthetic slings gained in popularity [1]. That said, data regarding the success and complications of retropubic suspensions were mostly expert opinion, cases series, or underpowered randomized trials until the last decade when two large randomized trials comparing the Burch urethropexy to suburethral slings were published [2, 3]. This chapter will review the retropubic procedures for incontinence and the diagnosis and management of complications that arise from retropubic urethropexy procedures.

Overview of Retropubic Procedures for Incontinence

Retropubic urethropexy procedures generally include the Marshall Marchetti Krantz (MMK), the Burch colposuspension and the paravaginal defect repair. First described by Marshall in 1949,

E.R. Mueller, MD, MSME, FACS (✉)
Division of Female Pelvic Medicine and Reconstructive Surgery, Departments of Urology and Obstetrics/Gynecology, Loyola University Chicago Stritch School of Medicine, 2160 South First Avenue, Building 103, Suite 1004, Maywood, IL 60153, USA
e-mail: emuelle@lumc.edu

the MMK procedure [4] suspends sutures placed on each side of the bladder neck to the posterior aspect of the pubic bone. This is thought to stabilize the bladder neck and allow abdominal pressures that are being transmitted to the bladder to be equally transmitted to the proximal bladder neck, maintaining continence during stress activities.

The Burch urethropexy was described by John Burch in 1961 as being born out of necessity when the sutures he was trying to place during a MMK kept pulling out of the pubic bone periosteum [5]. After utilizing the arcus tendonious and Cooper's ligament as the point of fixation, he chose the latter based on its consistent presence and inherent strength.

First described by White in 1909 as a procedure for anterior vaginal prolapse repair, the paravaginal defect repair was based on White's cadaveric dissections that demonstrated that the "bladder stays in place because it rests upon a firm fibrous shelf stretched across between the pubic bones" [6]. The procedure was popularized for female stress incontinence when the authors reported that reattaching the detached and retracted levator ani fascia to the arcus tendineus resulted in a greater than 90% cure rate [7] but it does not have acceptable success rates to justify its use as a stress incontinence procedure at this time.

Surgical Techniques

All of the abdominal retropubic procedures require the patient to be prepped and draped in dorsal lithotomy so that the primary surgeon can have their nondominant hand in the vagina for definition of anatomy and counter-traction. A Foley catheter is passed into the urethra and kept in the sterile field. A Pfannenstiel or Cherney incision is made and the space of Retzius is entered. The surgeon slides their dominant surgical hand (fingers first and palm faced up) behind the pubic bone and with gentle downward traction the retropubic and lateral pelvic sidewalls are exposed.

The nondominant hand is placed into the vagina and gentle tugging on the Foley catheter identifies the bladder neck. A finger on each side of the balloon allows the apt surgeon to use the remaining fingers and thumb to tug on the catheter when needed. Typically, the surgeon starts on the contralateral side and the surgical assistant uses a sponge stick to provide countertraction by directing the midline away from the sidewall of interest. A swab mounted on a curved forceps is used to sweep the overlying periurethral vessels and fat towards the midline and at the same time the vaginal fingers are elevated towards the ceiling so that the white, glistening tissue of the vagina is exposed. The venous plexus that can be seen in the vaginal wall should be avoided as much as possible since these vessels can be the source of a significant amount of blood loss when sheared during dissection or suture placement.

The MMK cystourethropexy places 2–3 permanent sutures on each side of the bladder neck and mid-urethra. Each suture consists of two bites encompassing full thickness of the vaginal wall but not the vaginal epithelium. The nondominant fingers in the vagina provide the necessary tactile feedback. The vaginal fingers elevate the urethra to the back of the pubic symphysis and suture ends are placed into the pubic bone and periosteum. The assistant ties the sutures as the surgeon positions the urethrovesical junction. The intent is to elevate the vagina and not to constrict the urethra.

The Burch procedure has undergone modifications and most contemporary studies including the two randomized trials by Ward and Albo [2, 3] place 1–2 sutures of delayed absorbable or permanent suture 1–2 cm lateral

on each side of the urethrovesical junction. A second pair of sutures is placed 1 cm distal and lateral at the level of the mid-urethra. Each suture placement consists of two bites through the full thickness of the vaginal wall excluding the vaginal epithelium. The sutures are attached to the ipsilateral Cooper's ligament and tied to elevate the anterior vagina to a minimally retropubic position. A suture bridge of 2–3 cm is expected between the vaginal wall and Cooper's ligament. Again, the aim of the surgical procedure is to elevate the vaginal wall, not to constrict the bladder neck.

Numerous authors have described laparoscopic approaches to the Burch colposuspension [8–10]. While the dissection of the retroperitoneal space is similar, various materials have been used to attach the vaginal wall to Cooper's ligament including sutures, staples, spiral metal tacks, and mesh.

Surgical Success

In the fourth edition of the International Consultation on Incontinence published in 2009, Smith et al. reviewed all of the literature available on retropubic suspensions and the authors have concluded, based on level 1 evidence, that open retropubic Burch colposuspension can be recommended as an effective treatment for primary stress incontinence [11]. In contrast, the MMK cystourethropexy and the paravaginal defect repair are *not* recommended for the treatment of stress incontinence. The authors also state that laparoscopic Burch colposuspension is not recommended for routine treatment but may be considered in patients undergoing concurrent laparoscopic surgery for other reasons. In contrast, the American Urological Society 2009 Guidelines for Surgical Management of Stress Urinary Incontinence state that open retropubic and laparoscopic suspension along with injectables, mid-urethral slings and pubovaginal slings, although not equivalent, may be considered for the uncomplicated women with stress incontinence [12].

Complications

Burch Colposuspension

Two large randomized trials comparing the open Burch colposuspension to tension-free vaginal tape and to the fascial sling were published in 2002 and 2007, respectively [2, 3]. The studies randomized 475 women to Burch colposuspension thus providing a solid basis for understanding complications that arise when a large number of surgeons are performing the procedure. Ward et al. [13] enrolled women from 14 urogynecology and urology centers in the United Kingdom. Women were randomized to the open Burch colposuspension or the tension-free mid-urethral sling. Exclusion criteria included current need for, or previous history of, surgery for pelvic organ prolapse (POP). One hundred and forty six women underwent the Burch urethropexy. Women in the Ward-Hilton study had the following intra-operative and postoperative complications reported at 6 months: urinary tract infection (32%), de novo detrusor overactivity on urodynamics (11%), wound infection (7%), voiding disorder (7%), bladder injury (2%), deep vein thrombosis (2%), and incisional hernia (2%). There were no reports of vascular injury or retropubic hematoma in this series. The need for patient catheterization decreased over time, but remained substantial with 8% of women requiring catheterization after 6 months. Interestingly, there was no statistically significant difference in rates of catheterization and voiding dysfunction compared to TVT.

In 2004, the authors reported the 2-year follow-up data. Of the 146 women randomized to Burch urethropexy, 5 (3.4%) underwent surgery for stress incontinence, 7 (4.8%) surgery for POP, and 5 (3.4%) had an incisional hernia repair. At 2 years, 4 (2.7%) women continued to catheterize and 3 (2.1%) continued to have symptoms of UTI. On physical exam, the number of women with vault/cervical prolapse increased from 21% preoperatively to 63% at 24 months; 18% of the women with POP were symptomatic. Over the same 2-year time period, vault/cervical prolapse rates increased from 16 to 29% in the TVT arm. In summary, when compared to TVT, Burch colposuspension at 24 months resulted in higher rates of enterocele, voiding dysfunction, and need for catheterization and a 4% lower rate of UTI.

In the Stress Incontinence Surgical Efficacy Trial (SISTEr) involving nine surgical centers in the United States, women were randomized to an open Burch colposuspension or autologous rectus fascial sling. A total of 329 women received a Burch colposuspension; however, 48% of the women had concomitant procedures for POP. The following adverse events were reported in women who underwent the Burch colposuspension: cystitis (50%), new-onset urge incontinence (3%), incidental cystotomy (3%), surgical wound complications requiring surgery (2.4%), voiding dysfunction >6 weeks (2%), recurrent cystitis leading to diagnostic cystoscopy (1.5%), bleeding (1%), ureteral injury (1%), incidental vaginotomy (0.5%), ureteral vaginal fistula (0.5%), erosion of suture into the bladder (0.5%), and pyelonephritis (0.5%). In summary, compared to a rectus fascial sling, a Burch colposuspension resulted in lower rates of success for stress incontinence and lower rates of cystitis, urge incontinence, and voiding dysfunction. In this study, women often received a concomitant POP procedure.

Marshall-Marchetti-Kranz Procedure

Complications related to the MMK procedure are similar to those mentioned for the Burch colposuspension. In a 1988 review of the literature, Mainprize and Drutz summarized the occurrence of postoperative complications in 2,712 patients as follows: wound complications (5.5%), urinary tract infection (3.9%), osteitis pubis (2.5%), direct injury to the urinary tract (1.6%), ureteral injury (0.1%). Of course, this data is limited and, with the exception of osteitis pubis, direct comparisons to the Burch data obtained in a randomized trial would not be advised [14].

Approach to Specific Complications

Urinary Tract Infections

Women who undergo surgical treatment for stress incontinence will most often develop symptoms that are consistent with or mistaken for a urinary tract infection. The rates are highest in the first 6 months but do remain between 2 and 9% 24 months after surgery [3, 13]. As a result, it is sensible to require that women with a history of urinary tract infections be free of infection prior to undergoing surgery. Women with symptoms of urinary tract infection (urgency, frequency, burning with urination) would benefit by having urine cultures obtained prior to antibiotic treatment to allow for more specific antibiotic treatment but also to document when the symptoms occur with negative cultures. Nonbacterial etiologies include lower urinary tract inflammation, urethral irritation, and irritative voiding symptoms associated with urethral obstruction.

Possible etiologies or recurrent or persistent UTI included incomplete emptying, bacterial colonization from instrumentation, and a foreign body in the urinary tract (Fig. 10.1). Women who require catheterization (intermittent or indwelling) should be placed on "treatment" doses of antibiotics once they have stopped using catheters since bacterial colonization occurs often within days of catheter use. Data from the SISTEr trial demonstrate that cystitis rates are highest in the first 6 weeks after surgery [15]. When compared to self-voiders with a cystitis rate of 6%, women who have intermittent or indwelling catheters have higher (23% and 13%, respectively) rates of cystitis. In addition, women who undergo voiding trials with postvoid residual measurements are often catheterized 2–3 times prior to being discharged thus increasing their risk of colonizing the urinary tract.

When UTIs also present with systemic signs such as fever, chills, and flank pain, upper tract imaging is warranted. The specific imaging depends on the question that needs to be answered. For example, in women presenting with febrile UTI and flank pain following an isolated retropubic urethropexy the imaging question may be "does this patient have ureteral reflux or obstruction" and a voiding cystourethrogram and renal ultrasound can be ordered. For patients with concomitant prolapse repair, upper tract imaging to assess ureteral patency and cystoscopy to rule-out bladder foreign body or cystotomy would be indicated.

Urge Incontinence

In the Ward study, 91% of women reported symptoms of bothersome urge incontinence prior to Burch urethropexy which decreased postprocedure to 34% at 6 months and 2 years. On urodynamic testing, the number of women who developed unstable detrusor contractions increased from 1% pre-op to 10% 6-months following a Burch colposuspension. Similarly, persistent urge incontinence was found in 18% of women enrolled in the Burch arm of the SISTEr trial and new-onset urge incontinence remained low at 3%.

Possible etiologies of de novo urge incontinence include UTI, obstructive voiding, and the presence of a foreign body in the lower urinary tract. In women whose symptoms persist after 6 weeks and post-void residuals are normal, conservative treatment for urge incontinence can be considered including anticholinergics and behavior modifications. A woman who is not responsive or whose symptoms appear severe might benefit from a cystoscopic examination to rule-out the presence of a foreign body in the lower urinary tract. Women, who have undergone a laparoscopic Burch procedure and have evidence of a foreign body in the bladder, may have undergone the procedure using metal helical "tackers" to suspend the bladder neck (Fig. 10.2). These are often placed or migrate into the bladder causing symptoms. If operative notes are not available, then an anterior/posterior and lateral plain X-ray will allow visualization of the offending material.

Uterine or Vaginal Vault Prolapse

In his initial description of the surgical procedure, Burch reported the surgical complication of uterine or vaginal vault prolapse. As described previously, 18% of women developed symptomatic prolapse and 4.8% underwent surgical correction over the 24 months of the Ward–Hilton study [13]. This is believed to be due to the anterior orientation of the vaginal apex. As a result, all women undergoing surgical correction of stress incontinence should have a complete physical exam including the evaluation of vaginal topography ideally in the standing-straining position. Women, who demonstrate apical or uterine

Fig. 10.1 (**a**) Cystoscopic view of a stone at the bladder neck in a patient with pelvic pain and UTIs following a Burch procedure. (**b**) Prolene suture and stone following surgical removal (photographs courtesy of Howard Goldman, MD, Cleveland Clinic, OH)

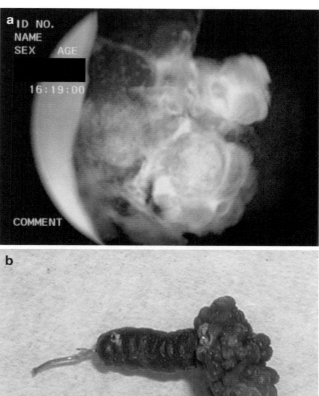

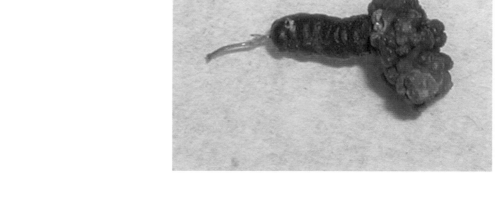

Fig. 10.2 Cystoscopic view of a metal tacker placed during a laparoscopic Burch colposuspension (photograph courtesy of Howard Goldman, MD, Cleveland Clinic, OH)

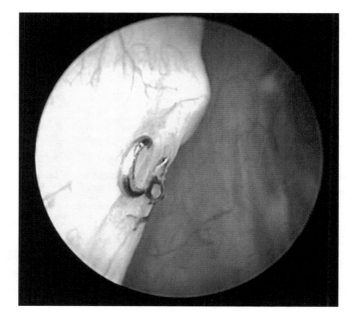

descent of greater than 3 cm from optimal position with Valsalva effort, would more likely benefit from a synthetic or autologous suburethral sling since they have not been shown to increase the risk of POP. When a patient is undergoing treatment of POP following an incontinence procedure, care should be taken to not "over-correct" the apical support since this may result in incontinence.

Voiding Dysfunction

Rates of voiding dysfunction following retropubic suspensions vary based on the definitions used, duration of the studies and whether women with preexisting voiding dysfunction were excluded from enrollment. The Ward–Hilton study [13] defined a woman as having voiding dysfunction when two of these three measurements were found on 6-month postoperative urodynamic studies (UDS): peak flow <15 mL/s, maximum voiding pressure >50 cm H_2O, and residual volume >100 mL. Of the women who underwent postoperative UDS, 7% were diagnosed with a voiding dysfunction. Thirty-three percent of women required catheterization (suprapubic, urethral, or intermittent) a week after surgery and this continued to diminish over time to 13% at 1 month, 8% at 6 months, and 2.7% at 24 months. There were no reports of surgical intervention for voiding dysfunction.

The SISTEr trial also had a gradual return to self-voiding in women undergoing the Burch procedure. While only 56% of women passed their first voiding trial the authors reported low rates (2%) of voiding dysfunction >6 weeks after surgery and no surgical revisions for voiding dysfunction in the 329 women who had undergone Burch procedure. As the series above demonstrate, most voiding dysfunction resolves by 6 weeks and can be treated conservatively with intermittent or indwelling catheterization. In addition, many patients may benefit by undergoing pelvic therapy specifically aimed at pelvic floor relaxation techniques [16].

When obstructive voiding symptoms persist, patients may benefit by filling cystometry and pressure-flow studies to determine if the etiology is obstructive or due to decreased detrusor function. In centers with fluoroscopy, imaging can be helpful. A cystoscopy at the same time would rule-out suture placement in the urethra (although this is a rare phenomena). The etiology is typically obstructive from sutures pulling the bladder neck; sutures placed distally resulting in urethral kinking or scarring of the bladder neck to the back of the pubic bone.

Women who clearly demonstrate obstruction on UDS should be considered for an urethrolysis. In women who have physical exam findings of an indentation of the anterior vaginal wall where sutures have been placed, we consider a transvaginal urethrolysis. A midline vaginal incision is made near mid-urethra and carried to the level of the bladder neck. The dissection continues using sharp and blunt dissection as if making the sling tunnels for a rectus fascial sling. Tissue that is adherent to pubic bone is swept lateral to medial using the surgeon's index finger. Since it is customary in our practice to use a permanent suture, we can palpate the suture as it travels from the proximal urethra and bladder neck to its attachment on the pubic bone (MMK) or Cooper's ligament (Burch). A scissors is then guided to the level of the sutures behind the pubic bone by the surgeon's index finger and the sutures are transected on each side.

In woman who are clearly obstructed and have failed a transvaginal urethrolysis or who do not have a palpable indentation at the level of the bladder neck, a retropubic urethrolysis can be performed. A Pfannenstiel incision is made and carried to the level of the fascia which is incised 2 cm proximal to the back of the pubic bone. As when placing the sutures, the surgeon's nondominant hand is placed into the vagina to assist in locating the sutures which are transected. If the anterior bladder remains fixed to the back of the pubic bone then this is carefully dissected until the bladder neck and urethra are sufficiently freed to restore a normal degree of mobility.

Anger et al. reported on a retrospective review of 16 women who had symptoms of overactive bladder and/or obstruction following a Burch urethropexy [17]. The study consisted of 7 women who had a vaginal approach and 9 who underwent the retropubic approach. The groups were

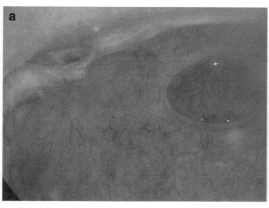

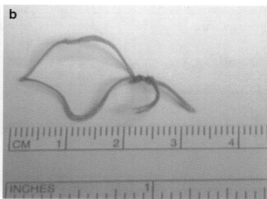

Fig. 10.3 (a) Cystoscopic view of suture in the right lateral wall of the bladder placed during open Burch colposuspension 3 years prior. Early postoperative course complicated by osteitis pubis requiring removal of the left sided suspension sutures. (b) Removal of the right bladder wall suture resulted in resolution of suprapubic pain at rest and ambulation (photographs courtesy of Howard Goldman, MD, Cleveland Clinic, OH)

not equivalent since 43% in the vaginal group and 55% of the women in the retropubic group performed self-catheterization. Success rates for a return to normal voiding were 66% with the vaginal approach and 100% with retropubic. The authors also reported that overactive symptoms were improved in the retropubic group compared to the transvaginal. They hypothesize that the inability to transect the most proximal sutures through the transvaginal route might result in the lower rates of symptom improvement. That said, most surgeons would agree that the transvaginal approach is less morbid and worth attempting as first-line treatment.

Intraoperative Hemorrhage

One of the most anticipated intraoperative complications during a retropubic urethropexy is intraoperative hemorrhage. There are numerous vessels that run alongside the bladder and within the vaginal wall. Vaginal wall vessels that are visible can usually be avoided when placing the sutures and if punctured will often stop bleeding once they are tied in place. When brisk bleeding does occur, direct pressure held for 5 min (by the clock) is often sufficient. Attempts to use metal clips often result in additional shearing of vaginal wall vessels. When packing is insufficient, agents such as gelfoam/thrombin or fibrin glue may be necessary. Of course, bleeding can be minimized by assuring that exposure to the retroperitoneal space is adequate and reviewing the simple steps of checking patient and surgeon positioning, light and retractor placement along with incision length.

Osteitis Pubis

Osteitis pubis is an inflammatory disease of the pubic symphysis and its surrounding attachments. It occurs in 1–2.5% of MMK procedures but can also occur in any procedure that is in the retropubic space (Fig. 10.3). Symptoms include pubic pain that may be localized to the pubis or radiate to the lower abdomen and thigh. Often patients adopt a limp and wide-based gait. The diagnosis can be aided by the use of MRI which can distinguish between osteitis pubis and pelvic osteomyelitis [18]. Medical management includes rest, ice, nonsteroidal anti-inflammatory drugs, physical therapy, and the use of steroids. Patients who are refractory to medical management may benefit by surgical removal of the offending sutures (Fig. 10.3).

Summary

With the advent of synthetic mid-urethral slings, the retropubic suspensions are often referred to as a procedure of historical interest. However as we continue to deal with the complications from surgical mesh placed in a transvaginal route, there remains a role for this procedure in the armamentarium of the well-versed pelvic surgeon.

References

1. Anger JT, Weinberg AE, Albo ME, et al. Trends in surgical management of stress urinary incontinence among female Medicare beneficiaries. Urol. 2009;74:283–7.
2. Ward KL, Hilton P, UK and Ireland TVT Trial Group. A prospective multicenter randomized trial of tension-free vaginal tape and colposuspension for primary urodynamic stress incontinence: two-year follow-up. Am J Obstet Gynecol. 2004;190:324–31.
3. Albo ME, Richter H, Brubaker L, et al. Burch colposuspension versus fascial sling to reduce urinary stress incontinence. N Engl J Med. 2007;356:2143–55.
4. Marshall VF, Marchetti AA, Krantz KE. The correction of stress incontinence by simple vesico-urethral suspension. Surg Gynecol Obstet. 1949;88:509.
5. Burch J. Urethrovaginal fixation to Cooper's ligament for correction of stress incontinence, cystocele and prolapse. Am J Obstet Gynecol. 1961;81:281–90.
6. White GR. A radical cure by suturing lateral sulci of vagina to the white line of the pelvic fascia. J Am Med Assoc. 1909;21:1707.
7. Richardson AC, Edmonds PB, Williams NL. Treatment of stress urinary incontinence due to paravaginal fascial defect. Obstet Gynecol. 1981;57:357–62.
8. Wallwiener D, Grischke E, Rimbach S, et al. Endoscopic retropubic colposuspension: "Retziusscopy" versus laparoscopy—a reasonable enlargement of the operative spectrum in the management of recurrent stress incontinence? Endosc Surg Allied Technol. 1995;3:115–8.
9. Ross J. Two techniques of laparoscopic Burch repair for stress incontinence: a prospective, randomized study. J Am Assoc Gynecol Laparosc. 1996;3:351–7.
10. Zullo F, Palomba S, Piccione F, et al. Laparoscopic Burch colposuspension: a randomized controlled trial comparing two transperitoneal surgical techniques. Obstet Gynecol. 2001;98:783–8.
11. Smith ARB, Dmochowski R, Hilton P, et al. Surgery for urinary incontinence in women. In: Abrams P, Cardoza L, Khoury S, et al. 4th ed. Plymouth: Health Publication; 2009.
12. Appell R, Dmochowski RR, Blaivas J, et al. American Urological Association Guidelines for the surgical management of stress incontinence: 2009 update. Plymouth: American Urological Association, Education and Research Inc.; 2009.
13. Ward K, Hilton P, United K, et al. Prospective multicentre randomised trial of tension-free vaginal tape and colposuspension as primary treatment for stress incontinence. BMJ. 2002;325:67.
14. Mainprize TC, Drutz HP. The Marshall-Marchetti-Krantz procedure—a critical review. Obstet Gynecol Surv. 1989;43:724–9.
15. Chai T, Albo M, Richter H, et al. Complications in women undergoing Burch colposuspension versus autologous rectus fascial sling for stress urinary incontinence. J Urol. 2009;181:2192–7.
16. Smith PP, Appell RA. Functional obstructed voiding in the neurologically normal patient. Curr Urol Rep. 2006;7:346–53.
17. Anger JT, Amundsen CL, Webster GD. Obstruction after Burch colposuspension: a return to retropubic urethrolysis. Int Urogynecol J Pelvic Floor Dysfunct. 2006;17:455–9.
18. Knoeller SM, Uhl M, Herget GW. Osteitis or osteomyelitis of the pubis? Acta Orthop Belg. 2006;72:541.

Complications of Biologic and Synthetic Slings and Their Management

11

Laura Chang-Kit, Melissa Kaufman, and Roger R. Dmochowski

Introduction

Female stress urinary incontinence (SUI) is estimated to affect 49% of community dwelling women [1], although true prevalence is unknown. Patient underreporting due to social embarrassment or fear as well as differences in the definition of SUI between studies contribute to the probable substantial underestimation of SUI patients [2, 3]. The financial impact of SUI is exceptional with one report estimating the healthcare burden of SUI at over US $16 billion dollars per year [4].

Slings are currently the most popular procedure for the surgical correction of female SUI. Sling surgery involves placement of graft material at the level of the bladder neck and proximal third of urethra (pubovaginal sling [PVS]) or midurethra (midurethral sling [MUS]). Numerous techniques and graft materials (autologous fascia, allograft, xenograft, and synthetic) have been developed over several decades for sling placement.

This chapter will focus on the diagnosis, evaluation, and management of complications specific to sling placement. Nonurologic perioperative consid-erations and complications (for example anticoagulation and risks of anesthesia) are discussed elsewhere in this book and will not be addressed in this chapter.

Use of Slings for Stress Urinary Incontinence

According to Medicare data, by 2001, PVS was the leading anti-incontinence procedure for SUI performed in the USA, surpassing more traditional retropubic needle suspensions and anterior urethropexies [5]. In the last decade however, *midurethral polypropylene slings have emerged as the most commonly performed sling procedure across the USA and Europe.* MUS sling use has expanded secondary to the short operative time, minimal morbidity, rapid convalescence, technical ease, and reproducibility of the procedures, as well as their long-term efficacy and durability [6].

Undoubtedly, *the most commonly used and evaluated material for PVS is autologous fascia, which has shown excellent efficacy and longevity* [7]. Cadaveric fascia has been used with more limited efficacy and durability and thus its use has dramatically declined [8]. Xenografts such as porcine dermis, porcine small intestinal submucosa, and bovine pericardium have also been used, with the most studied xenograft being porcine dermis. Synthetic bladder neck slings have fallen out of favor due to the tendency to extrude through the vagina or perforate into the lower urinary tract [9]. Therefore, this chapter will focus

L. Chang-Kit, MD (✉) • M. Kaufman, MD
R.R. Dmochowski, MD, FACS
Department of Urological Surgery, Vanderbilt University School of Medicine, A1302 Medical Center North, Nashville, TN 37232, USA
e-mail: laurachangkit@yahoo.com

on the autologous fascia PVS procedure and its complications as representative of the generalized experience with biologic slings.

MUS can be placed through a transvaginal, suprapubic, or transobturator approach. In general, these slings are composed of type I synthetic polypropylene monofilamentous mesh, with a pore size between 75 and 150 μm. This pore size is critical to allow fibrous tissue in-growth as well as leukocyte and macrophage entry in order to reduce bacterial colonization. Single-incision slings (aka "mini-slings") are the newest generation of MUS, which require only one vaginal incision without any entry or exit incisions. Unlike their predecessors, the mini-slings are meant to be entirely placed and stay within the pelvis, without any incorporation of the anterior abdominal wall or inner thigh musculature. As the data on these mini-slings is still limited, these will not be discussed in this chapter.

Mechanism of Action

The understanding of how slings correct SUI continues to evolve. In general, the aim of any SUI surgery is to augment the urethral closure pressures to prevent involuntary urinary leakage when there are increases in abdominal pressures [10]. PVSs are placed without any added tension and are thought to work by a combination of mechanisms: (1) to create a suburethral supporting hammock at the bladder neck and proximal urethra, which acts as a backboard against which the urethra is compressed during periods of increased intra-abdominal pressures (imitating the "hammock theory of continence") and (2) to stabilize the bladder neck and proximal urethra in an "intra-abdominal" position (reducing hypermobility) such that pressure transmission is maximized [11]. In addition, autologous fascia PVS can be purposely tensioned to compress and/or obstruct the urethra in cases of severe intrinsic sphincter deficiency (ISD) such as in decentralizing neuropathic conditions.

MUSs are also placed in a "tension-free" fashion and are thought to stabilize the midurethral complex, where the urethral closure pressure is maximal [12]. If the posterior wall of the urethra is not well supported, "shear forces" during periods of intra-abdominal pressure can cause the anterior wall of the urethra (attached to the pubic bone by pubourethral ligaments and endopelvic fascia) to move independently of the posterior wall, allowing urine leakage [13]. Another mechanism proposes that the MUS obstructs the downward movement of the urethra, in effect, kinking the urethra during stress maneuvers [14].

Indications and Contraindications

A 2006 prospective study by Petri et al. examined the reasons for 328 complications requiring surgical reintervention after tension-free slings in four European urogynecology centers [15]. Incorrect indication for the initial procedure was determined to be the second most common cause of complications (38%), after poor surgical technique (45%). It is therefore important to review the indications and contraindications for sling placement.

The PVS is considered the gold standard for management of all forms of SUI and is effective in patients with and without hypermobility [16]. It is favored in patients with loss of proximal urethral closure from neuropathic conditions, prior surgery or radiation, and in those with recurrent incontinence after prior failed anti-incontinence surgery [17]. It is also useful in cases of tissue loss such as in urethrovaginal fistulas or after urethral diverticulectomy. The MUS has replaced the PVS as the primary procedure for uncomplicated female SUI. The MUS has also been used effectively in recurrent SUI as well as with concomitant cystocele [7].

Patients with untreated low compliance bladders or urge urinary incontinence without stress incontinence are unsuitable candidates for ANY sling procedure. Interestingly, patients with mixed incontinence who demonstrate both detrusor overactivity and SUI on urodynamic studies often have resolution of their overactive bladder symptoms with satisfactory resolution of their SUI [18, 19].

According to the 2009 American Urological Association (AUA) Female Stress Urinary

Incontinence Guideline Update Panel, *synthetic sling surgery for SUI is contraindicated with a concurrent urethrovaginal fistula, urethral erosion, intraoperative urethral injury, and/or urethral diverticulum.* These patients are considered higher risk for subsequent urethral erosion, vaginal extrusion, urethrovaginal fistula, and foreign body granuloma formation. Autologous fascia and alternative biologic slings are preferred in these patients for the treatment of concomitant SUI [20].

Patient comorbidities must also be considered when choosing the type of sling to employ. In patients at high risk for abdominal wound complications (e.g., morbidly obese, history of steroid use, previous abdominal wall reconstruction), it is our practice to avoid harvesting rectus fascia for PVS in favor of either fascia lata, or porcine dermis. We also tend towards biologic rather than synthetic slings in patients with estrogen deficiency, previous surgery, or history of pelvic radiation, as well as in very young patients (<30 years old), because of the suspected increased risk of late complications such as erosion into the lower urinary tract. For young women who desire future vaginal deliveries, sling placement in general is a controversial topic and it is our practice to certainly avoid placement of synthetic slings in this population.

Incidence of Sling Complications

One estimate of the overall complication rate of patients undergoing SUI surgery from 1988 to 2000 using a US national database was 13%, with PVS having the lowest complication rate [21]. The overall incidence of complications is difficult to determine and current reported statistics likely underestimate the true incidence. Discrepancies in the accepted definition of "complication" as well as lack of long-term follow-up make tracking complications virtually impossible, compounded by the *highly variable reporting of complications* [15]. In addition, there are no requirements for mandatory reporting of complications in the US, and there exists *no mandatory central database for any procedure.* Surgical

complications related to medical devices can be voluntarily reported to the US Food and Drug Administration (FDA) Manufacturer and User Facility Device Experience (MAUDE) database; however this is unquestionably underutilized for a myriad of reasons.

In October 2008, the FDA issued a public notification about surgical mesh used in transvaginal SUI and pelvic organ prolapse (POP) surgeries [22]. This was prompted by a 3-year collection of over 1,000 reports of complications related to surgical mesh, with the most frequent being erosion through vaginal epithelium, infection, pain, urinary problems, and recurrence of prolapse and/or incontinence. Perforations into bowel, bladder, and blood vessels during insertion were also reported. In the three years following the 2008 public health notification, another 2,874 mesh-related reports were collected. Based on these findings and after review of the current literature, the FDA issued a safety communication about transvaginal mesh placement for POP in July 2011. Although 1,371 of these reports were associated with SUI repairs, the FDA Obstetrics and Gynecology Devices Panel comprehensively reviewed the use of surgical mesh for SUI procedures in September 2011. The Panel determined that first generation retropubic and transobturator MUSs were safe and effective but that second generation single-incision slings required further clinical studies as current evidence is limited. For now, the FDA continues to evaluate the safety and effectiveness of surgical mesh devices used in any pelvic floor surgery.

Classification of Complications

The first standardized classification and terminology system for complications arising from the insertion of synthetic and biological materials in female pelvic floor surgery was recently reported by the International Continence Society (ICS)/International Urogynecological Association (IUGA) (Table 11.1 and Fig. 11.1) [23]. Each complication is classified according to three aspects: category, time, and site. The aim of the classification is to improve communication amongst providers

Table 11.1 Recommended terminology in the joint International Continence Society/International Urogynecological Association classification of complications related to insertion of surgical prostheses and grafts in female pelvic floor surgery (adapted from ref. [23])

Terms used	Definition
Prosthesis	A fabricated substitute to assist a damaged body part or to augment or stabilize a hypoplastic structure
A: Mesh	A (prosthetic) network fabric or structure
B: Implant	A surgically inserted or embedded prosthesis
C: Tape (sling)	A flat strip of synthetic material
Graft	Any tissue or organ for transplantation. This term will refer to biological materials inserted
A. Autologous grafts	From the woman's own tissues, e.g., dura matter, rectus sheath, or fascia lata
B. Allografts	From postmortem tissue banks
C. Xenografts	From other species, e.g., modified porcine dermis, porcine small intestine, bovine pericardium
Complication	A morbid process or event that occurs during the course of a surgery that is not an essential part of that surgery
Contraction	Shrinkage or reduction in size
Prominence	Parts that protrude beyond the surface (e.g., due to wrinkling or folding with no epithelial separation)
Separation	Physically disconnected (e.g., vaginal epithelium)
Exposure	A condition of displaying, revealing, exhibiting or making accessible, e.g., vaginal mesh visualized through separated vaginal epithelium
Extrusion	Passage gradually out of a body structure or tissue
Compromise	Bring into danger
Perforation	Abnormal opening into a hollow organ or viscus
Dehiscence	A bursting open or gaping along natural or sutured line

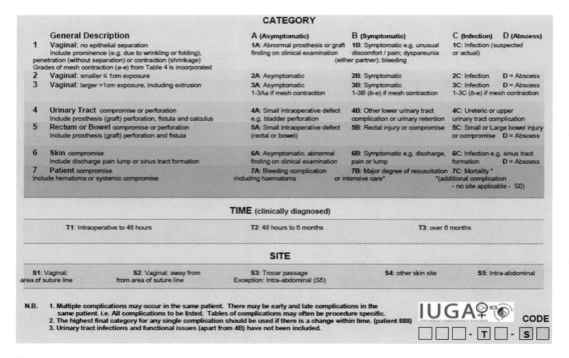

Fig. 11.1 A classification of complications related directly to the insertion of prostheses (meshes, implants, and tapes) or grafts in female pelvic floor surgery (figure adapted from ref. [23])

and allow standardization of research registries. Suggested changes to current terminology include avoidance of the term "erosion," in favor of the terms "extrusion" or "perforation" when referring to mesh exposures in the vagina or lower urinary tract. Interobserver and intraobserver reliability of the classification is yet to be tested, and widespread adoption is not yet accomplished. As all currently published references use the older nomenclature, this chapter will reflect this to avoid any potential discord in data.

Intraoperative Complications

Autologous Fascia Harvest Site

Autologous fascia is harvested from either the rectus fascia (through a Pfannenstiel incision) or fascia lata. The Pfannenstiel incision has a low incisional hernia rate of 0–2% [24]; however, incisions extending lateral to the edge of the rectus sheath may predispose to hernias and nerve entrapment [25]. It is important to adequately mobilize the abdominal fascia from the underlying rectus and overlying subcutaneous tissue in order to perform a tension-free fascial closure. If a tension-free closure is not possible, our patients have been successfully primarily closed using biological grafts or synthetic mesh with the assistance of general surgery. In obese patients, or patients with expected severe abdominal fascial scarring, fascia lata harvest can be a good option, with minimal morbidity [26, 27]. Pain on walking, limping, and wound pain can occur, but these symptoms usually last less than 1 week [27, 28]. Use of a fascial stripper can reduce morbidity [29]. To avoid seroma development, placement of a subcutaneous drain should be considered if a large suprafascial space was created during mobilization of the fascia. If employed, we usually remove this drain the morning following surgery. In order to reduce the risk of wound complications (as well as sling failure), patients are instructed to avoid lifting objects more than 5 lb in weight for 6 weeks and to avoid smoking. They should also aim to control conditions which increase intra-abdominal pressure (e.g., asthma or chronic allergies).

Hemorrhage

Significant bleeding during procedures for SUI is infrequent and transfusion rates range from 1 to 4% [20]. Major vascular injuries to iliac, femoral, obturator, and epigastric vessels during sling surgery have been reported in the literature and the FDA MAUDE database [30, 31]. Pelvic vessels coursing through the retropubic space, along the pelvic sidewall, and within the vascular pedicle of the bladder can also be injured during dissection or passage of trocars. Solid knowledge of the relative pelvic anatomy and adherence to good surgical technique are paramount in avoiding perioperative hemorrhage.

Preoperative correction of any bleeding diatheses is important prior to any pelvic surgery. The American College of Chest Physicians Patients publishes evidence-based guidelines on the perioperative management of patients who are chronically anticoagulated [32]. Perioperative consultation with the medical service regularly managing the anticoagulation can help balance the risk of hemorrhage with the risk of a thrombotic event.

During vaginal dissection, the source of bleeding can be difficult to identify and control due to lack of direct visualization. During dissection of the vaginal flap from the underlying pubocervical fascia, it is uncommon to encounter significant bleeding if the dissection planes are correct. Initial hydrodissection of the vaginal flap with either injectable saline or lidocaine with epinephrine generally helps to better elucidate this plane. This dissection is more difficult in patients with prior vaginal surgery or radiation who may have severe scarring and thinning of their vaginal wall. Bleeding at this stage signifies an excessively deep incision through the pubocervical fascia into the detrusor or urethra. If this occurs, the dissection should continue in the proper surgical plane and small areas of bleeding can be gently controlled with bipolar cautery.

Blind entry into the retropubic space through the endopelvic fascia either transvaginally with scissors or suprapubically with needles or trocars can lead to considerable bleeding. Perforating scissors should be directed towards the ipsilateral shoulder, with the tips curved away from the bladder. As with curved trocars, if directed too laterally, vessels located on the lateral side of the pelvis can be injured [33]. It is not unusual for some venous bleeding to occur on initial perforation of the endopelvic fascia, and this generally settles spontaneously. Significant retropubic bleeding can usually be quelled by quickly placing the sling and closing the vaginal mucosa. Further tamponade is gained with vaginal packing. Very rarely is the exact source of bleeding identified transvaginally due to poor exposure and visualization; however, this is usually unnecessary to control bleeding. In addition to vaginal compression, placement of a urethral foley catheter with an overinflated balloon on traction at the bladder neck has been described to help tamponade bleeding [34].

Bleeding that is unresponsive to these maneuvers implies major vessel injury and warrants open exploration of the retropubic space or embolization. Initial management includes communicating with anesthesia about the situation, ensuring adequate availability of blood products, and excellent exposure and lighting. Possible intraoperative consultation with a vascular surgeon should be considered. Pelvic bleeding is especially problematic to control because of the confined working space, depth of field, potential for rapid, massive bleeding, and close proximity and high anatomic variation of important structures. Abdominal access to the retropubic space is obtained via a low midline incision, while maintaining vaginal pressure using vaginal packing and manual compression of the anterior vaginal wall up against the pubic symphysis. The retropubic hematoma may be significant, and after initial evacuation of the hematoma, pelvic packing and compression may be required to allow subsequent localization of the bleeding. Vascular control can be accomplished by repairing larger vessels with 4-0 or 5-0 permanent sutures such as Prolene, whereas en bloc ligation is performed with absorbable 3-0 Vicryl sutures.

Hemostatic agents such as gelfoam or surgical can be applied over slowly oozing areas if no definite bleeding vessels are identified. If bleeding still cannot be controlled, the pelvis can be packed and the patient brought back for a second laparotomy 48 h later, after resuscitation.

Arterial embolization in pelvic fractures is effective in controlling retroperitoneal hemorrhage with an efficacy rate of 81–100% and low complication rate [35, 36]. It has also been successfully used in controlling venous bleeding after pelvic surgery following failed open attempts where bleeding could not be localized [37]. This option is particularly valuable if the patient is anticipated to have extensive abdominal or pelvic scarring from previous surgeries or radiation. The patient should be adequately stabilized for transfer to the interventional radiology suite prior to leaving the operating room.

Urinary Tract Injury

During any procedure for SUI, the urinary tract is at high risk for direct injury. Several studies estimate the rate of urinary tract injury during retropubic MUS procedures on patients without a prior history of surgical treatment to be about 7% [38–40]. However, in patients with a prior pelvic surgical history, urinary tract injury rates can remarkably approach 37–70% [38, 39]. Although urinary tract injury with transobturator MUS is reported to be <0.5% [41], suspicion must remain high. Immediate intraoperative detection and management of these injuries can mitigate a myriad of possible debilitating complications such as vesicovaginal fistula or urethral erosion.

Detection of Urinary Tract Injury

Performance of *intraoperative cystourethroscopy in all patients undergoing sling surgery in order to detect intraoperative urinary tract injuries is considered standard of practice according to the 2009 AUA guidelines* [20]. A rigid or flexible cystoscope should be used to inspect the bladder and urethra prior to the conclusion of the procedure. Optimal visualization of the female urethra is accomplished by using a short beak rigid cystoscope or flexible fiberoptic cystoscope. If a rigid

Fig. 11.2 Cystoscopic view of Stamey needle perforating anterior bladder wall during autologous fascia pubovaginal sling procedure

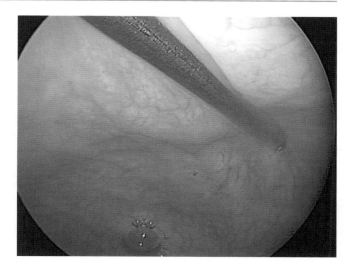

cystoscope is used, a 70° lens provides the best surveillance of the bladder, bladder neck, and ureteral orifices. The bladder must be examined while full, with special attention being paid to the bladder base between the 2 and 10 o'clock positions, where most injuries occur.

Ureteral patency can be assessed by visualizing efflux of previously administered IV indigo carmine or methylene blue from the ureteral orifices. An obvious yet occasionally overlooked confounder at this stage is the history of a unilaterally absent or poorly functioning renal unit. If ureteral patency is in question, a retrograde pyelogram can be conducted.

Bladder and Urethral Injury

Injury to the bladder and urethra typically occurs during vaginal dissection or during trocar passage (Fig. 11.2). Careful adherence to the planes of dissection cannot be overemphasized, especially in patients with vaginal scarring from previous surgery. Perforation of the endopelvic fascia should be carried out only after the bladder has been fully drained, with a urethral foley catheter or metal sound directing the urethra away from the perforating scissors, and with the tips of the scissors directed towards the ipsilateral shoulder, curving away from the bladder. In general, perforating instruments should be kept in close proximity to the respective bony landmarks in order to avoid entry into the bladder or abdominal cavity.

Bladder or urethral injury during vaginal dissection or perforation of the endopelvic fascia with scissors can be repaired with a watertight closure using two layers of absorbable suture, followed by catheter drainage for 5–7 days. This injury does not necessarily preclude placement of the autologous fascial sling at the same sitting, depending on patient comorbidities such as prior radiation and size of injury. In these cases, postponement of the PVS and/or possible tissue interposition graft such as a Martius flap can be considered. Placement of a synthetic MUS at the time of an intraoperative urethral injury is contraindicated, due to the higher risk of urethral erosion [20].

A 2009 Cochrane review of MUS examined 18 trials which compared the retropubic vs. transobturator approaches. There was a significantly higher rate of bladder perforation in the retropubic approaches 5.5% vs. 0.3% in the transobturator approaches (relative risk 0.14, 95% confidence interval 0.07–0.26) [30]. Several studies have also identified surgical inexperience as an independent risk factor for bladder perforation during MUS surgery [42, 43]. If the bladder is perforated during needle placement either during a MUS or PVS procedure, the needle is removed and repassed in the correct trajectory. These injuries do not require primary closure, but catheter drainage for 48–72 h is well advised to allow adequate healing.

Ureteral Injury

Ureteral injury during transvaginal SUI procedures are rare and are usually reported in conjunction with concomitant prolapse repairs. During transvaginal operations, the distal third of the ureter is at highest risk. If ureteral injury is suspected after cystoscopy, intraoperative retrograde pyelogram should be conducted to better assess ureteral integrity. Delayed ureteral injuries can present with flank pain, fever, and wound leakage. Appropriate imaging includes CT urography or retrograde pyelogram. The advantage to retrograde pyelography is that ureteral stenting, if necessary, can be conducted at the same time. Occasionally, the presence of a retroperitoneal urinoma will require percutaneous drainage.

If the ureter is obstructed or kinked, removal of the offending device (suture or needle) should follow and an indwelling ureteral double J stent placed. Partial transection or perforation of the ureter can also be managed with a temporary indwelling stent. Complete transection of the ureter requires formal ureteroneocystotomy.

Bowel Injury

Bowel injury during urinary incontinence procedures has been reported [40, 44] and usually occurs in patients with previous abdominal surgery [45–47]. Bowel injury can occur during entry into the retropubic space during PVS or during trocar passage during MUS. The highest reported risk of bowel complications (1%) is actually with retropubic MUS procedures [20]. Even without history of prior abdominal surgery, awake patients undergoing retropubic MUS procedures can be at risk of bowel perforation if a Valsalva maneuver is undertaken during trocar passage [48]. Placement of the patient in Trendelenberg position prior to trocar passage may reflect the bowel contents cranially and help prevent direct injury. In patients with suspected dense intraabdominal scarring, preoperative assessment with imaging may assist with operative planning. Sling options which do not involve the retropubic space should strongly be considered.

Injuries diagnosed intraoperatively can be closed primarily if there is no significant contamination of the peritoneal cavity, without the need for bowel diversion. Delayed diagnosis is not uncommon however, and complications such as abscess, sepsis, and even death can result [49]. Interestingly, initial symptoms and signs can be nonspecific, consisting of mild leukocytosis, low-grade fever, general malaise, ileus, and abdominal pain [48]. This can progress to emesis, severe suprapubic or abdominal pain and leakage of bile, or fecal material from wound sites. Early CT imaging and general surgery consultation is recommended. Almost all of these patients will require laparotomy, repair of the bowel injury, and possible bowel resection and/or bowel diversion.

Postoperative Complications

Voiding Dysfunction

The true incidence of voiding dysfunction and iatrogenic bladder outlet obstruction (BOO) after sling surgery is unknown owing to underdiagnosis, misdiagnosis, lack of standard definitions, and underreporting. A literature review from 1966 to 2001 by Dunn et al. reported rates of voiding dysfunction of 4–10% following PVS, and 2–4% following transvaginal tape (TVT) procedures [50]. A recent Cochrane review involving 14 trials of MUS showed postoperative voiding dysfunction occurred significantly less frequently with the transobturator route than with the retropubic route (4% vs. 7%) [30]. In most patients, postoperative voiding dysfunction is transient and resolves with conservative treatments such as catheter drainage or short-term pharmacological therapy. Surgery may be required for patients with severe or prolonged voiding dysfunction refractory to these conservative treatments.

Evaluation of Voiding Dysfunction

Patients with persistent voiding dysfunction after sling surgery must be evaluated with a focused history, physical examination, urinalysis and culture, and cystoscopy. A postvoid residual volume should be documented. We also utilize the AUA

Symptom Index in order to compare preoperative and postoperative symptoms and bother. Important factors in the history include preoperative and postoperative storage and voiding symptoms, the temporal relationship of the surgery to the symptoms, and type of sling surgery. Preoperative urodynamic data or flow studies become particularly useful when evaluating postoperative voiding complaints. Physical examination should evaluate for signs of a hyperelevated, fixed bladder neck or urethra, urethral hypermobility, stress incontinence, new or worsened pelvic organ prolapse, and vaginal erosion of mesh. Urine studies are critical to rule out urinary tract infection (UTI). Cystoscopy is essential to evaluate for stones, eroded sling, or suture material and other urinary tract injury or pathology including a hypersuspended bladder neck or midurethra, fibrosis, diverticula, or fistula.

Urodynamic evaluation provides useful information about sensation, bladder capacity, compliance, stress incontinence, detrusor overactivity, and coordination of sphincter activity. However, the role of urodynamic studies to evaluate for female BOO is controversial. The diagnosis of female BOO is problematic for a number of reasons. First, there is no accepted "gold standard" nomogram for female BOO, although several nomograms exist. Secondly, some female patients void primarily by pelvic floor relaxation, with barely any rise in their intravesical pressures and with possible Valsalva maneuvers. These patients can be obstructed by a very slight increase in urethral closure pressures. These women may not generate a significant contraction on urodynamic studies, but are still obstructed. Thirdly, although the classic urodynamic "high pressure-low flow" pattern indicative of BOO in men confirms the diagnosis of BOO in women, if present, its absence does not rule out obstruction. To date, there are no consistent preoperative parameters or urodynamic findings which predict success or failure of urethrolysis for BOO [51]. Indeed, patients who have failed to generate a detrusor contraction and those with nondiagnostic urodynamic studies have had the same outcome after urethrolysis as those patients who demonstrated the classic "high pressure-low flow" pattern [52].

How then should the diagnosis of female BOO after sling surgery be made? The diagnosis is obvious in patients with absolute prolonged urinary retention, or who produce the classic urodynamic pattern of obstruction. However, without these, in patients who had normal preoperative voiding function, a culmination of the history, physical exam, temporal relationship of the surgery to the symptoms, and supporting cystoscopic findings should raise the suspicion of BOO.

Urinary Retention and Obstruction

Presentation

Iatrogenic obstruction secondary to sling surgery is the most common cause of female BOO [53], which presents with storage symptoms such as frequency, urgency, and urge incontinence along with obstructive voiding symptoms and elevated PVR. Interestingly, in a study of 51 women undergoing urethrolysis, 75% presented with storage (irritative) symptoms, 61% with voiding (obstructive) symptoms, 55% with de novo urge incontinence, and 24% with persistent retention [54]. Therefore, patients complaining of de novo postoperative storage symptoms, even in the absence of voiding symptoms, should be evaluated for possible obstruction.

Transient Retention

Temporary urethral obstruction can be caused by postoperative edema of the bladder neck or urethra. Retention after nonradical pelvic surgery may also be attributed to a lack of urethral relaxation due to increased sympathetic response to pain, local irritation, anxiety, and trauma [55]. Other possible causes for postoperative retention include use of narcotic or anticholinergic medications, constipation, immobility, and retropubic hematomas. A successful strategy which settles most cases of postoperative retention is to address all the reversible risk factors, while instituting short-term (typically a few days) urethral catheter drainage or clean intermittent catheterization (CIC). Patients should be counseled preoperatively about the potential need for catheterization postoperatively. In complex cases of urethral reconstruction where a PVS is employed, placement of both a urethral and suprapubic catheter may be useful.

Prolonged Retention and Obstruction

The incidence of postoperative retention lasting more than a month or requiring intervention has been reported in 8% of patients following PVS surgery without concomitant prolapse repair, and 3% of women after synthetic MUS placement [20]. Several studies have sought to identify definite risk factors for postoperative obstruction; however, conclusions from these studies are limited by small sample size. Women who void with no or minimal detrusor pressure and who undergo PVS or MUS may be at increased risk of postoperative retention [56, 57], although other studies have not found this same association [58].

Once the diagnosis of obstruction is established or suspected, surgical options for management of prolonged obstruction include incision of the sling, transvaginal urethrolysis, retropubic urethrolysis, suprameatal transvaginal urethrolysis, and interposition grafts. Urethral dilation and attempts to loosen an obstructing PVS with traction on the dilator in the very early postoperative period can be successful. However, multiple attempts are not advised due to the potential for urethral scarring. Urethral dilation after TVT has been successfully used [59]. We do not advocate use of dilation techniques for synthetic mesh MUS because of the risk of urethral erosion.

Timing of Surgical Intervention

The timing of surgical intervention is debated in the literature and is dependent on the type of procedure, symptom severity, patient bother, and expectation of outcome. Historically, expectant management with catheter drainage for up to 3 months has been used in patients with obstructive voiding symptoms after PVS as 98% resolved without surgical intervention [19]. This is thought to allow sufficient retropubic scarification and fibrosis, which may explain low rates of recurrent SUI after urethrolysis. Longstanding BOO may cause irreversible bladder dysfunction, however, even after successful urethrolysis [60]. Earlier lysis of PVS and MUS

$(6 \pm 3.2$ months vs. 33 ± 20.1 months) has been recently shown to be a predictor of overall improvement with no difference in SUI [61]. In our experience, significant incomplete emptying and urinary retention after 4–6 weeks usually requires operative intervention.

Midurethral Sling Incision

This 3-month waiting period is generally not applied to MUSs. After these slings, 66–100% of temporary voiding dysfunction resolves by 6 weeks [59, 62], and most patients will empty fairly normally after 72 h. If the transvaginal incision of the MUS is conducted within 7–10 days, there is little tissue in-growth into the sling, and the procedure can be done with minimal manipulation. Although this can be done in the office setting under local anesthetic, we prefer the more controlled setting of the operating room where vaginal exposure can be maximized. The vaginal wall is infiltrated with local anesthetic and the suture used to close the vaginal wall is opened. The sling can usually be easily visualized. A right-angle clamp is then placed behind the sling and the sling is loosened by either downward traction or spreading of the right-angle clamp. Caution must be taken to avoid urethral injury when passing the clamp between the urethra and an overtensioned sling. If the sling is already incorporated into the tissue or has been in place for more than 2 weeks, it may be cut in the midline. We prefer to excise the cut ends of the sling as well as remove any suburethral portion to prevent any potential protrusion through the vaginal wall closure rather than leaving them in situ.

Pubovaginal Sling Incision

A more formal transvaginal sling incision is required for PVS. Sling incision has comparable success rates (84–100%) without the longer operative time and potential morbidity of a formal urethrolysis [52, 58, 63, 64]. We begin with cystourethroscopy of the urethra, bladder, and bladder neck. A 30° lens scope with a short beak allows examination of the urethra for signs of sling erosion or hypersuspension. The inverted-U vaginal flap is first hydrodissected and then dissected off the pubocervical fascia to the level of the bladder neck. A metal urethral sound or

Table 11.2 Results of urethrolysis

References	No. of patients	Type of urethrolysis	Time to urethrolysis (months)	Overall success (%)	Rate of stress urinary incontinence (%)
Foster and McGuire [74]	48	Transvaginal	26	65	0
Nitti and Raz [52]	42	Transvaginal	54	71	0
Cross et al. [75]	39	Transvaginal	11	72	3
Goldman et al. [76]	32	Transvaginal	14	84	19
Webster and Kreder [66]	15	Retropubic	8	93	13
Scarpero et al. [62]	24	Retropubic	9	92	18
Petrou et al. [65]	32	Suprameatal	Not reported	67	3
Carr and Webster [54]	54	Mixed	15	78	14

cystoscope can be placed in the urethra to better expose the proximal urethra and area of the sling. The sling is then dissected off the underlying pubocervical fascia such that a right-angle clamp can be placed behind the sling. An Allis clamp placed on the sling and pulled downward can facilitate dissection. If there is too much scarring in the midline to isolate the sling, this can be done laterally. The sling is lifted off the pubocervical fascia and incised. We always perform cystoscopy after any sling manipulation to ensure no urinary tract injury and to assess for residual anatomic obstruction.

In patients who fail transvaginal sling incision, urethrolysis can be performed either by a transvaginal or retropubic approach, with success rates ranging from 65 to 84%. Generally, we use transvaginal urethrolysis as a primary procedure, and retropubic urethrolysis as a secondary procedure due to the increased morbidity of the latter. Transvaginal suprameatal urethrolysis has also been described [65]; however, success rates are lower than for the transvaginal and retropubic methods. This technique is not as widely used and will not be described in this section. Success rates and rates of recurrent SUI for transvaginal, retropubic, and suprameatal urethrolysis are outlined in Table 11.2.

Transvaginal Urethrolysis

An inverted U-shaped anterior vaginal wall flap is created with the apex at the midurethra and base at the bladder neck (Fig. 11.3). The dissection is taken along the plane of pubocervical fascia up to the pubic bone laterally. The endopelvic fascia is

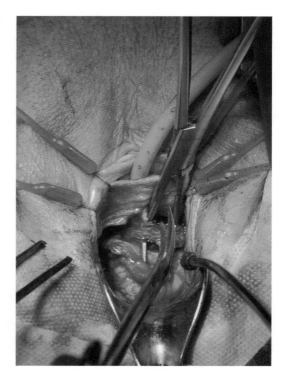

Fig. 11.3 Transvaginal urethrolysis demonstrating midline incision of synthetic midurethral sling (MUS)

perforated sharply with Metzenbaum scissors to enter the retropubic space. Blunt and sharp dissection is used to free the urethra from its attachments to the pubic bone. Any scar or sling encountered in the retropubic space is divided. The urethra is freed proximally to the bladder neck. Occasionally, if adequate vesicourethral mobility cannot be achieved, urethrolysis may be completed from a retropubic approach [62].

Retropubic Urethrolysis

The technique of retropubic urethrolysis has been described by Webster and Kreder [66]. A low midline or Pfannenstiel incision is made and the retropubic space of Retzius developed. All retropubic and prevesical adhesions are sharply incised and all visible suspension sutures and sling materials are cut. All the attachments to the pubic symphysis are released. If there is significant scarring and fibrosis, the dissection can be extended laterally to the ischial tuberosities, creating a paravaginal defect. If this occurs, a formal paravaginal repair involving reapproximation of the paravaginal fascia to the arcus tendineous fascia pelvis is performed. Adequate vesicourethral mobility is determined by observation of free flow of urine from the urethral meatus on application of a Crede maneuver. In the original description, an pedicled omentum flap is routinely interposed between the urethra and pubic bone to prevent readherence.

Failed Urethrolysis

Persistent obstruction following urethrolysis is thought to be due to inadequate vesicourethral mobilization, recurrent periurethral fibrosis, and retropubic scarring or a concomitant resuspension procedure [67]. Scarpero et al. reported on the efficacy of repeat urethrolysis after failed initial urethrolysis. Twenty-four women with persistent urethral obstruction underwent aggressive dissection to free all periurethral and retropubic attachments. Retropubic urethrolysis was performed in 12 (50%), transvaginal in 10 (42%), and 2 (8%) patients had combined techniques. The success rate was 92% with the recurrent SUI rate of 18% being comparable to other published rates after primary urethrolysis. This supports the use of aggressive repeat urethrolysis after failed primary urethrolysis.

De Novo Urgency

Anti-incontinence surgery may cure or aggravate urge symptoms and lead to de novo urgency and detrusor overactivity. This aspect of anti-inconti-

nence surgery is unpredictable and a major cause of patient dissatisfaction. A meta-analysis of studies from December 2002 to June 2005 of patients undergoing sling surgery without concomitant prolapse repair estimated median rates of de novo urge incontinence to be 9% in PVS groups and 6% in MUS groups [20]; however, the MUS groups were not separated according to route. In the Cochrane review by Ogah and Cody, there was no statistical difference in de novo urgency and urge incontinence between transobturator and retropubic MUS groups in the 14 trials compared (7% vs. 6% respectively, RR 1.08, 95% CI 0.75–1.56) [30], but the confidence interval was wide. These symptoms can persist long term. Kuuva and Nilsson reported a de novo urgency rate of 4.7% in 129 women, 6 years after TVT implantation [68].

It is important to remember that storage symptoms such as de novo urgency, without incomplete emptying, may be a manifestation of urethral obstruction [54]. If diagnosed, relief of obstruction is the primary goal of treatment, while urge symptoms may be alleviated by antimuscarinic therapy. In the absence of obstruction (or any other reversible anatomic cause of the urgency such as sling erosion), initial treatment of urgency and urge incontinence consists of fluid management, timed voiding, and antimuscarinic medications. Most patients will have cure or control of their symptoms with these conservative measures. Refractory cases can be treated with surgical procedures such as sacral neuromodulation and peripheral nerve stimulation, and in more extreme cases, augmentation cystoplasty. Prior to consideration of augmentation, intradetrusor injection of botulinum toxin type A can be trialed.

Erosion/Extrusion

Prior to the recently published ICS/IUGA joint terminology and classification system, the term "erosion" was widely used to indicate the finding of material within the lumen of the urinary tract and "extrusion" referred to the finding of exposed material within the vaginal canal. These terms

Fig. 11.4 Cystoscopic view of synthetic MUS erosion into proximal urethra

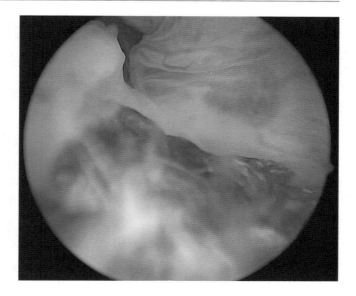

will be used in this section, to avoid any miscommunication of the published literature.

Erosion

Previous series estimated the urethral erosion rate for autologous slings to be <0.003% and for synthetic slings 0.02% [69]. Updated data suggest a higher erosion rate for synthetic slings between 2 and 4% [20]. Underreporting and variability in terminology likely cause underestimation of this complication in the literature. At our institution, we have noticed an alarming increase in the number of referrals for urinary tract erosions from surgical mesh especially over the last 5 years [70].

Urinary tract erosion can be a devastating complication for patients and in our experience always requires primary surgical management. It is unclear whether erosions represent missed intraoperative perforations into the urinary tract or result from passive migration of the material into the urinary tract postoperatively. Intraoperative cystoscopy during sling surgery is considered standard of care in order to identify intraoperative urinary tract injuries [20]. Potential contributing factors to urethral erosion include compromised urethral blood supply (from radiation or estrogen deficiency), excessive sling tension, extensive dissection too close to the urethra with subsequent devascularization, missed intraoperative urethral injury, and traumatic catheterization or dilation postoperatively.

Patients can present with irritative and obstructive voiding complaints, urinary incontinence, hematuria, recurrent UTIs, and pain. Diagnosis is often delayed; Amundsen et al. reported mean of 9 months from sling placement to diagnosis of urethral erosion [71]. Definitive diagnosis is made endoscopically. Autologous and allograft sling urethral erosion is usually managed with excision of the part of the sling which has eroded and simple closure of the urethra [9]. Synthetic mesh erosions typically mandate open exploration, removal of all the exposed material, closure of the urinary tract, placement of an interposition graft material, and adequate postoperative drainage. Most erosions involve the urethra and bladder walls (Figs. 11.4 and 11.5) and will require a complex surgical approach [70] (Fig. 11.6). Occasionally, small intravesical erosions can be treated with endoscopic scissor or laser excision and/or ablation. In our experience, after initial repair, 40% of patients will require a secondary procedure and two thirds will have incontinence postoperatively [70]. Due to complex nature of these repairs, preoperative counseling should emphasize realistic goals of anatomical and functional outcomes.

Fig. 11.5 Cystoscopic view of synthetic MUS erosion into lateral bladder wall

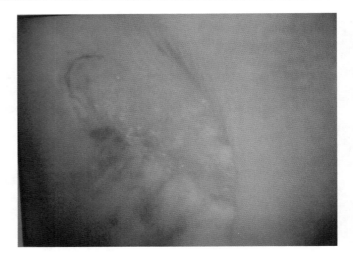

Fig. 11.6 Transvesical excision of synthetic MUS which was eroded into bladder base

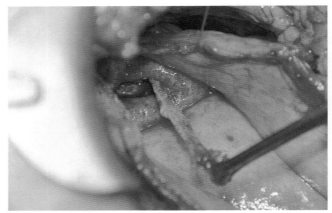

Extrusion

The incidence of extrusion of synthetic slings into the vagina is 2–9% [20]. Extrusions may result from subclinical or overt infection, wound dehiscence, unrecognized vaginal wall perforation, devascularized vaginal flaps, wound compromise secondary to early local trauma (such as early intercourse), or the physical properties of the graft itself. Several earlier types of mesh were taken off the market due to high rates of encapsulation and subsequent extrusion [72, 73].

Patients are typically symptomatic and may present with malodorous vaginal discharge, vaginal pain, dyspareunia, vaginal spotting, and partner discomfort during intercourse. Patients also frequently report that they can palpate mesh in the vagina. The extruded mesh is often palpable

and visible on physical exam and can be associated with granulomatous tissue (Fig. 11.7).

Unlike erosions into the urinary tract, management of mesh extrusion is usually straightforward and is associated with a high success rate and resolution of symptoms. Small extrusions can be initially treated conservatively with the application of topical estrogen creams to promote healing of the vaginal mucosa over the extruded material. These should only be observed for a brief period of time before considering surgical intervention. Larger extrusions and those failing conservative treatment can be treated by raising vaginal flaps and covering the exposed mesh. We prefer to excise the extruded sling before covering the defect with the vaginal flaps to prevent future extrusions.

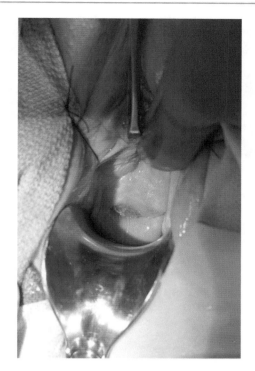

Fig. 11.7 Synthetic MUS exposure in vagina

Recurrent UTI

Four percent to 15% of patients undergoing sling procedures report UTIs [20], and 8% of women undergoing urethrolysis after sling surgery presented with recurrent UTI [54]. However, there are inconsistencies in the detection and reporting of UTI after SUI procedures. A patient presenting after a routine sling procedure with typical symptoms of a UTI such as frequency, urgency, and hematuria should be evaluated with a history, physical exam, urinalysis, and urine culture. Routine dipstick may be difficult to interpret immediately postoperatively, especially if the patient is being catheterized. A short course of antibiotics can be instituted empirically while awaiting culture results.

Patients with severe, ascending, or systemic symptoms (such as abdominal or flank pain, fever) and persistent or recurrent UTI warrant more thorough investigation. This includes a full history, physical exam, and appropriate urine and blood studies including cultures. Cross-sectional imaging and cystoscopy are essential in diagnos-

ing sources of infection such as abscess, upper urinary tract obstruction, stones, foreign bodies, erosion of slings, or other occult bladder diseases. Postvoid residual measurement and urodynamic studies can be used to rule out obstruction as a cause of the recurrent UTI.

Conclusion

Sling surgeries for female SUI are widely performed with generally high rates of success and low rates of morbidity and mortality. Complications from these procedures are likely underreported in the literature because of variability of definitions, lack of mandatory reporting vehicles, and the need for studies with longer follow-up. Enthusiasm for minimally invasive MUSs have substantially increased the number of sling surgeries performed, as well as increased the number of and variability in the practitioners implanting these devices. Many complications can be prevented by first ensuring that the indication for the particular type of sling is appropriate, and second, by adhering to good surgical technique. Patients must be well counseled preoperatively about all the potential risks of the procedure, as well as the realistic expected outcomes. Practitioners should remain attentive to patient symptoms postoperatively, in order to promptly identify potential complications.

References

1. van Geelen JM, Hunskaar S. The epidemiology of female urinary incontinence. Eur Clin Obstet Gynecol. 2005;1:3.
2. Luber KM. The definition, prevalence, and risk factors for stress urinary incontinence. Rev Urol. 2004; 6:S3.
3. Milsom I, Altman D, Lapitan MC, et al. Epidemiology of urinary and fecal incontinence and pelvic organ prolapse. In: Abrams P, Cardozo L, Khoury S, Wein A, editors. Incontinence. 4th ed. Paris: Health Publication; 2009. p. 64–78.
4. Wilson J, Brown JS, Shin GP, Luc KO, Subak LL. Annual direct cost of urinary incontinence. Obstet Gynecol. 2001;98:398.
5. Anger JT, Weinberg AE, Albo ME, Smith AL, Kim J, Rodriguez LV, et al. Trends in surgical management

of stress urinary incontinence among female medicare beneficiaries. J Urol. 2009;74(2):283–7.

6. Virkud A. Management of stress urinary incontinence. Best Pract Res Clin Obstet Gynaecol. 2011;25(2): 205–16.

7. Smith ARB, Dmochowski R, Hilton P, et al. Surgery for urinary incontinence in women. In: Abrams P, Cardozo L, Khoury S, Wein A, editors. Incontinence. 4th ed. Paris: Health Publication; 2009. p. 1193–272.

8. O'Reilly KJ, Govier FE. Intermediate term failure of pubovaginal slings using cadaveric fascia lata: a case series. J Urol. 2002;167:1356.

9. Blaivas JG, Sandhu J. Urethral reconstruction after erosion of slings in women. Curr Opin Urol. 2004;14:335–8.

10. Nitti V, Blaivas J. Chapter 60: urinary incontinence: epidemiology, pathophysiology, evaluation, and management overview. In: Wein A, editor. Campbell-Walsh urology, vol. III. 9th ed. Philadelphia: Saunders Elsevier; 2007.

11. Blaivas JG, Rutman M, Walsh R. How and why incontinence surgery works. In: Cardozo L, Staskin D, editors. Textbook of female urology and urogynecology, vol. II. 3rd ed. London: Informa Healthcare; 2010. p. 635–42.

12. Westby M, Asmussen M, Ulmsten U. Location of maximum intraurethral pressure related to urogenital diaphragm in the female subject as studied by simultaneous urethrocystometry and voiding urethrocystography. Am J Obstet Gynecol. 1982;144(4): 408–12.

13. Tash J, Staskin DR. Artificial graft slings at the midurethra: physiology of continence. Curr Urol Rep. 2003;4:367–70.

14. Fritel X, Zabak K, Pigne A, Demaria F, Benifla JL. Predictive value of urethral mobility before suburethral tape procedure for urinary stress incontinence in women. J Urol. 2002;168(6):2472–5.

15. Petri E, Niemeyer R, Martan A, Tunn R, Naumann G, Koelbl H. Reasons for and treatment of surgical complications with alloplastic slings. Int Urogynecol J Pelvic Floor Dysfunct. 2006;17(1):3–13.

16. Chaikin DC, Rosenthal J, Blaivas JG. Pubovaginal fascial sling for all types of stress urinary incontinence: long term analysis. J Urol. 1998;160:1312–6.

17. Oh SJ, Stoffel J, Mcguire EJ. Pubovaginal sling. In: Wein A, Kavoussi L, Novick A, Partin A, Peters C, editors. Campbell-Walsh urology (Ch 67), vol. III. 9th ed. Philadelphia: Saunders Elsevier; 2007.

18. Langer R, Ron El R, Newman M, et al. Detrusor instability following colposuspension for stress incontinence. Br J Obstet Gynaecol. 1988;95:607–10.

19. Morgan Jr TO, Westney OL, McGuire EJ. Pubovaginal sling: 4-year outcome analysis and quality of life assessment. J Urol. 2000;163:1845–8.

20. Appell R, Dmochowski RR, Blaivas J, et al. Guideline for the surgical management of female stress urinary incontinence: 2009 update. Atlanta: American Urological Association; 2009.

21. Taub DA, Hollenbeck BK, Wei JT, Dunn RL, McGuire EJ, Latini JM. Complications following surgical intervention for stress urinary incontinence: a national perspective. Neurourol Urodyn. 2005;24(7):659–65.

22. US Food and Drug Administration. US Food and Drug Administration Alerts and Notices (Medical Devices) website. October 2008. http://www.fda.gov/MedicalDevices/Safety/AlertsandNotices/Public HealthNotifications/ucm061976.htm. Accessed Oct 2008.

23. Haylen BT, Freeman RM, Swift SE, et al. IUGA/ICS joint terminology and classification of the complications related directly to the insertion of prostheses (meshes, implants and tapes) and grafts in female pelvic floor surgery. Neurourol Urodyn. 2011;30:2–12.

24. Kisielinski K, Conze J, Murken AH, Lenzen NN, Klinge U, Schumpelick V. The Pfannenstiel or so called "bikini cut": still effective more than 100 years after first description. Hernia. 2004;8(3):177–81.

25. Luijendijk RW, Jeekel J, Storm RK, Schutte PJ, Hop WC, Drogendijk AC, et al. The low transverse Pfannenstiel incision and the prevalence of incisional hernia and nerve entrapment. Ann Surg. 1997;225(4): 365–9.

26. Latini JM, Brown JA, Kreder KJ. Abdominal sacral colpopexy using autologous fascia lata. J Urol. 2004; 171(3):1176–9.

27. Latini JM, Lux MM, Kreder KJ. Efficacy and morbidity of autologous fascia lata sling cystourethropexy. J Urol. 2004;171(3):1180–4.

28. Wheatcroft SM, Vardy SJ, Tyers AG. Complications of fascia lata harvesting for ptosis surgery. Br J Ophthalmol. 1997;81(7):581–3.

29. Chibber PJ, Shah HN, Jain P. A minimally invasive technique for harvesting autologous fascia lata for pubo-vaginal sling suspension. Int Urol Nephrol. 2005;37(1):43–6.

30. Ogah J, Cody JD. Minimally invasive synthetic suburethral sling operations for stress urinary incontinence in women. Cochrane Database Syst Rev. 2009; CD006375.

31. Zilbert AW, Farrell SA. External iliac artery laceration during tension-free vaginal tape procedure. Int Urogynecol J Pelvic Floor Dysfunct. 2001;12:141.

32. Douketis JD, Berger PB, Dunn AS, et al. The perioperative management of antithrombotic therapy: American College of Chest Physicians Evidence-Based Clinical Practice Guidelines (8th edition). Chest. 2008;133:299S–399.

33. Muir TW, Tulikangas PK, Fidela Paraison M, Walters MD. The relationship of tension-free vaginal tape insertion and the vascular anatomy. Obstet Gynecol. 2003;101:933.

34. Katske FA, Raz S. Use of Foley catheter to obtain transvaginal tamponade. Urology. 1987;26:18.

35. Papakostidis C, Kanakaris N, Dimitriou R, Giannoudis PV. The role of arterial embolization in controlling pelvic fracture haemorrhage: a systematic review of the literature. Eur J Radiol. 2012;81(5):897–904.

36. Tanizaki S, Maeda S, Hayashi H, Matano H, Ishida H, Yoshikawa J, et al. Early embolization without external fixation in pelvic trauma. Am J Emerg Med. 2012;30(2):342–6.
37. Anchala PR, Resnick SA. Treatment of postoperative hemorrhage with venous embolization. J Vasc Interv Radiol. 2010;21(12):1915–7.
38. Jeffry L, Deval B, Birsan A, Soriano D, Daraï E. Objective and subjective cure rates after tension-free vaginal tape for treatment of urinary incontinence. Urology. 2001;58(5):702–6.
39. Deval B, Levardon M, Samain E, Rafii A, Cortesse A, Amarenco G, et al. A French multicenter clinical trial of SPARC for stress urinary incontinence. Eur Urol. 2003;44(2):254–8; discussion 258–9.
40. Hodroff MA, Sutherland SE, Kesha JB, Siegel SW. Treatment of stress incontinence with the SPARC sling: intraoperative and early complications of 445 patients. Urology. 2005;66(4):760–2.
41. Daneshgari F, Kong W, Swartz M. Complications of mid urethral slings: important outcomes for future clinical trials. J Urol. 2008;180:1890.
42. Stav K, Dwyer PL, Rosamilia A, Schierlitz L, Lim YN, Lee J. Risk factors for trocar injury to the bladder during mid urethral sling procedures. J Urol. 2009; 182(1):174–9.
43. McLennan MT, Melick CF. Bladder perforation during tension-free vaginal tape procedures: analysis of learning curve and risk factors. Obstet Gynecol. 2005;106(5 Pt 1):1000–4.
44. Kobashi K, Govier F. Perioperative complications: the first 140 polypropylene pubovaginal slings. J Urol. 2003;170:1918–21.
45. Leboeuf L, Tellez CA, Ead D, Gousse AE. Complication of bowel perforation during insertion of tension-free vaginal tape. J Urol. 2003;170:1310–1.
46. Castillo OA, Bodden E, Olivares RA, Urena RD. Intestinal perforation: an infrequent complication during insertion of tension-free vaginal tape. J Urol. 2004;2004(172):1364.
47. Meschia M, Busacca M, Pifarotti P, De Marinis S. Bowel perforation during insertion of tension-free vaginal tape. Int Urogynecol J Pelvic Floor Dysfunct. 2002;13:263–5.
48. Rooney KE, Cholhan HJ. Bowel perforation during retropubic sling procedure. Obstet Gynecol. 2010;115(Pt 2):429–31.
49. US Food and Drug Administration. Manufacturer and User Facility Device Experience database; 2007.
50. Dunn JS, Bent AE, Ellerkman RM, Nihira MA, Melick CF. Voiding dysfunction after surgery for stress incontinence: literature and survey results. Int Urogynecol J. 2004;11:353–8.
51. Shah S, Nitti V. Diagnosis and treatment of obstruction following incontinence surgery—urethrolysis and other techniques. In: Cardozo L, Staskin D, editors. Textbook of female urology and urogynecology,

vol. II. 3rd ed. London: Informa Healthcare; 2010. p. 749–62.
52. Nitti V, Raz S. Obstruction following anti-incontinence procedures: diagnosis and treatment with transvaginal urethrolysis. J Urol. 1999;161:1535–40.
53. Gomelsky A, Scarpero HM, Dmochowski RR. Sling surgery for stress urinary incontinence in the female: what surgery, which material? AUA Update Series. 2003;22:266.
54. Carr LK, Webster GD. Voiding dysfunction following incontinence surgery: diagnosis and treatment with retropubic or vaginal urethrolysis. J Urol. 1997;157: 821–3.
55. Fitzgerald MP, Brubaker L. The etiology of urinary retention after surgery for genuine stress incontinence. Neurourol Urodyn. 2001;30:13–21.
56. Miller EA, Amundsen CL, Toh KL, Flynn BJ, Webster GD. Preoperative urodynamic evaluation may predict voiding dysfunction in women undergoing pubovaginal sling. J Urol. 2003;169:2234–7.
57. Weinberger MW, Ostergard DR. Postoperative catheterization, urinary retention and permanent voiding dysfunction after polytetrafluoroethylene suburethral sling placement. Obstet Gynecol. 1996;87:50–4.
58. McLennan MT, Melick CF, Bent AE. Clinical and urodynamic predictors of delayed voiding after fascia lata suburethral sling. Obstet Gynecol. 1998;92:608–12.
59. Mishra VC, Mishra N, Karim OMA, Motiwala HG. Voiding dysfunction after tension-free vaginal tape: a conservative approach is often successful. Int Urogynecol J. 2005;16:210–5.
60. Leng WW, Davies BJ, Tarin T, Sweeney DD, Chancellor MB. Delayed treatment of bladder outlet obstruction after sling surgery: association with irreversible bladder dysfunction. J Urol. 2004;172(4 Pt 1): 1379–81.
61. South MM, Wu JM, Webster GD, Weidner AC, Roelands JJ, Amundsen CL. Early vs late midline sling lysis results in greater improvement in lower urinary tract symptoms. Am J Obstet Gynecol. 2009; 200(5):564.e1–5.
62. Scarpero HM, Dmochowski RR, Nitti VW. Repeat urethrolysis after failed urethrolysis for iatrogenic obstruction. J Urol. 2003;169:1013–6.
63. Goldman HB. Simple sling incision for the treatment of iatrogenic urethral obstruction. Urology. 2003;62: 714–8.
64. Kusuda L. Simple release of pubovaginal sling. Urology. 2001;57(2):358–9.
65. Petrou SP, Brown JA, Blaivas JG. Suprameatal transvaginal urethrolysis. J Urol. 1999;161:1268–71.
66. Webster GD, Kreder KJ. Voiding dysfunction following cystourethropexy: its evaluation and management. J Urol. 1990;144:670–3.
67. Starkman JS, Scarpero HM, Dmochowski RR. Methods and results of urethrolysis. Curr Urol Rep. 2006;7(5):384–94.

68. Kuuva N, Nilsson CG. Long-term results of the tension-free vaginal tape operation in an unselected group of 129 stress incontinent women. Acta Obstet Gynecol Scand. 2006;85(4):482–7.

69. Leach GE, Dmochowski RR, Appell RA, et al. Female stress urinary incontinence clinical guidelines panel summary report on surgical management of female stress urinary incontinence. The American Urological Association. J Urol. 1997;158:875.

70. Changkit L, Dmochowski RR. Functional outcomes after repair of mesh erosion into the lower urinary tract [abstract]. In: Paper presented at Society of Urodynamics and Female Urology winter meeting, Phoenix, AZ, 1–5 March 2011.

71. Amundsen CL, Flynn BJ, Webster GD, et al. Urethral erosion after synthetic and nonsynthetic pubovaginal slings: differences in management and continence outcome. J Urol. 2003;170:134–7.

72. Yamada BS, Govier FE, Stefanovic KB, Kobashi KC. High rate of vaginal erosions associated with the mentor ObTape. J Urol. 2006;176(2):651–4.

73. Bafghi A, Benizri EI, Trastour C, Benizri EJ, Michiels JF, Bongain A. Multifilament polypropylene mesh for urinary incontinence: 10 cases of infections requiring removal of the sling. BJOG. 2005;112(3): 376–8.

74. Foster HE, McGuire EJ. Management of urethral obstruction with transvaginal urethrolysis. J Urol. 1993;150(5 Pt 1):1448–51.

75. Cross CA, Cespedes RD, English SF, et al. Transvaginal urethrolysis for urethral obstruction after anti-incontinence surgery. J Urol. 1998;159: 1199–201.

76. Goldman HB, Rackley PR, Appell RA. The efficacy of urethrolysis without resuspension for iatrogenic urethral obstruction. J Urol. 1999;161(1):196–8.

Complications of Female Urethral Reconstructive Surgery

Jerry Blaivas and Dorota Borawski

Introduction

Female urethral reconstruction is an uncommon surgery used to repair female urethral strictures and fistulas. Because of the rarity of these operations, complications have not been well described in the literature. Complications can be categorized as intraoperative and postoperative. Postoperative can be further divided into general complications common to all pelvic surgery, which will not be discussed here, and those that are specific to urethral reconstruction. Those complications include: (1) early or late postoperative wound complications from the graft or flap harvest site, (2) stricture or fistula recurrence, (3) de novo postoperative incontinence, (4) de novo or recurrent urethral obstruction, and (5) de novo detrusor overactivity.

Since almost all of the patients who undergo urethral reconstruction represent complications or failures of the operation that caused the problem in the first place, the same preoperative principles apply to both the primary and secondary procedures. Prior to reconstructive surgery, the surgeon should perform a thorough preoper-

ative assessment, tailor surgery to fundamental principles of surgical technique, and be familiar with a variety of different techniques to minimize the chance of complications. The best means of managing complications is to prevent them from occurring in the first place.

Preoperative Assessment

Many complications related to urethral reconstructive surgery are preventable, particularly because the elective nature of most female urethral reconstructive surgery permits appropriate preoperative surgical planning.

Minimizing the risk of preoperative complications involves multiple steps beginning with a detailed history and physical examination of the urethral defect, assessment of urethral sphincter and detrusor function, and exclusion of concomitant vesicovaginal or ureterovaginal fistula, as well as ureteral obstruction. Almost all patients who require urethral reconstruction have had prior surgery, so it is important to either obtain the operative reports or discuss the surgery with the previous surgeon. It is particularly important to know whether or not there is a foreign body such as mesh in or near the wound. One of our patients failed a urethral reconstruction because of retained mesh at the site of an urethrovaginal fistula. Neither the patient nor the surgeon even knew that a mesh sling had been done previously. This unfortunate case emphasizes the need for obtaining an accurate surgical history.

J. Blaivas, MD (✉)
Department of Urology, Weill Medical College
of Cornell University, 445 East 77th Street,
New York, NY 10075, USA
e-mail: jblvs@aol.com

D. Borawski, MD
SUNY Downstate Medical Center and the Institute
for Bladder and Prostate Research

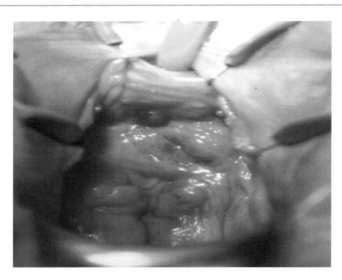

Fig. 12.1 Inspection of the anterior vaginal wall in a woman with a seemingly straightforward urethrovaginal fistula. She underwent a simple repair with vaginal wall flaps and a Martius flap, but the fistula recurred within 3 weeks. At secondary repair, a mesh sling was encountered and excised. Neither the patient nor the surgeon knew that mesh had been used in a prior anti-incontinence operation (courtesy of J.G. Blaivas)

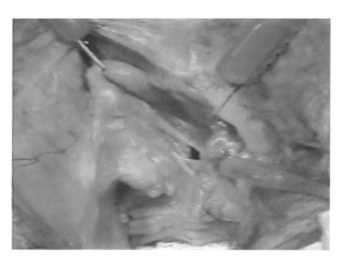

Fig. 12.2 Inspection of the anterior vaginal wall in a woman who had previously undergone an extensive urethral reconstruction after excision of a sterile periurethral abscess that formed after injection of calcium hydroxylapatite (Coaptite) for sphincteric incontinence refractory to two mesh slings. Despite the obvious stricture, she had severe sphincteric incontinence as well. At the time of surgery, after incising the stricture, the proximal urethra was only about 2 cm in length, just barely large enough to accept an autologous fascial sling (courtesy of J.G. Blaivas)

Preoperative physical examination should be performed with a comfortably full bladder. Particular attention should be paid to the health of the vaginal tissue. In patients with vaginal atrophy and postradiation changes, preoperative estrogen cream may improve the quality of vaginal tissue. A careful speculum examination of the entire vaginal mucosa should assess the presence of any sling erosion, granulation tissue, drainage from a sinus tract, fistula, and scarring of the anterior vaginal wall, all of which are tell-tale signs of mesh erosion.

In cases of urethral damage from previous vaginal or urethral surgery, the vaginal tissue is often scarred, fibrotic, and ischemic. The extent of urethral tissue loss, the integrity of the vaginal tissue, adequacy of the vasculature, and the need for advancement,

Fig. 12.3 Voiding cystourethrogram in this patient confirms a distal urethral stricture. There is almost no possibility of sphincteric injury during reconstructive surgery that is limited to the distal urethra, so either a ventral or dorsal approach may be considered (courtesy of J.G. Blaivas)

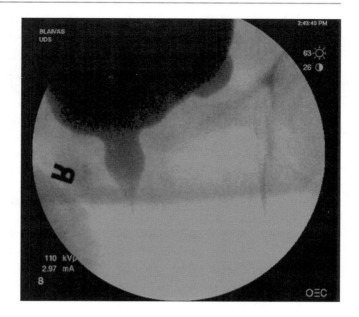

lateral or pedicle skin flaps, should be assessed preoperatively (Figs. 12.1 and 12.2). Bimanual pelvic exam should focus on the presence of urethral masses, pelvic organ prolapse, and the position of the urethrovaginal junction. When incontinence is observed from the urethral meatus, and a fistula suspected, the examination should be repeated with a finger occluding the meatus to observe leakage from the fistula itself.

Videourodynamics may show urethral obstruction, sphincteric incontinence, low bladder compliance, impaired detrusor contractility, or detrusor overactivity secondary to urethral damage. The voiding cystourethrogram (VCUG) is a critical component in preoperative evaluation of the diseased urethra. In patients with urethral obstruction, VCUG assesses the site, and for those with strictures, the length and location in relation to the bladder neck. If the urethral stricture is located at the distal third of the urethra or the meatus, imaging typically reveals ballooning of the bladder neck on voiding (Fig. 12.3).

Other imaging techniques like MRI and delayed CT with contrast may be useful to distinguish abscess, cyst, tumor, and urethral diverticulum in patients with periurethral masses, to assess foreign bodies and to rule out additional injury to the urinary tract following pelvic trauma.

Cystourethroscopy will confirm a urethral stricture, the presence of a foreign body, including suture or sling material, and evaluate the extent of the fistula. It can also evaluate the remainder of the urethra, particularly the length, viability, and sphincteric function of the proximal urethra.

Principles of the Surgical Technique

The choice of surgical technique is dictated by a number of factors including (1) the experience and expertise of the surgeon, (2) the desires of the patient, (3) the patient's age and comorbidities, (4) lower urinary tract and renal function, (5) the presence of concomitant conditions such as pelvic organ prolapse or abdominal or pelvic disease requiring surgical correction, (6) prior abdominal and pelvic surgical procedures, and (7) sexual function.

1. *The surgeon*: Urethral reconstruction ranges from simple ventral incision and meatotomy for distal urethral strictures to full-length dorsal buccal grafts for longer strictures to neourethral reconstruction with local vaginal

wall flaps reinforced with Martius flaps and occasionally, gracilis, thigh, or rectus flaps. Few of these procedures are learned in residency or fellowship; most of the expertise is garnered over decades of experience in tertiary referral centers. In our judgment, the most demanding part of the expertise is decision making both before and during the surgery. With the exception of proximal dorsal buccal mucosal grafts for strictures and ventral bladder neck reconstruction, the technical aspects of the surgery are usually straightforward. With these caveats in mind, it is up to the individual surgeon to decide whether he or she possesses the requisite surgical expertise for each individual patient. In some instances, referral to a reconstructive expert is prudent.

2. *The patient*: For practical purposes, the damaged urethra presents one or more of three potential problems—incontinence, urethral obstruction, and pelvic pain. Surgical treatment of incontinence and pain is entirely elective; whereas, untreated urethral obstruction may portend urinary retention or upper tract damage and even renal failure. Further, the success rate for treating urethral obstruction and sphincteric incontinence is very high—over 90%, while the success rate for pelvic pain and overactive bladder is far less. Keeping these facts in mind, it is important that the patient be apprised of the pros and cons of surgical intervention and that the decision about how to proceed is based on realistic expectations for success, failure, and complications.

3. *Patient age and comorbidities*: Age and comorbidities are a factor insofar as the patient's life expectancy and ability to withstand the morbidity of surgery that could last as long as 4–6 h, although excessive blood loss is rarely encountered.

4. *Urinary tract function*: It is axiomatic that lower urinary tract function is an essential component of decision making in planning surgery. As a general rule, we believe it is most prudent to treat sphincteric incontinence as part of the reconstructive procedure, although some surgeons prefer a staged operation. Low bladder compliance and detrusor overactivity often improve after successful surgery, so they are not addressed at the same time except in rare circumstances when due to multiple surgeries or radiation. In these instances, urinary diversion rather than urethral reconstruction might be considered (Fig. 12.4).

5. *Concomitant conditions*: When concomitant conditions such as pelvic organ prolapse or vesicovaginal fistula are present, they should be repaired at the same time as the urethral reconstruction, but it is not usually necessary to repair vesicoureteral reflux unless there is a clear-cut anatomic cause or if there are symptomatic recurrent upper urinary tract infections. Ureteral obstruction or reflux due to sling complications is best handled at the time that the sling is removed.

6. *Prior surgery*: It is important to know what prior pelvic surgeries the patient has undergone, particularly if mesh has been used for prior repairs. As a general rule, as much mesh as can be safely removed should be taken; when that is not feasible, it is important that all mesh be at least removed from the urethra and bladder when there has been erosion. In patients complaining of pain, it is best to remove all mesh from the affected side whenever possible, but this can be extremely challenging in patients who have undergone TOT repairs.

7. *Sexual function*: It is essential that the patient's desires about future sexuality be discussed and incorporated into surgical planning and informed consent. The literature about sexual complications of urethral reconstructions is rudimentary at best, but dyspareunia can occur after any of these operations. When maintaining sexual function is a factor, special attention must be paid to insuring adequate vaginal size of at least two loose finger breaths to a depth of at least 8 cm.

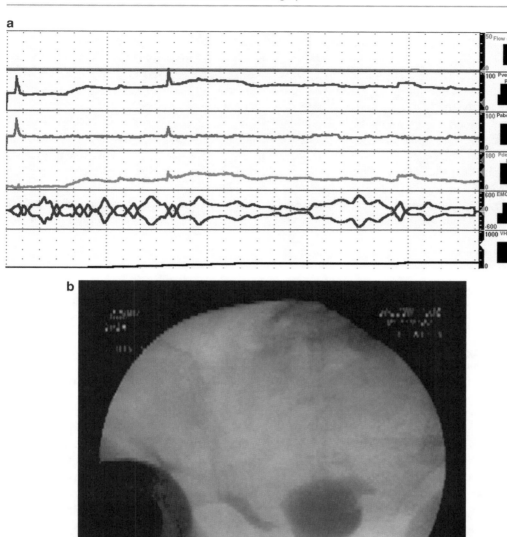

Fig. 12.4 Videourodynamic study in a 72-year-old woman who underwent anterior prolapse repair and TVT sling complicated by colovesical and urethrovaginal fistula. She subsequently underwent unsuccessful attempts at surgical repair of these defects and presented with refractory urge incontinence as well as sphincteric incontinence and colovesical fistula. She had arthritis that precluded self-catheterization through the urethra. Because of the findings described below, she underwent continent urinary diversion instead of another attempt at lower urinary tract reconstruction. (**a**) Urodynamic tracing demonstrates severe low bladder compliance (2 mL/cm H$_2$O) at a bladder volume of only 50 mL. Note that each time infusion is stopped, detrusor pressure falls. (courtesy of J.G. Blaivas). (**b**) Cystogram reveals a tiny bladder with right vesicoureteral reflux. The colovesical fistula and sphincteric incontinence was not visualized (courtesy of J.G. Blaivas)

Surgical Techniques

Before proceeding with the vaginal incision, it is critical to choose the site and shape of the initial incision for the urethral reconstruction. We have previously described several methods of urethral reconstruction, and in the majority of the cases, the repair can be accomplished with a single transvaginal operation [1].

All surgical approaches follow the same rules: fine sharp dissection is preferable and homeostasis is maintained. Sharp dissection permits the development of correct planes and excision of the dense fibrotic tissue and may prevent inadvertent injury to the sphincter. The urethra should be opened proximal enough to clearly see the extent of the urethral stricture. In addition to aiding in visualization, attention to homeostasis may prevent hematoma and breakdown of the sutures lines. When excessive bleeding is encountered, pressure should be applied until the bleeding stops or bleeding vessels individually clamped and sutured or coagulated. Frantic efforts to control hemorrhage without clearly identifying the bleeding vessels leads to unnecessary injury to adjacent organs.

In preparing for vaginal surgery, the patient is placed in a dorsal lithotomy position with steep Trendelenburg. Draping should permit access to the vagina as well as abdominal area (when concomitant surgery is planned). At the onset of surgery, the bladder is drained via a transurethral catheter and palpation of the balloon allows identification of the bladder neck. If suprapubic cystotomy, pubovaginal sling, or rectus muscle graft is planned, these should be done prior to the vaginal reconstructive surgery to avoid subsequent damage to the reconstruction during dissection for these procedures. For pubovaginal sling, though, the sutures should not be tied until the reconstruction has been completed so that tension can be judged.

In cases of minimal urethral disruption, such as a small urethrovaginal fistula, the defect can be circumscribed and closed over a catheter with tension-free, interrupted sutures of 3–4:O chromic catgut. An inverted U anterior vaginal wall flap is for closure. Closure of the wound can be accomplished with elevation of lateral vaginal flaps and closure in the midline, alternatively the U-shaped incision can be advanced.

If urethral damage is extensive and sufficient vaginal wall tissue exists, vaginal wall flaps may be considered. Flap-based urethroplasty techniques have been demonstrated to be effective and improve the outcome in the urethrovaginal fistulas and are the treatment of choice for most female urethral strictures [2–4]. In one such technique, the anterior vaginal wall can be mobilized and a rectangular incision around the urethral defect is made. A lateral vaginal wall flap is advanced to the midline, rolled over the catheter, and sutured in the midline without tension. However, if the extent of urethral injury and lack of vaginal tissue preclude simple repair, use of an advancement flap may be required. Another choice is to create a labia minora flap. An oval-shaped incision is made in an adjacent hair-free portion of the labia minora and carried through the underlying tissue and a pedicle is raised on a posterior- or anterior-based blood supply. This island flap is tunneled beneath the vaginal wall, rotated, and sutured over the catheter, so the vaginal epithelial surface creates the inner wall of the urethra. Rarely, it is not possible to close the defect in the vaginal wall primarily. In such instances, it is possible to create a labia majora flap to cover the wound. We have only needed a gracilis flap on one occasion and have never used any other major kind of flap (rectus, Singapore, etc.), but of course, those are available if needed [1].

Urethral damage associated with erosion of synthetic material poses unique considerations and the repairs can be even more challenging. Most authors agree that eroded synthetic slings require complete removal of the sling from the urethra and bladder. The literature on the surgical management of erosions suggests midline anterior vaginal wall incision at the erosion site, bilateral dissection into the retropubic space, and removal of the entire synthetic sling including sutures, and when possible, bone anchors if they were used [5]. In our experience, especially with transobturator techniques, attempting to remove all of the sling leads to difficult and morbid surgery and should probably be reserved for those who failed at first attempt. Once the sling has been excised, the urethra can usually be repaired primarily. If this is not feasible, any of the techniques described above may be considered.

For patients with urethral stricture, in our judgment, ventral urethroplasty using vaginal and labial skin flaps is the least morbid technique. This approach is utilized in patients with mid-to-distal urethral strictures and an intact bladder neck and urinary sphincter mechanism. However, ventral urethrotomy risks urethral sphincter damage and de novo urinary incontinence when the stricture involves the proximal urethra or when sphincteric incontinence was present preoperatively. In cases of documented preoperative sphincteric incontinence, the ventral approach offers easier access to the bladder neck and permits an easier concomitant anti-incontinence procedure.

Unlike the dorsal approach, ventral urethroplasty may redirect the urethra and the urinary stream posteriorly. Consequently, postoperative complaints of vaginally directed urinary stream after ventral urethroplasty that improved after 6 months have been reported [6].

Recently, several groups have proposed a dorsal onlay urethroplasty using buccal mucosa graft [7, 8], labia minora skin graft [9], or vestibular flap [10]. The dorsal technique has several advantages, but requires different surgical expertise, utilizing many of the surgical principles derived from urethral reconstruction in men. A surgical plane is developed between the urethra and overlying clitoral cavernous tissue. Care should be taken during the dissection of the dorsal urethra to avoid injury to the clitoral bulb, body or crura, and the clitoral neurovascular bundle and minimize excessive bleeding. The clitoro-urethrovaginal complex is supplied by pudendal

neurovascular bundles which arise from pelvic side walls and bifurcate into clitoral and perineal divisions. The clitoral neurovascular bundle ascends along the ischipubic ramus and adjacent clitoral crura on both sides, runs under the surface of the symphysis pubis in the midline, and then travels along the cephaled surface of the clitoral body towards the glans (Fig. 12.5). The nerves of the clitoral neurovascular bundle are not large enough to be seen on the MRI. However, the histological dissections show that they accompany the vessels [11].

From a practical standpoint, it is fairly straightforward to avoid these structures during the dissection. We are unaware of any reports of injury to the clitoral structures, nor have there been any reports of orgasmic changes. Our experience with five such operations corroborates these findings.

Not infrequently during the dissection troublesome bleeding is encountered, but we caution against blind coagulation or suture ligature. Positioning the graft on the dorsal surface preserves intact ventral midurethra and provides a better vascular bed for a graft. In our judgment, doing so minimizes the likelihood of requiring an incontinence procedure. However, unlike the ventral approach, dorsal dissection is infrequently performed in pelvic reconstructive surgery, and for most surgeons, the anatomy is not well known. Further, most pelvic surgeons are unfamiliar with the techniques of graft reconstruction which are done much more commonly in men.

Use of a Graft and Potential Complications

One of the challenges of urethral reconstructive surgery is achieving a long and stricture-free lumen that allows nonobstructive voiding and maintains continence. Due to the variable etiology of the urethral pathology, local tissue may not be available for the urethral repair. In cases of extensive posttraumatic or postsurgical urethral fibrosis, congenital malformations, and recurrent urethral strictures, reconstructing the urethra with

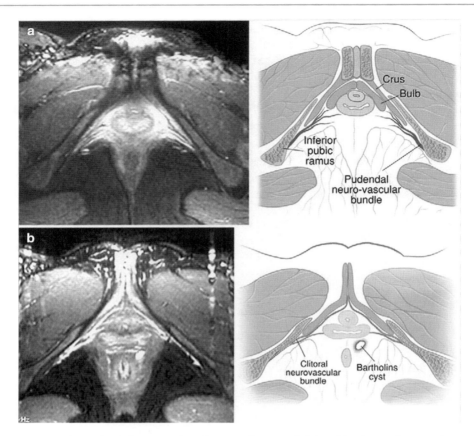

Fig. 12.5 (**a**) MRI of the clitoris in the axial section as seen on the left, shows divisions of the pudendal neuro-vascular bundle, which arises from the pelvic side wall and bifurcates into perineal and clitoral neurovascular bundle. Vascular component of the bundle and cavernous tissue are bright white due to fat saturation technique. Muscles and bone appear as dark structures. (**b**) On the right is an artist's rendition of the images. Reprinted with permission from the Journal of Urology [11]

a free graft provides an alternative to a vaginal flap or bladder flap.

Various graft urethroplasty techniques have been proposed in small series. These techniques can be complicated and require knowledge and experience with processing and tissue transfer.

Buccal mucosa grafts are commonly used in male urethral reconstructive surgery and have been shown to be successful in construction of the neourethra in female pediatric patients [12]. The buccal mucosa graft has been applied to female urethral strictures using both dorsal and ventral approaches [6–8, 13].

In our experience, buccal mucosa graft is an option in patients with previously failed reconstructive surgery and urethral stricture recurrence. It is also our treatment of choice for proximal urethral strictures in women who do not have a current or past history of sphincteric incontinence because we believe that there is no need for anti-incontinence surgery when the dorsal approach is used. Buccal mucosa has several advantages, is easy to harvest, is resilient to infection, and is already accustomed to a wet environment. Properties like elasticity and thick epithelium make it easy to handle [14]. It has the ability to form a conduit that closely resembles a normal functioning urethra with low risk of sacculation and diverticulum formation. In animal studies, extensive neovascularization in the subepithelial layer was evident 3 weeks after surgery, followed by inflammation and minimal fibrosis at 6 weeks [15]. Supple urethral coaptation can be accomplished by buccal mucosa graft and may play a role in achieving incontinence after urethral reconstruction [12]. The graft is harvested from the lateral cheek below the Stensen's duct opening which is identified adjacent to the second upper molar and typically measures between 2 and 2.5 cm wide and 2–4 cm in length depending on the amount of tissue needed. The graft is defatted and sutured to the urethrostomy. To maximize outcomes after free grafts, ensuring adequate vascularity of the donor bed is necessary. All fibrotic tissue has to be excised and the graft must be anastomosed to the recipient bed using monofilament absorbable sutures. In order to allow possible postoperative shrinkage of graft, it should be trimmed to larger size than urethral defect or stricture.

Complications associated with harvesting buccal mucosa graft are rare and have not been reported in any female case series. In male reconstructive surgery, complications reported include donor site wound pain, swelling, damage to parotid duct, postoperative perioral numbness, difficulty with mouth opening, and infection. According to data from male case series, 59% patients developed short-term numbness after surgery, which persisted in 16% beyond 1 year [16]. Complications of buccal grafts are uncommon; however, the possibility of a mental nerve neuropathy is unique to buccal graft surgery [17]. Injury to Stensen's duct is extremely rare and can be avoided by marking the buccal mucosa and careful closure of the donor site. When it is difficult to perform closure, some surgeons prefer to leave the harvest site open. If buccal mucosa graft is used ventrally and adequate periurethral tissue does not exist for coverage of the graft, it may be advisable to use well-vascularized tissue flaps to provide an adequate blood supply and prevent fistula formation. However, to our knowledge tissue flaps have not been utilized in dorsal approach.

Recently, Sharma described use of dorsal onlay lingual graft urethroplasty in 15 women with urethral stricture [18]. Lingual mucosa, harvested from lateral and ventral surfaces of the tongue, has similar tissue characteristics as buccal mucosa thick epithelium, high content of elastic fibers, thin lamina propria, and rich vasularization [19]. There were no functional limitations or intraoral complications at 1-year follow-up. Distinct advantages of harvesting lingual mucosa graft instead of buccal mucosa graft are avoidance of injury to parotid gland duct and mental nerve as well as no risk of the mouth deviation or lip retraction [18].

Intraoperative Complications

Intraoperative complications during urethral reconstructive surgery are rare based on our review of the literature. One case of intraoperative hemorrhage has been reported in early series by Elkins on 20 women who underwent repair of a vesicovaginal fistula involving the urethra with the anterior bladder flap technique and Martius flap. During total urethral reconstruction, a patient developed hemorrhage in the space of Retzius and required postoperative blood transfusion [20]. However, there is no surgery that spares the patient from potential risk of other complications like anesthesia or injury to adjacent organs such as bladder, ureter, or rectum. For bleeding that occurs during the dissection for creating vaginal flaps, we believe it is best to simply apply pressure with a pack unless there is an obvious bleeding vessel that can be coagulated or ligated. Bleeding that occurs from the retropubic space after entry from the vagina is best handled with the same approach. If bleeding seems excessive, we advise against trying to explore from the vaginal wound; rather, one or two 4×4 sponges or a lap pad should be inserted into the retropubic space through the vagina to tamponade the bleeding while other parts of the operation are continued. In thousands of reconstructive surgeries, we have never found it necessary to explore the retropubic space from above to control bleeding. Another potential source of excessive bleeding is during the dissection for the Martius flap which is discussed in section "Complications of Ancillary Procedures." It is possible to injure the distal ureter during a dissection for urethral reconstruction, but we have never seen this nor has it been reported. On two occasions, though, the ureter has been transected or avulsed in the course of removing mesh to which the ureter was adherent. One should be alert to the possibility of this complication whenever the dissection extends to the vicinity of the ureter or when traction is exerted on retropubic mesh. For that reason, it is always prudent to administer intravenous indigo carmine and check for ureteral patency by observing efflux of blue urine from each ureteral orifice through a cystoscope. When in doubt, retrograde pyelography should be done and a ureteral stent left in place if there appears to be an injury. In cases of avulsion or transaction of the ureter, immediate ureteroneocystotomy should be done.

Early Complications

All types of urethral reconstructive surgery share common complications like infection, flap necrosis, urinary retention, and postoperative bleeding, yet the overall incidence of major complications such as bleeding is very low. Complications related to the ancillary procedures like graft, flap, or sling placement are discussed below.

One of the earliest, but rare, complications of urethral reconstruction is wound infection and flap necrosis. Unrecognized infection may lead to the disruption of the suture lines, flap necrosis, and fistula formation; however, we could find no reports on this and none has ever occurred in our series.

Sharma et al. in a case series of 15 patients, who underwent dorsal onlay lingual mucosal graft urethroplasty for urethral stricture, reported one case of wound infection which was treated with antibiotics. The patient subsequently developed submeatal stenosis treated with monthly dilation [18].

Another potential complication is inadvertent traction on the catheter which occurred in one elderly patient in our series completely disrupting the repair. To prevent that, we routinely suture a Foley catheter to the anterior abdominal wall with a gentle loop in order to minimize tension on the urethra. Failure to maintain a correct position of the catheter may result in necrosis of the urethra. The urethral wound and the catheter should be checked frequently during postoperative care to ensure that there is no pressure on the suture line. Additionally, adequate bladder drainage should be maintained until the patient voids at 3 weeks postoperatively and VCUG does not show extravasation.

Another complication that may be encountered in the early postoperative period is urinary retention, but there are no reports of this in the literature that we reviewed and none has occurred in our series. If urinary retention were to occur, first check for meatal stenosis, and if present, a gentle attempt at urethral dilation should be done. If there is no obvious meatal stenosis, we recommend a gentle attempt at placement of a Foley catheter followed by trial of voiding after 2 weeks. If placement of the catheter is unsuccessful, a suprapubic catheter should be placed. If the patient fails the second voiding trial, we recommend cystoscopy, and if there is no obvious obstruction, videourodynamics. If urethral stricture is diagnosed, it should be dilated.

Late Complications

Because of the relatively small number of case series reported in the literature, available data cannot provide a consensus for management of various complications of urethral reconstructive surgery. In general, when urethral reconstruction is properly performed, it is associated with high long-term anatomic success rate and low complication rates. However, functional complications including overactive bladder and stress incontinence have been reported.

1. Postoperative sphincteric incontinence
Postoperative stress urinary incontinence is a result of unrecognized sphincteric incontinence before the procedure or a consequence of injury to the sphincter during dissection. In proximal urethral injuries postoperative incontinence rates may range between 44 and 80% unless a concomitant anti-incontinence surgery is performed [21].

Fig. 12.6 The completed repair with the Foley catheter sutured in place to prevent downward traction that could disrupt the wound (courtesy of J.G. Blaivas)

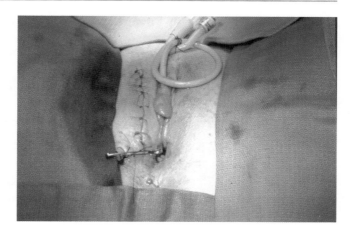

In the majority of studies, the criteria for incontinence following the reconstructive surgery are not specified leading to a likely underestimation of incidence.

In our previously published series of 74 patients who underwent vaginal flap urethroplasty, 62 women with preoperative incontinence underwent concomitant fascial pubovaginal sling placement. Successful anatomical repair was achieved in 93% patients and 87% considered themselves cured or improved with respect to incontinence. All patients with persistent postoperative stress incontinence were successfully treated by secondary procedures [1].

In our most recent case series of 9 women who underwent urethral stricture repair, 5 concomitant fascial slings were performed due to sphincteric incontinence. Postoperatively no urinary incontinence was reported and satisfactory outcome was achieved in all. Success or failure of anatomical repair and incontinence was assessed subjectively and objectively by validated questionnaires, physical examination, voiding diaries, and 24 h pad tests [22].

Recurrent sphincteric incontinence following urethral repair complicated by synthetic sling erosion is very common unless a concomitant anti-incontinence procedure is performed. Extensive scarring may preclude the successful repair, therefore some authors recommend a staged procedure to correct the incontinence [5].

Amundsen et al. reported persistent stress incontinence in 2 of 3 cases following synthetic sling removal, repair of the urethra, and Martius flap placement. All were treated with a second stage pubovaginal sling placement and injection of transurethral collagen. Interestingly, none of the patients after excision of the nonsynthetic sling required further anti-incontinence procedure. Clemens et al. reported 5 cases of recurrent postoperative stress incontinence in 6 patients who underwent removal of an eroded sling from the urethra or vaginal mucosa [23]. In our view documented preoperative sphincteric incontinence and compromised integrity of the sphincter during reconstruction are sufficient reasons to perform concomitant pubovaginal sling at the time of urethral reconstruction. First, harvesting of the fascial graft and placement of the sling around the urethra should be done, then the urethral reconstruction should be completed and, when necessary, the Martius flap is interposed between the reconstructed urethra followed by tensioning and tying the sling in place [24] (Fig. 12.6). When sphincteric incontinence develops after urethral reconstruction, treatment should be tailored to the patient. Of course any treatment at all is elective and some patients are not bothered enough to want to consider further treatment. In our judgment, the patient should be evaluated just as would be done if she had not had prior urethral reconstruction and, for us, that means a bladder questionnaire, diary, exam, uroflow, assessment of postvoid residual urine, videourodynamics, and cystoscopy. As a general rule, though, we defer this evaluation until about 3 months from the reconstructive surgery. If recurrent sphincteric incontinence is documented, we recommend a biologic sling, either autologous fascia or a xenograft or homograft. Ideally, the sling should be placed at a virgin site at the bladder neck, or the mid or proximal urethra. If the entire mid and proximal urethra has been reconstructed, it is possible to place the sling at the reconstructed urethra, but special care should be taken to not injure the urethra during the surgery. To this end we recommend that the plane of dissection around the urethra be accomplished sharply under direct vision with a scissor staying in a very superficial plane just beneath the vaginal epithelium. If there is any difficulty extending the dissection into the retropubic space, it should be opened from abdominal side and completed under direct vision. Depending on the nature of the prior reconstruction and the characteristics of the urethra, a Martius flap may be considered as well, placing it between the sling and reconstructed urethra. We do not recommend a synthetic sling in these circumstances.

2. Overactive bladder

Persistent or de novo overactive bladder symptoms can be problematic postoperatively. In our series of 74 women after urethral reconstruction, 16% of patients had severe urinary urgency or urge incontinence postoperatively, including those who underwent concomitant autologous pubovaginal sling placement [1]. The series by Onol et al. reports 2 cases of persistent urge incontinence in 17 women who underwent urethral stricture repair [6]. Similarly, Gormley et al. in their series counted 2 cases of persistent urge incontinence and 1 de novo urge incontinence among 12 women who had repair for urethral stricture [3].

The assessment of OAB symptoms should commence within days to weeks after their occurrence to look for remediable causes such as urinary tract infection, urethral obstruction, and incomplete bladder emptying.

Urinary tract infection should be treated with culture-specific antibiotics and urethral

obstruction and incomplete emptying ruled out by uroflow and measurement of postvoid residual urine. If symptoms persist after these conditions have been treated or excluded, empiric treatment can be tried, but if they prove unsuccessful after a month or so, we recommend cystoscopy and urodynamics to look for obstruction, foreign body, and stones. Patients with refractory OAB after 3 months or so, who underwent sling surgery as part of the reconstruction, are candidates for empiric sling incision or urethrolysis even if they appear unobstructed.

3. Urethral stricture

The strictures occurred after dorsal labia minora skin graft urethroplasty [9], dorsal lingual mucosa graft urethroplasty [18], ventral buccal mucosa graft urethroplasty [13], and all were distal to the initial reconstruction. In the first case, the patient reported recurrent urinary tract infections and lower urinary tract symptoms at 9 months after surgery. Meatal stenosis was diagnosed and treated with meatotomy and she was asymptomatic thereafter [9]. In another series, 2 patients presented with obstructive voiding symptoms at 3 months and lower urinary tract symptoms at 5 months follow-up [13, 18]. Both were found to have submeatal stenosis requiring urethral dilatations which resulted in complete resolution of symptoms at 12 months follow-up.

From our experience, urethral stricture may recur at 5 years or more after surgery. In 2 women from our recent case series who underwent vaginal flap urethroplasty, urethral recurrence was noted at 5 and 6 years. Subsequently both patients underwent successful urethral repair using dorsal buccal mucosa graft and were stricture-free at 12 and 15 months follow-up [22]. Both of these patients developed the recurrent stricture at the time of menopause, so it is possible that hormonal influences played a role in their genesis. To prevent recurrent strictures, we recommend that peri-menopausal and menopausal women be treated with topical estrogens. In a report by Gormley who described follow-up on 12 patients after vaginal flap urethroplasty for female stricture disease, 1 patient underwent repeat dilation 3 weeks after procedure due to narrowing of the bladder neck and another required cystoscopy with catheter insertion in the OR 58 months postoperatively [3].

Although most studies report good short-term success, long-term follow-up of every patient is recommended to avoid complications of unrecognized urethral stricture recurrence.

Unfortunately current sparse data are not enough to determine which factors may predispose a patient to stricture recurrence, thus allowing the employment of appropriate preventive measures. Inadequate fibrotic tissue excision due to failure to expose the urethra during surgery, ischemic changes, and wound contracture might possibly lead to stricture recurrence or narrowing of the urethra at a location different from the primary repair.

4. Sexual dysfunction

One of the possible adverse effects of urethral reconstruction is sexual dysfunction. From a theoretical standpoint, this is of particular concern after the dorsal dissection between the clitoris and urethra that is done for dorsal buccal mucosal graft urethroplasty which could damage the corporal bodies or nerves. To date, though, we are unaware of any reports of this complication. Further, we have specifically queried all of our patients who underwent this surgery about changes in sexual function, including orgasm and pain and none have suffered any negative sequelae.

Complications of Ancillary Procedures

After reconstruction of the severely damaged urethra, it is sometimes advisable to perform a concomitant pubovaginal sling and interpose a vascularized pedicle flap over the repair site. When an anti-incontinence procedure is deemed necessary, in the vast majority of cases, a Martius flap incorporating a labia majora fat pad can be successfully used. Other flaps include rectus abdominus muscle and gracilis myocutaneous flaps. Flaps improve vascularity of periurethral tissue bed, enhance granulation, separate the suture lines, and promote graft survival. For construction of a Martius flaps, a vertical incision is made over the labia majora and is carried down

through Scarpa's fascia. The fat pad is mobilized with attention to preserve the ventral blood supply from external pudendal artery or dorsal from internal pudendal artery. To minimize blood loss, it is important to incise Scarpa's fascia and dissect between it and the fat pad to create a flap. The fat pad is tunneled underneath the vaginal epithelium and sewn in place over the suture lines of the reconstructed urethra. To the inexperienced surgeon, the plane between Scarpa's fascia and the skin looks like a better plane. However, there are multiple, broad, flat veins from which bleeding is difficult to control, so that plane should be avoided.

If Martius flap is used, a penrose drain is traditionally left in for 24–48 h. The overall incidence of the complications attributable to Martius flap is low. In data by Elkins et al. on 35 women who underwent vesicovaginal and rectovaginal fistula repair with Martius graft, 2 had blood loss of more than 350 mL from the harvest site, 3 experienced cellulitis, and 2 dyspareunia due to narrowing of the vagina. However, in two circumstances of cellulitis and vaginal narrowing, closure of the vaginal mucosa over the flap was not possible and it was left to heal by secondary intention [2].

In our cumulative experience with urethral reconstructive surgery between 1983 and 2011, only 1 of 70 women who underwent vaginal flap repair with concomitant Martius graft required incision and drainage of the labial hematoma.

Serious hemorrhage can be prevented by careful dissection of the plane of fibroadipose tissue with avoidance of deep muscle tissue and attainment of meticulous hemostasis. Other complications of the labial flap may include an undesirable cosmetic effect, asymmetry, and impaired sensation at the harvest site [25].

Urinary retention, obstruction, urgency, and urge incontinence are well known complications after pubovaginal sling. The most recent AUA panel data reports 8% urinary retention rate after pubovaginal fascial sling placement without concurrent repair of prolapse. The rates of de novo urge incontinence and postoperative urge incontinence in patients with preexisting incontinence were 9% and 33%, respectively [26]. In our retrospective review of more than 500 women who underwent pubovaginal fascial sling procedure for stress incontinence, de novo urge incontinence occurred in 3% patients. Other complications such as wound infections, incisional hernia, or long-term urethral obstruction requiring surgery or intermittent catheterization each occurred in 1% of patients [27].

Conclusions

Urethral reconstruction in women is an uncommon surgery and as such complications are not well described in the literature. These can be minimized by a thorough preoperative work-up and preoperative planning. Intraoperative complications include hemorrhage and ureteral injury, though both are rare. Perioperative and postoperative complications include complications specific to graft or flap site, recurrence, incontinence, urethral obstruction, or detrusor overactivity. In our experience these complications are unusual and can be treated successfully. Because of the possibility of late recurrence of stricture, in our opinion long-term follow-up is mandatory.

References

1. Flisser AJ, Blaivas JG. Outcome of urethral reconstructive surgery in a series of 74 women. J Urol. 2003;169(6):2246–9.
2. Elkins TE, DeLancey JO, McGuire EJ. The use of modified Martius graft as an adjunctive technique in vesicovaginal and rectovaginal fistula repair. Obstet Gynecol. 1990;75(4):727–33.
3. Gormley EA. Vaginal flap urethroplasty for female urethral stricture disease. Neurourol Urodyn. 2010;29 Suppl 1:S42.
4. Tanello M, Frego E, Simeone C, Cosciani Cunico S. Use of pedicle flap from the labia minora for the repair of female urethral strictures. Urol Int. 2002; 69(2):95–8.
5. Amundsen CL, Flynn BJ, Webster GD. Urethral erosion after synthetic and non synthetic pubovaginal slings: differences in management and continence outcome. J Urol. 2003;170(1):134–7.
6. Onol FF, Antar B, Köse O, Erdem MR, Onol SY. Techniques and results of urethroplasty for female urethral strictures: our experience with 17 patients. Urology. 2011;77(6):1318–24.
7. Tsivian A, Sidi AA. Dorsal graft urethroplasty for female urethral stricture. J Urol. 2006;176(2):611–3.
8. Migliari R, Leone P, Berdondini E, De Angelis M, Barbagli G, Palminteri E. Dorsal buccal mucosa graft urethroplasty for female urethral strictures. J Urol. 2006;176(4 Pt 1):1473–6.
9. Rehder P. Dorsal urethroplasty with labia minora skin graft for female urethral strictures. BJU Int. 2010;106(8):1211.
10. Montorsi F, Salonia A, Centemero A, Guazzoni G, Nava L, DaPozzo LF, et al. Vestibular flap urethroplasty for strictures of the female urethra. Urol Int. 2002;69:12.
11. O'Connell HE, DeLancey JO. Clitoral anatomy in nulliparous, healthy, premenopausal volunteers using unenhanced magnetic resonance imaging. J Urol. 2005;173(6):2060–3.
12. Park JM, Hendren WH. Construction of female urethra using buccal mucosa graft. J Urol. 2001;166(2): 640–3.
13. Berglund RK, Vasavada S, Angermeier K, Rackley R. Buccal mucosa graft urethroplasty for recurrent stricture of female urethra. Urology. 2006;67(5): 1069–71.
14. Bhargava S, Chapple CR. Buccal mucosal urethroplasty: is it the new gold standard? BJU Int. 2004; 93(9):1191–3.
15. Souza GF, Calado AA, Delcelo R, Ortiz V, Macedo Jr A. Histopathological evaluation of urethroplasty with dorsal buccal mucosa: an experimental study in rabbits. Int Braz J Urol. 2008;34(3):345–51.
16. Dublin N, Stewart LH. Oral complications after buccal mucosal graft harvest for urethroplasty. BJU Int. 2004;94(6):867–9.
17. Kamp S, Knoll T, Osman M, Häcker A, Michel MS, Alken P. Donor-site morbidity in buccal mucosa urethroplasty: lower lip or inner cheek? BJU Int. 2005;96(4):619–23.
18. Sharma GK. Dorsal onlay lingual mucosal graft urethroplasty for urethral strictures in women. BJU Int. 2010;105(9):1309.
19. Simonato A, Gregori A, Lissiani A, Galli S, Ottaviani F, Rossi R, et al. The tongue as an alternative donor site for graft urethroplasty: a pilot study. J Urol. 2006;175(2):589–92.
20. Elkins TE, Ghosh TS, Tagoe GA, Stocker R. Transvaginal mobilization and utilization of the anterior bladder wall to repair vesicovaginal fistulas involving the urethra. Obstet Gynecol. 1992;79: 455–60.
21. Blaivas JG, Sandhu J. Urethral reconstruction after erosion of slings in women. Curt Opin Urol. 2004; 14(6):335–8.
22. Blaivas JG, Santos A, Tsui JF, Purohit RS, Weiss JP. Management of urethral stricture in women. Abstract number 1695 presented at the 2011 AUA under the "Urodynamics/ Incontinence/ Female Urology Podium".
23. Clemens JQ, DeLancey JO, Faerber GJ, Westney OL, Mcguire EJ. Urinary tract erosions after synthetic

pubovaginal slings: diagnosis and management strategy. Urology. 2000;56:589–94.

24. Blaivas JG, Heritz DM. Vaginal flap reconstruction of the urethra and vesical neck in women: a report of 49 cases. J Urol. 1996;155(3):1014–7.

25. Petrou SP, Jones J, Parra RO. Martius flap harvest site: patient self-perception. J Urol. 2002;167(5): 2098–9.

26. Dmochowski RR, Blaivas JM, Gormley EA, Juma S, Karram MM, Lightner DJ, et al. Update of AUA guideline on the surgical management of female stress urinary incontinence. J Urol. 2010;183(5):1906–14.

27. Blaivas JG, Chaikin DC. Pubovaginal fascial sling for the treatment of all types of stress urinary incontinence: surgical technique and long-term outcome. Urol Clin North Am. 2011;38(1):7–15, v.

Complications of Urethral Diverticulectomy

13

Alienor S. Gilchrist and Eric S. Rovner

Introduction

Urethral diverticulum (UD) is a rare condition and frequently can present diagnostic dilemmas to the clinician [1]. Once the correct diagnosis is made, surgical excision is the mainstay of definitive treatment. Although surgical treatment of urethral diverticula includes marsupialization, designed for a distal diverticula ostium, this review will focus on complications from the transvaginal approach for mid and proximal urethral diverticulum excision, as has been previously described. A full discussion of urethral diverticulectomy surgical technique is beyond the scope of this chapter, but specific points will be discussed where appropriate.

Prevention of Complications

Although most complications are treatable and reversible, the optimal scenario is to prevent or minimize potential for adverse outcomes.

This process begins in the preoperative period, initiated during the diagnostic evaluation and work-up. The typical evaluation of patients with a suspected UD consists of a history, physical examination, cystourethroscopy, and appropriate imaging, including voiding cystourethrograpy and magnetic resonance imaging as clinically indicated. For patients with lower urinary tract symptoms or incontinence, videourodynamic studies may be utilized to evaluate for the presence of stress incontinence, voiding dysfunction, and specifically for the presence of a closed, competent bladder neck at rest. With the presence of stress incontinence or an incompetent bladder neck, patients can be offered concomitant placement of an autologous fascial sling at the time of UD excision. Urine cytology, when positive, can assist in making the correct diagnosis of malignancy; however, negative cytology cannot rule out malignancy. In all cases, UDs should be sent for permanent pathologic evaluation following excision to evaluate for malignant tissue. Preoperative urine cultures are obtained to appropriately tailor preoperative antibiotics and decrease the risks of intraoperative and postoperative infection. The differential diagnosis of periurethral masses (Table 13.1) is extensive and includes Skene's gland abscess (Fig. 13.1), vaginal leiomyoma [2], and primary urethral cancer. Therefore, the importance of a correct diagnosis prior to undertaking surgical excision cannot be overemphasized.

A.S. Gilchrist, MD • E.S. Rovner, MD (✉)
Department of Urology, Medical University
of South Carolina, 96 Jonathan Lucas Street,
CSB 644, Charleston, SC 29425, USA
e-mail: rovnere@musc.edu

H.B. Goldman (ed.), *Complications of Female Incontinence and Pelvic Reconstructive Surgery,*
Current Clinical Urology, DOI 10.1007/978-1-61779-924-2_13, © Springer Science+Business Media, LLC 2013

Table 13.1 Differential diagnosis of a periurethral masses

Leiomyoma
Skene's gland abnormalities
Gartner's duct abnormalities
Vaginal wall cysts
Urethral mucosal prolapse
Urethral caruncle
Periurethral bulking agents
Malignancy
Endometriosis

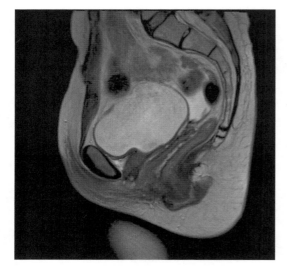

Fig. 13.1 Skene's gland abscess

Intraoperative Complications

Intraoperative complications related to anterior compartment vaginal surgery have been previously described and include, but are not limited to, bleeding and injury to the urinary tract.

Bleeding

The risk of bleeding during surgery can be minimized, but not entirely eliminated by good operative technique. Multiple blood vessels traverse the deep pelvis including large venous channels in the retropubic space. Named vessels in the obturator fossa along the pelvic sidewall including the iliac vessels and within the vascular pedicle of the bladder are at risk for injury, especially during passage of trocars or needles for concomitant pubovaginal sling. Major vascular injury can quickly lead to life-threatening hemorrhage if not recognized intraoperatively and may result in large retropubic hematomas postoperatively [3, 4]. Bleeding during the harvest of an adjuvant Martius flap is usually easily visualized and controlled with a combination of cautery, suture ligature, and direct compression. Labial hematomas have been reported with postoperative bleeding [5].

Bleeding during UD surgery can be problematic at times. The initial dissection of the vaginal flap from the underlying periurethral fascia should be associated with minimal bleeding. Bleeding encountered during this early dissection may indicate an excessively deep and incorrect surgical plane. In this circumstance, immediate recognition and reevaluation is necessary to avoid inadvertent entry into the urethral diverticulum or urinary tract and to minimize bleeding. Following identification of this situation, dissection should proceed in the proper surgical plane; in reoperative surgery, however, this may be difficult to identify.

Another common site of bleeding during transvaginal UD surgery occurs when traversing the endopelvic fascia for placement of a pubovaginal sling. Entry into the retropubic space from the transvaginal side or placement of the suprapubic needles or trocars from the abdominal side may be associated with copious bleeding as the endopelvic fascia is perforated. If the bleeding continues and is brisk, the vagina can be packed. It can be very helpful to manually elevate the anterior vaginal wall and compress it anteriorly against the posterior symphysis pubis for several minutes using the surgeon's hand, sponge stick, or a retractor. These maneuvers will effectively tamponade bleeding in the retropubic space. Packing and compression will result in adequate control in the majority of cases; if not, the surgeon should expeditiously complete the procedure, close the incisions, and pack the vagina [6]. Brisk bleeding that does not respond to manual compression for an extended period of time may suggest a major vessel injury and mandates retropubic exploration.

Urinary Tract Injury

Urethra

The Foley catheter is usually seen following complete excision of UD. The urethra can be reconstructed over as small as a 14F Foley catheter without long-term risk of urethral stricture and should be closed in a watertight fashion with absorbable suture [7]. The closure should be tension-free. Uncommonly, a UD may extend circumferentially around the urethra and require segmental resection of the involved portion of the urethra and complex reconstruction [8, 9].

Ureter

Ureteral injury during UD surgery is rare, but may occur with a large or proximal UD extending beyond the bladder neck and below the trigone. In these instances, cystoscopic placement of ureteric catheters prior to the dissection may aid in ureteral identification. Virtually all of these injuries can be identified by intraoperative cystoscopy. The administration of intravenous vital dyes such as indigo carmine permits obvious visualization of ureteral efflux confirming ureteral patency. Suspected ureteral injuries are confirmed by retrograde pyeloureterography. Ureteral transection requires ureteroneocystostomy.

Bladder

Intraoperative bladder injury may occur during dissection of a large UD extending proximal to the bladder neck and under the bladder (Fig. 13.2), or alternatively, may occur with passage of a ligature carrier through the retropubic space if placing a pubovaginal sling.

Injury to the bladder during UD excision is diagnosed intraoperatively by careful endoscopic examination of the bladder and bladder neck with a 70° lens following UD dissection and/or passage of the ligature carrier. The bladder should be filled and then examined to ensure that a small injury does not go unrecognized in a fold of the bladder wall.

To avoid injury during ligature carrier passage, the urethra should be clearly palpated, the bladder drained, and the pelvic anatomy well delineated. If a bladder injury is noted intraoperatively, the

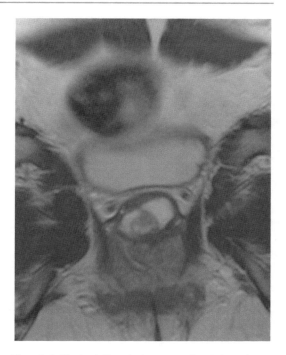

Fig. 13.2 Urethral diverticulum extending below trigone

ligature carrier should be removed and reinserted. Bladder perforation from a ligature carrier usually does not require primary closure.

Injury to the bladder floor during UD dissection requires cystoscopic examination to assess the extent of the injury and intravenous dyes should be administered to confirm ureteral integrity. Small cystotomies may be closed in layers with absorbable sutures transvaginally. More extensive injuries involving the trigone or more proximal bladder may require transabdominal repair. Postoperative drainage of the bladder with a Foley will help avoid urinoma, fistula formation, and pelvic abscess.

Postoperative Complications

Careful adherence to the principles of transvaginal urethral diverticulectomy should minimize postoperative complications (Table 13.2). Nevertheless, complications may arise (Table 13.3). One small series suggested that large diverticula (>4 cm) or those associated with a lateral or horseshoe

Table 13.2 Principles of transvaginal urethral diverticulectomy

Mobilization of a well-vascularized anterior vaginal wall flap(s)
Preservation of the periurethral fascia
Identification and excision of the neck of the UD or ostia
Removal of entire UD wall or sac (mucosa)
Watertight urethral closure
Multilayered, nonoverlapping closure with absorbable suture
Closure of dead space
Preservation or creation of continence

Table 13.3 Complications of transvaginal urethral diverticulectomy (adapted from Dmochowski [32])

Complication (% range of reported incidence)
Urinary incontinence (1.7–16.1%)
Urethrovaginal fistula (0.9–8.3%)
Urethral stricture (0–5.2%)
Recurrent UD (1–25%)
Recurrent UTI (0–31.3%)
Other
Hypospadias/distal urethral necrosis
Bladder or ureteral injury
Vaginal scarring or narrowing: dyspareunia, etc.

configuration may be associated with a greater likelihood of postoperative complications [10]. In a larger series, risk factors for failure or poor functional outcome included horseshoe or circumferential configuration or a previous (failed) surgical intervention. Large or more complex UD typically require greater dissection and more involved reconstruction. Common complications include recurrent urinary tract infections (UTIs), urinary incontinence, or recurrent UD, while urethrovaginal fistula is a more rare but devastating complication.

Incontinence

Stress Urinary Incontinence

Patients with preoperative symptomatic stress urinary incontinence (SUI) in association with UD can be offered simultaneous anti-incontinence surgery. Preoperative videourodynamics may be helpful in evaluating the anatomy of the UD,

assessing the competence of the bladder neck, and confirming the diagnosis of SUI. In patients with SUI and UD, Ganabathi and others have described excellent results with concomitant needle bladder neck suspension [7, 11], although such needle suspensions are rarely done anymore. More recently, pubovaginal autologous fascial slings have been utilized in patients with UD and SUI with satisfactory outcomes [1, 12, 13]. The role of synthetic midurethral slings, however, has not been well defined in this population and current AUA guidelines recommend against using synthetic material in this setting [14]. Placement of synthetic material adjacent to a fresh suture line following diverticulectomy in the setting of potentially infected urine may place the patient at higher risk for subsequent urethral erosion and vaginal extrusion of the sling material as well as urethrovaginal fistula formation and foreign body granuloma formation [14].

Significant postoperative de novo SUI may occur in between 7 and 16% of individuals undergoing urethral diverticulectomy surgery without a concomitant anti-incontinence surgery [5, 15, 16]. However, Lee et al. noted at least minor de novo SUI in 49% of patients following urethral diverticulectomy, the majority of which was minor and did not require additional therapy [17]. Only 10% of these individuals underwent a subsequent SUI operation. Risk factors for de novo SUI may include the size of the diverticulum (>30 mm) and more proximal location [16]. Ljungqvist et al. correlated de novo SUI with wide diverticulum excision in addition to size and location [5]. De novo SUI may arise from the extensive suburethral dissection required for a large UD and the more proximal UD location may compromise the urethral sphincter and bladder neck anatomical support and the sphincter mechanism [16]. Alternatively, large UD at the bladder neck may cause obstruction [18] and occult SUI may be unmasked after removing the obstructing UD [19].

Management of de novo postoperative SUI is undertaken after allowing postsurgical inflammation to subside. Autologous pubovaginal sling is a reasonable option in this setting. Synthetic materials such as midurethral polypropylene slings must be used judiciously in this setting, however, as safety data are lacking. Repeat preoperative imaging may be helpful in excluding a recurrent or persistent UD, or urethrovaginal fistula prior to surgery [5].

Urinary Urgency and Urge Incontinence

Stav et al. reported rates of urgency-frequency symptoms decreased significantly postoperatively from 60 to 16% and noted complete resolution of urge incontinence [16]. Other series, however, have demonstrated rates of postoperative urgency of 54% [20] and de novo urge incontinence in 36% of patients [5]. These symptoms may be managed expectantly postoperatively; nonetheless continual symptoms postoperatively may herald UD persistence or recurrence or de novo urethral obstruction. Importantly, urinary incontinence following UD excision should be evaluated to rule out the presence of urethrovaginal or vesicovaginal fistula.

Urethrovaginal Fistula

A urethrovaginal fistula located beyond the sphincteric mechanism should not be associated with symptoms other than perhaps a split urinary stream and/or vaginal voiding. As such, an asymptomatic distal urethrovaginal fistula may not require repair, although some patients may request repair. Conversely, a proximal fistula located at the bladder neck or at the midurethra in patients with an incompetent bladder neck will likely result in considerable symptomatic urinary leakage. These patients should undergo repair with consideration for the use of an adjuvant tissue flap such as a Martius flap to provide a well-vascularized additional tissue layer. The actual timing of the repair relative to the initial procedure is controversial, but should allow for tissue inflammation to subside. Meticulous attention to surgical technique, good hemostasis, avoidance of infection, preservation of the periurethral fascia, and a well-vascularized anterior vaginal wall flap, combined with a multilayered closure and nonoverlapping suture lines, should minimize the potential for postoperative urethrovaginal fistula formation [19].

Recurrent Symptoms

While complete resolution of obstructive and irritative urinary symptoms after UD excision may occur [16], some patients will have persistence or recurrence of their preoperative symptoms postoperatively. Ljungqvist et al. noted reoperation (but not necessarily extent of the primary operation) was the greatest clinical factor associated with residual symptoms postoperatively [5]. These symptoms may be from the surgery itself, and if so, may resolve over time. Alternatively, the finding of a UD following a presumably successful urethral diverticulectomy may occur as a result of incomplete excision of the initial lesion, or as a result of a new UD. Such symptoms should be investigated.

Recurrent Urethral Diverticulum

Recurrence of UD may be due to incomplete removal of the UD, inadequate closure of the urethra, failure to close residual dead space, excessive tension on the repair, infection, or other technical factors [19, 21]. Lee noted recurrent urethral diverticulum in 8/85 patients at follow-up of between 2 and 15 years from the initial UD resection [22], while Ljungqvist et al. reported recurrence in 11/68 patients over a 26-year follow-up [5]. The risk of recurrence of UD following transvaginal excision may be related to the complexity of the anatomical configuration. Han et al. reported no recurrent UD in 17 patients with simple UD, but of the 10 patients with circumferential UD, recurrence was noted in 6 (60%) [15]. Notably in this series, secondary procedures were not as successful in completely removing the UD. Ockrim et al. similarly cured all 19 patients presenting with simple urethral diverticula on the first attempt, but the 11 patients with complex anatomical configurations required a total of 17 procedures for success [18]. Ingber reported a 10% reoperation rate for UD recurrence which was associated with proximal UD location, multiplicity, and prior urethral vaginal surgery [20]. Recurrent UD after failed prior surgeries may lead to more complex, circumferential involvement [8]. Repeat urethral diverticulectomy surgery can be challenging due to altered anatomy, scarring, and the difficulty in identifying the proper anatomic planes. Prevention of recurrence, especially in reoperative UDs, includes the use of a Martius flap, while MRI remains invaluable in surgical planning to ensure complete excision [18, 23]. Complications such as fistula and recurrence of the UD are more common in reoperative cases [5].

Urethral Stricture

Urethral strictures are rare following UD excision; Rovner noted urethral stricture in 1/44 patients and Ljungvqist in 1/27 patients [5, 8]. It may result from closing the urethra too tightly or reconstructing it over too small a sound or in one instance, postoperative catheter dislodgement [8]. Additionally, poorly vascularized periurethral tissues can result in ischemic strictures postoperatively. A Martius flap should be considered intraoperatively to provide a healthy graft and assist in stricture prevention. A urethral stricture may be managed postoperatively with urethral dilation. Rarely is open reconstruction with urethroplasty necessary.

Recurrent Urinary Tract Infections

UTIs may persist following UD excision and may be due to recurrence or other etiologies. Ingber et al. found 23% of patients reported having three or more infections in the last year of follow-up after urethral diverticulectomy [20]. In a series of 30 patients, Ockrim found the incidence of recurrent UTIs decreased from 17 to 3% [18]. Recurrent UTI work-up can be undertaken once recurrent UD has been excluded.

Pain

Urethral pain and/or severe pelvic pain was significantly relieved or resolved in all patients following diverticulectomy in one series [8]. Romanzi found resolution of preoperative urethral pain in

all but 2 patients postoperatively [1]. Nonetheless, urethral pain may persist despite surgical intervention. Ockrim et al. reported persistent pain in 2 patients, despite repeat diverticulectomy including skeletalizing the urethra [18]. Persistent postoperative urethral and pelvic pain, in the absence of UD recurrence, may be secondary to postsurgical changes, long-standing chronic inflammation of the periurethral tissues from the prior UD, or multifactorial in etiology and may ultimately require a multimodal treatment approach.

Dyspareunia

Dyspareunia is one of the classic presenting symptoms of UD. In two larger series of UD patients with preoperative dyspareunia rates of 54% and 56%, rates dropped to 10% and 8%, respectively [16, 18]. Persistent or de novo dyspareunia postoperatively may result from postsurgical changes, including vaginal scarring and narrowing, especially in patients undergoing reoperation. Vaginal narrowing can be prevented by harvesting a wide-based vaginal flap, thereby avoiding subsequent devascularization and contracture. Romanzi et al. reported dyspareunia resulting from the Martius flap and labial point tenderness on the harvest side [1]. Patients should be counseled appropriately regarding possible postoperative persistence of this symptom and be well informed of the possible sequelae of the Martius flap harvest. Similar to persistent urethral and pelvic pain, postoperative management of dyspareunia may require a multimodal approach.

Hypospadias/Distal Urethral Necrosis

For those utilizing the Spence-Duckett marsupialization procedure, distal urethral necrosis and/or hypospadias are both possible complications.

Malignant Lesions

Malignant and benign tumors may be found in urethral diverticula. Approximately 10% of urethral diverticulectomy specimens may demonstrate histopathological abnormalities including metaplasia, dysplasia, or frank carcinoma which require long-term follow-up or additional therapy [24]. The most common malignant pathology in UD is adenocarcinoma, followed by transitional cell and squamous cell carcinomas [24, 25], which is in direct contrast to primary urethral carcinoma in which the primary histologic type is squamous cell carcinoma. Nonexcisional therapy of UD such as marsupialization or endoscopic incision can be combined with a biopsy to rule out malignancy [26]. Although it is interesting to speculate, it has not been conclusively demonstrated that any particular preoperative imaging modality such as ultrasound or MRI can reliably and prospectively diagnose a small malignancy arising in a UD [27]. There is no consensus on proper treatment in these cases, and recurrence rates are high with local treatment alone [25]. When considering curative therapy, it is unclear whether extensive surgery including cystourethrectomy with or without adjuvant external beam radiotherapy is superior to local excision followed by radiotherapy [28]. However, pelvic exenteration may offer the highest likelihood of prolonged disease-free interval [29].

Stones

Calculi within UD are not uncommon and may be diagnosed in 4–10% of cases [1, 30, 31] and are most likely due to urinary stasis and/or infection. This may be suspected by physical exam findings or noted incidentally on preoperative imaging. The presence of a stone will not significantly alter the evaluation or surgical approach and it can be removed with the UD specimen at the time of surgery.

References

1. Romanzi LJ, Groutz A, Blaivas JG. Urethral diverticulum in women: diverse presentations resulting in diagnostic delay and mismanagement. J Urol. 2000; 164:428.
2. Shirvani AR, Winters JC. Vaginal leiomyoma presenting as a urethral diverticulum. J Urol. 2000; 163:1869.
3. Rajan S, Kohli N. Retropubic hematoma after transobturator sling procedure. Obstet Gynecol. 2005; 106:1199.
4. Walters MD, Tulikangas PK, LaSala C, Muir TW. Vascular injury during tension-free vaginal tape procedure for stress urinary incontinence. Obstet Gynecol. 2001;98:957.
5. Ljungqvist L, Peeker R, Fall M. Female urethral diverticulum: 26-year followup of a large series. J Urol. 2007;177:219.
6. Ficazzola M, Nitti VW. Complications of incontinence procedures in women. In: Taneja S, Smith RB, Ehrlich RM, editors. Complications of urologic surgery: prevention and management. 3rd ed. Philadelphia: WB Saunders; 2001;482–498.
7. Ganabathi K, Leach GE, Zimmern PE, Dmochowski R. Experience with the management of urethral diverticulum in 63 women. J Urol. 1994;152:1445.
8. Rovner ES, Wein AJ. Diagnosis and reconstruction of the dorsal or circumferential urethral diverticulum. J Urol. 2003;170:82.
9. Tamada S, Iwai Y, Tanimoto Y, Ito S, Yoshida N, Kawashima H, et al. Urethral diverticula surrounding the urethra in women: report of 2 cases. Hinyokika Kiyo. 2000;46:639.
10. Porpiglia F, Destefanis P, Fiori C, Fontana D. Preoperative risk factors for surgery female urethral diverticula. Our experience. Urol Int. 2002;69:7.
11. Lockhart JL, Ellis GF, Helal M, Pow-Sang JM. Combined cystourethropexy for the treatment of type 3 and complicated female urinary incontinence. J Urol. 1990;143:722.
12. Faerber GJ. Urethral diverticulectomy and pubovaginal sling for simultaneous treatment of urethral diverticulum and intrinsic sphincter deficiency. Tech Urol. 1998;4:192.
13. Swierzewski III SJ, McGuire EJ. Pubovaginal sling for treatment of female stress urinary incontinence complicated by urethral diverticulum. J Urol. 1993; 149:1012.
14. Dmochowski RR, Blaivas JM, Gormley EA, et al. Update of AUA guideline on the surgical management of female stress urinary incontinence. J Urol. 2010; 183:1906.
15. Han DH, Jeong YS, Choo MS, Lee KS. Outcomes of surgery of female urethral diverticula classified using magnetic resonance imaging. Eur Urol. 2007; 51:1664.
16. Stav K, Dwyer PL, Rosamilia A, Chao F. Urinary symptoms before and after female urethral diverticulectomy—can we predict de novo stress urinary incontinence? J Urol. 2008;180:2088.
17. Lee UJ, Goldman H, Moore C, et al. Rate of de novo stress urinary incontinence after urethal diverticulum repair. Urology. 2008;71:849.
18. Ockrim JL, Allen DJ, Shah PJ, Greenwell TJ. A tertiary experience of urethral diverticulectomy: diagnosis, imaging and surgical outcomes. BJU Int. 2009; 103:1550.
19. Patel AK, Chapple CR. Female urethral diverticula. Curr Opin Urol. 2006;16:248.

20. Ingber MS, Firoozi F, Vasavada SP, et al. Surgically corrected urethral diverticula: long-term voiding dysfunction and reoperation rates. Urology. 2011;77:65.

21. Aspera AM, Rackley RR, Vasavada SP. Contemporary evaluation and management of the female urethral diverticulum. Urol Clin North Am. 2002;29:617.

22. Lee RA. Diverticulum of the female urethra: postoperative complications and results. Obstet Gynecol. 1983;61:52.

23. Lorenzo AJ, Zimmern P, Lemack GE, Nurenberg P. Endorectal coil magnetic resonance imaging for diagnosis of urethral and periurethral pathologic findings in women. Urology. 2003;61:1129.

24. Thomas AA, Rackley RR, Lee U, et al. Urethral diverticula in 90 female patients: a study with emphasis on neoplastic alterations. J Urol. 2008;180:2463.

25. Rajan N, Tucci P, Mallouh C, Choudhury M. Carcinoma in female urethral diverticulum: case reports and review of management. J Urol. 1993;150:1911.

26. McLoughlin MG. Carcinoma in situ in urethral diverticulum: pitfalls of marsupialization alone. Urology. 1975;6:343.

27. Chung DE, Purohit RS, Girshman J, Blaivas JG. Urethral diverticula in women: discrepancies between magnetic resonance imaging and surgical findings. J Urol. 2010;183:2265.

28. Patanaphan V, Prempree T, Sewchand W, et al. Adenocarcinoma arising in female urethral diverticulum. Urology. 1983;22:259.

29. Shalev M, Mistry S, Kernen K, Miles BJ. Squamous cell carcinoma in a female urethral diverticulum. Urology. 2002;59:773.

30. Ward JN, Draper JW, Tovell HM. Diagnosis and treatment of urethral diverticula in the female. Surg Gynecol Obstet. 1967;125:1293.

31. Ginesin Y, Bolkier M, Nachmias J, Levin DR. Primary giant calculus in urethral diverticulum. Urol Int. 1988;43:47.

32. Dmochowski R. Surgery for vesicovaginal fistula, urethrovaginal fistula, and urethral diverticulum. In: Walsh PC, Retik AB, Vaughan Jr ED, Wein AJ, editors. Campbell's urology. 8th ed. Philadelphia: WB Saunders; 2002.

Vesicovaginal and Urethrovaginal Fistula Repair

14

Michael Ingber and Ray Rackley

Introduction

A urogenital fistula is an abnormal communication between two structures which causes urine to leak into a space other than through the urethral meatus. Vesicovaginal fistulae represent the most common type of fistula encountered by pelvic surgeons today. In developed countries, the more common etiologies include pelvic surgeries for hysterectomy, incontinence, or pelvic reconstructive procedures [1]. In developing countries, pregnancy-related complications from obstructed labor result in ischemic injury to the bladder and vagina and can lead to very large fistulae that can be difficult to treat [2] (Table 14.1).

Regardless of the etiology, repair of vesicovaginal fistulae can be challenging, and complications can occur even when performed by expert surgeons. Patients with fistulae by their nature often have significant comorbidities that make them more prone to having complications. Furthermore, not only do tissue ischemia, inflammation, and devitalized tissue cause fistulae, but they also can

M. Ingber, MD (✉)
Department of Urogynecology, Saint Clare's
Health System, Denville, NJ 07834, USA

Department of Urology, Weill Cornell Medical College,
New York, NY, USA
e-mail: ingbermd@aol.com

R. Rackley, MD
Department of Urology, Cleveland Clinic,
Cleveland, OH, USA

be a limiting factor in proper management and cure. Controversies continue to exist with respect to the proper timing of treatment, route and method of surgery, and use of any adjuvant flaps. Nevertheless, several steps may be performed in order to minimize such perioperative issues. Herein we describe complications related to vesicovaginal and urethrovaginal fistulae and ways to prevent adverse outcomes from surgical repair.

Preoperative Considerations

Timing of Repair

Obstetrical fistulae typically have significant tissue ischemia due to prolonged pressure from the fetal head on the bladder wall. As such, most experts agree that waiting several months to fix such fistulae increases likelihood of success (Fig. 14.1). However, when to fix an iatrogenic fistula has been a subject of controversy for many years [3]. Each case should be managed individually, as both early repair and delayed repair may be successful in the appropriate circumstance [4–7]. In general, fistulae which are recognized within several days of injury should be immediately repaired. Delaying in cases of immediate recognition only causes additional psychological suffering, given the significant amount of leakage that patients will experience while waiting for repair. In cases where tissue edema and inflammation prevent successful repair, a waiting period of several weeks to months may be appropriate.

H.B. Goldman (ed.), *Complications of Female Incontinence and Pelvic Reconstructive Surgery*,
Current Clinical Urology, DOI 10.1007/978-1-61779-924-2_14, © Springer Science+Business Media, LLC 2013

Table 14.1 Causes of urogenital fistulae

Congenital
Acquired
Iatrogenic
Postoperative
Hysterectomy
Abdominal
Transvaginal
Laparoscopic
Incontinence procedures
Transvaginal slings
Retropubic
Laparoscopic
Prolapse procedures
Anterior colporrhaphy
Mesh kits
Sacrospinous/uterosacral fixation
Urethral diverticulectomy
Endoscopic procedures
Bowel and vascular surgeries
Radiation injury
Noniatrogenic
Pelvic malignancy
Obstructed labor
Trauma
Sexual injury
Infection
Foreign body

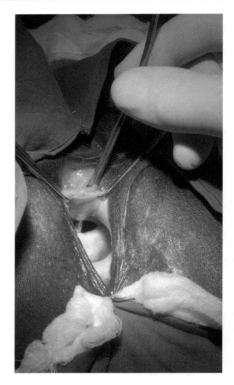

Fig. 14.1 Obstetric vesicovaginal fistulae are typically larger, due to prolonged tissue ischemia

Diagnostic Studies

Determining the location of severe vaginal urinary leakage is often the most challenging part of an incontinence evaluation. While voiding cystourethrograms and plain cystograms can often demonstrate the presence of a fistula, they often fail to demonstrate the exact location of vesicovaginal fistulae, as well as the presence of multiple fistulae (Fig. 14.2). Additionally, ureteral injury can be present in up to 12% of cases of vesicovaginal fistulae, and recognition of this preoperatively is essential [8]. CT Urography has largely replaced intravenous pyelography as a diagnostic modality of choice when evaluating upper tract damage or fistula. Cystoscopy is an essential component in the evaluation of any woman with unexplained or continuous incontinence.

Typically, cystoscopy can show a fistulous tract, or at least suggest fistula due to severe inflammatory changes (Fig. 14.3). Retrograde pyelogram at the time of cystoscopy can usually demonstrate ureteral extravasation of contrast (Fig. 14.4). Alternatively, CT Urography can show locations of urinary extravasation and often be diagnostic of ureterovaginal fistula (Fig. 14.5).

Approaches to Fistula Repair

Determining which route to perform fistula repair is of utmost importance in order to prevent untoward complications. Most fistula experts agree that the first attempt at repair is the most important surgery which can provide the surgeon with the opportunity to definitively repair the defect. Therefore, the first attempt should be the route in which the surgeon feels most comfortable with. There are some benefits, however, to choosing specific methods based on the type of fistula.

Fig. 14.2 Performing a careful examination is essential, as many patients have multiple fistulae which should all be addressed simultaneously during surgical repair. This patient had both a vesicovaginal and a urethrovaginal fistula

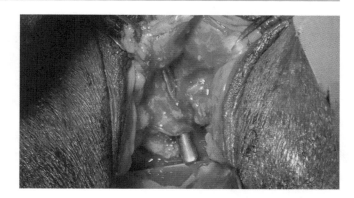

Fig. 14.3 Cystoscopic examination will often show a fistulous tract, or area of inflammation suspicious for vesicovaginal fistula

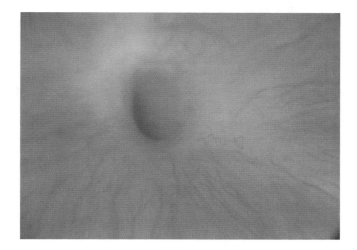

Fig. 14.4 Retrograde pyelogram demonstrating ureteral extravasation of contrast into vagina. With ureterovaginal fistulae, early ureteral stenting may avert need for ureteral reimplantation

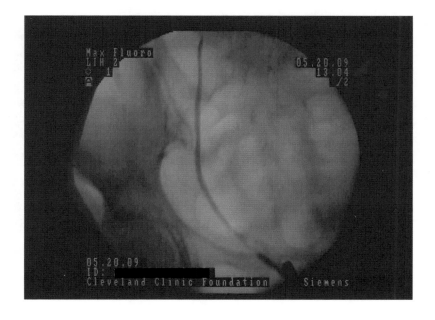

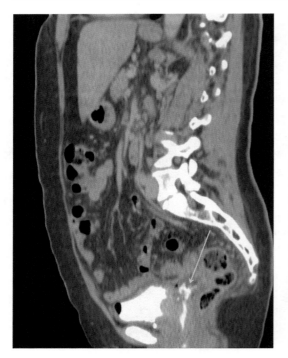

Fig. 14.5 CT Urography can be an excellent imaging modality when evaluating for presence of fistula. Here, a communication can be seen (*arrow*) between the distal ureter and vagina

Open Abdominal Repair

The abdominal route may be preferred in women who have poor vaginal access, ischemic tissue from radiation, or those in whom a laparoscopic approach is contraindicated. Women with multiple fistulae including other organs (i.e., enterovaginal fistulae) are often better served with an open abdominal approach. Large, well-vascularized adjuvant tissue flaps are a major advantage to open abdominal approaches and may decrease recurrence risk in such cases. Complications related to open repair include wound infection, incisional hernia, and increased bleeding risk.

Transvaginal Repair

Choosing a transvaginal route and avoiding intraperitoneal access is often a preferred method in most fistulae, provided that the surgeon has access to the site. Specifically, for distally located fistulae, the transvaginal route is recommended, as fistula repair can be performed in an outpatient setting. Some practitioners prefer the Latzko partial

colpocleisis to repair apical fistulae, as this method has rather high success rates [9–11]. Most women handle postoperative pain well with the transvaginal route. Complications specific to the transvaginal route include vaginal shortening and vaginal stenosis which may lead to dyspareunia.

Laparoscopic and Robotic-Assisted Laparoscopic Repair

Several authors have described laparoscopic and robotic-assisted laparoscopic repair of vesicovaginal fistulae [12]. The advantage of utilizing robotic technology is the ability to have excellent magnified views of the repair, along with the ability to suture for those surgeons not experienced in laparoscopic suturing techniques. Robotic and laparoscopic repairs are often a preferred route in apical fistulae that are unable to be reached vaginally, as they provide superior visualization to defects in this area when compared to the open route. One potential disadvantage that could lead to increased risk for recurrence is the difficulty in obtaining an interposed omental flap, although peritoneal flaps are typically easy to obtain during laparoscopic repair.

In a recent report, authors compared intraoperative data and outcomes of 12 robotic-assisted repairs to 20 open surgical repairs [13]. All subjects in the robotic group and 90% of those in the open cohort were managed successfully. Not surprising, mean blood loss was significantly less in the robotic group (88 mL vs. 170 mL, $p < 0.05$). Mean hospital stay was also shorter in the robotic group (3.1 vs. 5.6 days, $p < 0.05$). In the authors' experience, laparoscopic and robotic-assisted repairs can typically be discharged home after a 23 h stay. Neither group had a significant difference in complication rate. Complications relevant to laparoscopic repair include port-site hernias, bowel injury, and adjacent organ injury.

Intraoperative Considerations

Because of the already present poor tissue conditions that led to development of a fistula in the first place, intraoperative complications can be relatively common during fistula surgery.

Fig. 14.6 Permanent sutures should never be used during fistula repair. Similarly, absorbable suture knots should be tied external to the bladder mucosa, in order to prevent fistula recurrence and stone formation, as in this patient

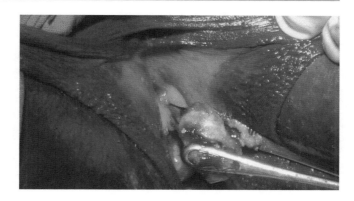

Complications During Dissection

Many fistulae are surrounded by significant inflammation, which can lead to excessive bleeding and poor visualization intraoperatively. Careful dissection is of utmost importance when performing repair, as the surgeon must obtain several layers of closure to prevent recurrence. Complications may occur if the initial dissection of the vaginal epithelium is too deep, and additional layers of closure are unattainable. Excess bleeding may result when improper tissue planes are entered. In cases where flaps are too thin for a good watertight closure, adjuvant tissue flaps utilizing omentum (in abdominal repair) or a Martius flap (in vaginal repair) are crucial.

The authors do not routinely excise the entire fistula tract. Nevertheless, in cases of prior malignancy or in postradiation fistulae, one should obtain a biopsy to ensure that there is no malignancy at the site of the fistula. Any nonviable tissue should always be removed in order to obtain better healing. Avoidance of cautery is important, as excess cautery can compromise blood supply to tissue flaps and jeopardize healing. Hence, significant bleeding should be controlled with interrupted suture.

Complications related to adjacent organ injury are relatively uncommon. If the ureters are close to the repair, they should be stented initially. Ureteral injury may be a result of cautery injury or sharp dissection and should be recognized immediately. A small ureteral defect may be repaired primarily. However, extensive cautery injury, or full transection, typically requires reimplantation in order to prevent ureteral leak or

stricture formation. Injury to the bowel may occur during transperitoneal repair, either immediately from dissection injury, or 1–2 weeks following repair due to cautery injury. Patients with prior pelvic radiation may have more inflammation, resulting in additional adhesions, and can be more prone to such injuries.

Closure

Choosing the proper suture is extremely important in minimizing complications. Closure of the bladder or urethral defect should be performed with absorbable suture such as 3-0 polygalactin or 3-0 chromic. If knots are tied on the intravesical side, a patient may be predisposed to developing calcifications or infections due to delayed absorption when exposed to urine. Nonabsorbable suture should never be used during fistula repair, as permanent suture material can lead to infections and stone formation within the bladder (Fig. 14.6). Additional layers such as a pubocervical fascial layer should also be closed with absorbable suture so that suture lines are non-overlapping. Once fully closed, the repair should be tested for water-tightness by instilling saline. Any sites of leakage along the suture line should be oversewn with additional suture to ensure complete closure.

Adjuvant Flaps

Providing an additional layer of closure should be considered when a three-layer closure is not able to be performed, or when tissue quality may compromise proper healing. Interposed tissue flaps should be secured with absorbable suture at least 1–2 cm beyond the site of repair. Complications related to harvesting flaps are relatively minimal and are typically limited to bleeding from the site of where the flap was obtained. One study evaluated eight women who underwent Martius flap surgery and questioned subjects on appearance of the harvest site and any postoperative complications [14]. Three (38%) women felt the appearance of the flap site was different from the contralateral labia. At 1 year after the procedure, one patient (13%) complained of dyspareunia, three (38%) patients had intermittent discomfort in the harvest area, and five patients (62%) complained of permanently decreased sensation or numbness at the harvest site. Another study evaluating mostly obstetrical urethrovaginal and vesicovaginal fistulae, however, showed decreased incidence of dyspareunia as well as recurrence after Martius interposition [15].

Omental flaps are an excellent source of adjuvant tissue during transabdominal repair and can occasionally be accessible during transvaginal repair in posthysterectomy vesicovaginal fistulae. The blood supply to omental flaps are based upon the right or left gastroepiploic artery, although the right gastroepiploic is both larger and more caudal, allowing for better reach distally during intra-abdominal fistula repair. Regardless, tissue interposition should be determined based on the quality of repair. All patients should be counseled about potential use of flaps and the complications specific to the site of tissue interposition.

Postoperative Complications

Not unexpectedly, the most common complication encountered after vesicovaginal and urethrovaginal fistula repair is recurrence of the fistula. With a complete preoperative workup, attention to basic fistula principles, and careful surgical repair, recurrence rates can be minimal. Should a recurrence occur, management can be via any route.

To a woman suffering from continuous incontinence from a fistula, persistence of urinary incontinence despite a properly repaired fistula can be devastating. Stress incontinence may occur after both transvaginal and transabdominal fistula repair if the dissection disrupts the ligamentous support of the urethra or the sphincteric mechanism. In several series, the rate of stress incontinence after fistula repair ranges from 4 to 33% after surgery and are likely higher in obstetrical fistula [16, 17]. Risk factors of stress incontinence after fistula surgery include involvement of the urethra, small bladder capacity, large fistula, and need for extensive vaginal reconstruction [18]. In women with vesicovaginal fistula and concomitant stress incontinence, a simple midurethral sling may be performed provided that the urethral dissection is well away from any fistula repair. However, in the setting of any periurethral dissection during fistula repair, it is the authors' preference that any therapy for stress incontinence wait until after total healing occurs after fistula surgery.

Urinary tract infection is a relatively common complication of fistula repair postoperatively, as instrumentation of the urinary bladder itself can predispose a woman to infection. Studies evaluating antibiotic use during and after fistula repair are limited to obstetric fistula. In a review of single-dose gentamicin vs. extended postoperative antibiotics during 722 obstetric fistula repairs in Ethiopia, Muleta et al. showed no difference in rates of postoperative infection [19]. Regardless of postoperative antibiotic use, sterilization of the urine prior to repair is of utmost importance, as preoperative urinary tract infection may increase the likelihood of fistula recurrence [20]. The authors occasionally use a low-dose antibiotic such as nitrofurantoin while patients await repair not only to prevent perioperative urinary tract infection, but also to decrease tissue edema and inflammation which allows for easier repair.

Urinary urgency may occur after any vaginal surgery which involves dissection around the urethra and the bladder. Rates of postoperative urinary urgency are difficult to determine due to the few studies that have used urinary urgency as an outcome. However, in one small study evaluating 20 genitourinary fistulae, seven (35%) developed urinary urgency postoperatively. Because de novo urgency can be an irritative complication, it should be discussed preoperatively with patients.

Fig. 14.7 Urethrovaginal fistula can affect the external sphincter and simple repair of the defect may still result in chronic incontinence. This patient required autologous fascial sling to correct the resulting stress incontinence after fistula repair (courtesy Howard B. Goldman, MD)

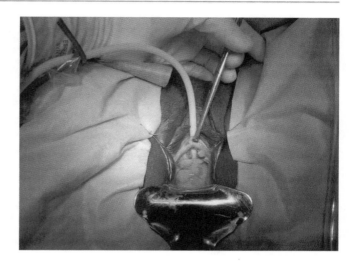

It is the authors' preference to offer patients anticholinergic therapy during the healing phase when catheters are present to minimize uninhibited detrusor contractions. Rarely, patients may have persistent urinary urgency even several months after repair. When such a complication occurs, urodynamic investigation to ensure no evidence for bladder outlet obstruction is essential. Long-term treatment of the urgency may be required in some patients.

Vaginal shortening is more common with apical fistulae when the Latzko partial colpocleisis is utilized. However, when done appropriately, only 1–2 cm of vaginal length is compromised, and this should not be an issue. Typically, women can remain sexually active without major problems with dyspareunia even when significant vaginal shortening occurs [21]. Nevertheless, vaginal shortening should be mentioned when counseling women who are sexually active, as women may recognize the change in anatomy with deep penetration of their partner.

Urethrovaginal Fistula

In developed countries, urethrovaginal fistulae are most commonly a result of previous vaginal surgery. Symptoms are variable as are techniques for repair. Like vesicovaginal fistula, complications specific to urethrovaginal fistula most commonly involve recurrence, with 10% of primary repairs recurring in a recent series [22]. Knowing the location and number of the fistulae are extremely important.

Because of the proximity of the urethral sphincter, patients with urethrovaginal fistula that occur within the proximal and/or middle urethra are prone to development or worsening of stress urinary incontinence after repair (Fig. 14.7). In the aforementioned study, of 71 subjects undergoing repair, 37 (52.1%) developed stress incontinence after repair [22]. Some surgeons advocate the use of autologous fascia in order to correct stress incontinence during urethrovaginal fistula repair [23, 24], but the authors typically prefer to wait until any fistula repair is complete. Once several months of healing has occurred, if the incontinence remains, it may be assessed, and a synthetic or autologous sling may be placed if necessary.

Conclusion

Vesicovaginal and urethrovaginal fistulae are conditions which require extensive preoperative planning, experience-driven intraoperative judgment, and close outpatient follow-up. When basic principles of fistula repair are followed, complications may be minimized, and subsequently, chances of a successful repair can be maximized.

References

1. Lafay Pillet M, Leonard F, Chopin N, et al. Incidence and risk factors of bladder injuries during laparoscopic hysterectomy indicated for benign uterine pathologies: a 14.5 years experience in a continuous series of 1501 procedures. Hum Reprod. 2009;24(4): 842–9.
2. Muleta M. Obstetric fistula in developing countries: a review article. J Obstet Gynaecol Can. 2006;28(11): 962–6.
3. Blaivas J, Heritz D, Romanzi L. Early versus late repair of vesicovaginal fistulas: vaginal and abdominal approaches. J Urol. 1995;153(4):1110–2.
4. Shelbaia AM, Hashish NM. Limited experience in early management of genitourinary tract fistulas. Urology. 2007;69(3):572–4.
5. Badenoch D, Tiptaft R, Thakar D, et al. Early repair of accidental injury to the ureter or bladder following gynaecological surgery. Br J Urol. 1987;59(6): 516–8.
6. Persky L, Herman G, Guerrier K. Non-delay in vesicovaginal fistula repair. Urology. 1979;13:273.
7. Blandy J, Badenoch D, Fowler C, et al. Early repair of iatrogenic injury to the ureter or bladder after gynecological surgery. J Urol. 1991;146(3):761–5.
8. Goodwin W, Scardino P. Vesicovaginal and ureterovaginal fistulas: a summary of 25 years of experience. J Urol. 1980;123:370–4.
9. Tancer M. The post-total hysterectomy (vault) vesicovaginal fistula. J Urol. 1980;123(6):839–40.
10. Ansquer Y, Mellier G, Santulli P, Bennis M, Mandelbrot L, Madelenat P, et al. Latzko operation for vault vesicovaginal fistula. Acta Obstet Gynecol Scand. 2006;85(10):1248–51.
11. Dorairajan L, Khattar N, Kumar S, et al. Latzko repair for vesicovaginal fistula revisited in the era of minimal-access surgery. Int Urol Nephrol. 2008; 40(2):317–20.
12. Hemal AK, Kolla SB, Wadhwa P. Robotic reconstruction for recurrent supratrigonal vesicovaginal fistulas. J Urol. 2008;180(3):981–5.
13. Gupta NP, Mishra S, Hemal AK, Mishra A, Seth A, Dogra PN. Comparative analysis of outcome between open and robotic surgical repair of recurrent supratrigonalvesico-vaginal fistula. J Endourol. 2010; 24(11):1779–82.
14. Petrou SP, Jones J, Parra RO. Martius flap harvest site: patient self-perception. J Urol. 2002;167(5): 2098–9.
15. Rangnekar NP, Imdad Ali N, Kaul SA, Pathak HR. Role of the martius procedure in the management of urinary-vaginal fistulas. J Am Coll Surg. 2000;191(3): 259–63.
16. Holme A, Breen M, MacArthur C. Obstetric fistulae: a study of women managed at the Monze Mission Hospital, Zambia. BJOG. 2007;114(8):1010–7.
17. Zambon JP, Batezini NS, Pinto ER, Skaff M, Girotti ME, Almeida FG. Do we need new surgical techniques to repair vesico-vaginal fistulas? Int Urogynecol J Pelvic Floor Dysfunct. 2010;21(3):337–42.
18. Browning A. Risk factors for developing residual urinary incontinence after obstetric fistula repair. BJOG. 2006;113(4):482–5.
19. Muleta M, Tafesse B, Aytenfisu HG. Antibiotic use in obstetric fistula repair: single blinded randomized clinical trial. Ethiop Med J. 2010;48(3):211–7.
20. Ayed M, El Atat R, Hassine LB, Sfaxi M, Chebil M, Zmerli S. Prognostic factors of recurrence after vesicovaginal fistula repair. Int J Urol. 2006;13(4): 345–9.
21. Occhino JA, Trabuco EC, Heisler CA, Klingele CJ, Gebhart JB. Changes in vaginal anatomy and sexual function after vaginal surgery. Int Urogynecol J Pelvic Floor Dysfunct. 2011;22(7):799–804.
22. Pushkar DY, Dyakov VV, Kosko JW, Kasyan GR. Management of urethrovaginal fistulas. Eur Urol. 2006;50(5):1000–5.
23. Blaivas JG, Purohit RS. Post-traumatic female urethral reconstruction. Curr Urol Rep. 2008;9(5): 397–404.
24. Golomb J, Leibovitch I, Mor Y, Nadu A, Ramon J. Fascial patch technique for repair of complicated urethrovaginal fistula. Urology. 2006;68(5):1115–8.

Complications of Transvaginal Bladder Neck Closure

David A. Ginsberg

Indications

The indication for an adult woman to undergo a transvaginal BNC is an eroded and destroyed bladder neck/urethra secondary to a chronic, indwelling catheter. While the indication for the initial catheter placement may be varied, the chain of events leading to this scenario is usually quite similar. The catheter is usually placed for refractory urinary incontinence or retention, usually of neurogenic etiology but not necessarily.

The common clinical scenario that results in an incompetent, eroded urethra is initiated with the simple decision to manage a patient with an indwelling catheter. With long-term catheter use, female patients may experience urethral erosion, which often leads to urinary leakage around the catheter. This erosive reaction is often further exacerbated by the caregivers' decision to use a larger catheter size and inflate the balloon with larger volumes of water. The hope is that this will minimize leakage around the catheter; however, this often results in further urethral erosion. Erosion can be so severe that catheters cannot be maintained in the bladder and spontaneously fall out. In addition, a poorly secured catheter that is

traumatically pulled out over and over can also contribute to urethral injury. If severe enough, the urethra becomes overly patulous and a urethral indwelling catheter cannot be maintained. The urethra can be wide enough and short enough that one or two fingers can be inserted directly into the bladder [1]. In addition, the erosion can be severe enough that when a finger is inserted into the urethra, the undersurface of the pubic symphysis is directly palpated as there is no remaining urethral tissue anteriorly. Because of the length of the urethra, this is rarely an issue in the male patient; the analogous reaction in the male to long-term catheter usage would be a traumatic hypospadias.

For these women there are few options besides use of pads/diapers. There is no female version of a condom catheter and many of these patients are not interested in or physically unable to undergo lower urinary reconstruction due to their disability. Placement of a suprapubic catheter (SP) is a nice option for these patients, and by itself, may be sufficient to control leakage of urine per the eroded urethra [2]. However, depending on the degree of the erosion and damage, leakage may still occur per the urethra despite continuous drainage per the SP tube. For these patients, options include placement of an obstructing sling or BNC. Sling placement is nice in that it does not permanently close the bladder neck; however, these outlets are often so damaged that there is not an adequate amount of urethral damage to allow for sling placement. Approaches for BNC include transvaginal and transabdominal.

D.A. Ginsberg, MD (✉)
Department of Urology, Keck School
of Medicine of USC, USC Institute of Urology,
1441 Eastlake Avenue, NOR 7416, Los Angeles,
CA 90033-9178, USA
e-mail: rovnere@musc.edu

H.B. Goldman (ed.), *Complications of Female Incontinence and Pelvic Reconstructive Surgery*,
Current Clinical Urology, DOI 10.1007/978-1-61779-924-2_15, © Springer Science+Business Media, LLC 2013

The transabdominal approach is often done in conjunction with some type of LUT reconstruction, is more invasive than a vaginal procedure, and has been reported to have lower rate of post-op leak/fistula formation. The alternative is a transvaginal approach which is often done in conjunction with SP tube placement; it is less invasive but may be a more challenging procedure for surgeons less experienced with vaginal surgery [3].

Complications

There is essentially one primary complication associated with BNC which is continued leakage and formation of a vesicovaginal fistula (VVF) between the attempted closure site and anterior vaginal wall. The fistula rate after the initial surgery ranges between 0 and 100% and is summarized in Table 15.1. The various surgical techniques described are fairly similar and are based on several essential principals: (1) complete mobilization of the urethra/bladder neck off the supporting pelvic ligaments; (2) resection of necrotic tissue down to healthy, viable tissue before closure is attempted: (3) multilayered closure; (4) mobilization of a large anterior vaginal wall flap to advance over the BNC.

Depending on the degree of erosion, it is possible that BNC may occur close to the ureteral orifices. It is important that the ureteral orifices are identified prior to BNC to minimize risk of damage. Certainly there is a theoretical risk of ureteral injury at the time of BNC, though that has not been previously described in the literature.

Table 15.1 Bladder neck closure fistula rate

References	Patients	Fistula rate (%)
Zimmern et al. [1]	6	0
Nielsen and Bruskewitz [10]	5	20
Eckford et al. [11]	50	22
Levy et al. [3]	4	50
Andrews and Shah [2]	8	50
Stoffel and McGuire [12]	8	87.5
Ginger et al. [4]	2	100
Rovner et al. [5]	11	9

The remainder of this chapter will focus on steps to minimize the risk of forming a fistula after transvaginal BNC peri-operatively as well as how to manage the problem if a fistula does occur.

Pre-op

There is unfortunately little that can be done pre-operatively to enhance success postoperatively in these patients. One important decision the surgeon should make is whether or not to perform BNC at all, and if so, via which approach. Levy et al. reviewed their experience with 12 patients, all of whom underwent BNC for urethral injury secondary to long-term indwelling catheters [3]. The first four patients all underwent a primary transvaginal approach. Of those, two succeeded and the other two failed a total of five transvaginal attempts to close the bladder neck, resulting in a success rate of 50%. Both of these patients ultimately underwent successful BNC with a combined abdominal and vaginal approach. The next ten patients (eight new patients and the two that had failed the prior transvaginal attempts) underwent combined abdominal and vaginal approach with 100% success. The authors' recommendation at the time was that a purely transvaginal approach may not be optimal if the operating surgeon does not have extensive experience performing transvaginal surgery. This manuscript was published in 1994 and one would hope that more urologic surgeons are comfortable with transvaginal surgery. However, if that is not the case, then use of an abdominal approach should be considered. There are few studies that evaluated outcomes using multiple approaches; however, a study by Ginger et al. revealed a 11% leakage rate in 26 patients undergoing a transabdominal BNC compared to a 100% leakage rate in the two patients in their study that underwent transvaginal BNC [4].

Poor nutrition is one issue that could be improved preoperatively. Rovner et al. correctly state that many of these patients often have multiple medical comorbidities and poor nutritional status at baseline [5]. Poor nutrition has been shown to impact wound healing, increase susceptibility to infection, and place the patient at increased risk for pulmonary complications, prolonged hospitalization, and mortality [6]. However, preoperative nutritional supplementation appears to only be valuable in severely malnourished patients; in all other patients, surgery does not need to be delayed [7].

Intra-op

To minimize risk of postoperative failure and leak, there are several surgical steps that should be emphasized. Initially, two incisions are made. One is made circumferentially around the external urethra meatus. The other incision, along the anterior vaginal wall, allows for the dissection of a wide, anterior vaginal wall flap when beginning the procedure. This flap is advanced once the BNC is complete past the area of repair, thus minimizing the presence of overlapping suture lines. Prior to closing the bladder neck, appropriate mobilization is necessary. This includes transection of the urethra completely off the pubourethral ligament dorsally and the urethropelvic ligaments and remaining attachments laterally. Optimal mobility of the bladder neck is extremely important. Without mobility the closure of the bladder neck itself is very challenging. Prior to closing the urethra/bladder neck, all necrotic tissue should be resected down to viable tissue. This often results in resecting all if not the entire urethra. Thus, mobility allows the surgeon to pull the bladder neck out towards you with stays; thus making the actual closure of the bladder neck less challenging. In addition, with adequate mobility of the closed bladder neck, it can be mobilized anteriorly away from the vaginal wall closure. After closing the bladder neck in two layers, I will tag the sutures. The needle attached to those BNC sutures can then be brought through the undersurface of the pubic symphysis or even the anterior abdominal wall. Without adequate mobility the surgeon is unable to get to this area and the closed bladder neck cannot be easily maneuvered upwards in the appropriate direction. If successful, the suture line of the BNC is essentially mobilized anteriorly, well away from the vaginal wall. Theoretically, this will help minimize formation of the fistula if the initial repair is not watertight.

Closure of the bladder neck with multiple layers is certainly an important step and several techniques have been described. Zimmern et al. used an initial vertical and anterior–posterior layer followed by a second layer placed transversely in perivesical fascia and detrusor muscle superficially [1]. Rovner et al. described a modification of this technique using a posterior urethral flap (Fig. 15.1). Once the bladder neck has been fully mobilized, the dorsal urethra is bivalved into the anterior bladder wall for 2–3 cm. The bivalved posterior urethral flap is then rotated cephalad and secured to the anterior bladder wall. That suture line is subsequently rotated upwards to the retropubic space, behind the pubic symphysis [5]. It should be noted that use of an adjuvant flap or graft placement is not usually required for primary repairs; these techniques are more commonly seen for patients requiring redo surgery for postoperative fistula after failure of primary BNC [4].

Post-op

Without appropriate postoperative management, even the best of repairs will break down, resulting in formation of a VVF. The importance of optimal drainage post-op in these patients cannot be overemphasized. Ginger et al. noted a significant association between poor post-op catheter care and persistent leakage [4]. A total of 29 patients in their series underwent retropubic BNC, with eight of these patients continuing to have persistent urinary leakage post-op. This was directly attributable to catheter mismanagement in seven of the eight patients. An appropriately sized suprapubic tube should be placed, secured, and optimally drained postoperatively to help ensure healing of the suture line along the closed bladder neck.

In addition to poor drainage, residual detrusor overactivity can negatively impact the healing process. Even with a catheter in place allowing for continuous bladder drainage, patients can

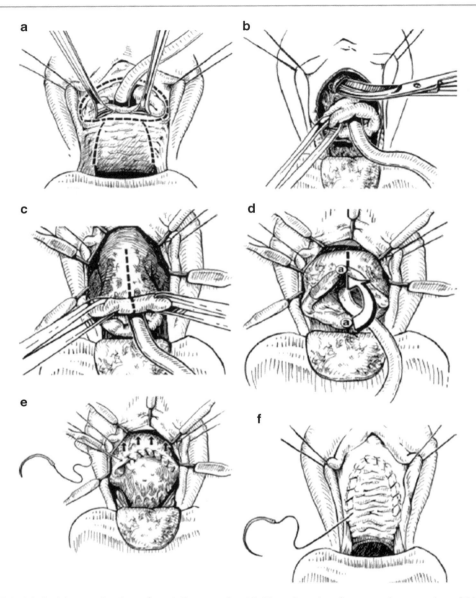

Fig. 15.1 (a) Incision made circumferentially around urethra with arms extending proximally to develop anterior vaginal wall flap. (b) Urethra is freed from its attachments as the urethropelvic and pubourethral ligaments are divided. (c) Dorsal urethra bivalved up to bladder neck. (d) Ventral urethra flap rotated up to edge of bivalved urethra. (e) Closure of bladder beck. With rotation of flap in a cephalad direction, the suture line rotates under the symphysis pubis. (f) Anterior vaginal wall advanced and vaginal wall closed with no overlapping suture lines

have residual detrusor overactivity. The bladder's natural response to a detrusor contraction is relaxation of the bladder neck and a spontaneous void. If the bladder neck has been surgically closed, this only leads to increased pressure on the suture line and greater risk of postoperative failure. Anticholinergics are thus an important part of the postoperative management of these patients and should be started immediately postoperatively. Theoretically, peri-operative injection of botulinum toxin A into the detrusor muscle could be used in the hopes of completely eliminating any postoperative detrusor overactivity [8]. The clinical uses of botulinum toxin A in urology continue to be explored and expanded; however, this actual use has yet to be documented.

Fistula Diagnosis

The diagnosis of a post-BNC fistula is fairly straightforward and can be done either radiographically or on examination. A leak at the closure site may be suggested at the postoperative visit if the patient complains of continued urinary leakage vaginally; however, a lack of leakage does not mean that the BNC has adequately healed. All patients should have a cystogram 2–3 weeks postoperatively to adequately assess the quality of the repair. If a residual leak is noted, then continued catheter drainage could be considered. The theory with a posthysterectomy VVF is that prolonged catheter drainage can be successful and lead to closure if the patient is dry with the catheter in place and is unlikely to succeed if the patient continues to leak per the fistula site despite continuous catheter drainage. This has not been evaluated in post-BNC leaks, but it is likely that the theory and healing process is similar—if urine continues to leak through a hole (i.e., the fistula site), then that hole will not heal.

If the cystogram is equivocal or if a patient returns complaining of leakage despite a previously noted negative cystogram, then direct examination may be helpful in identifying a fistula. As opposed to most posthysterectomy fistulae, which tend to be deep towards the vaginal vault and can be challenging to identify on examination, these fistulae are not deep in the vault and are often easy to see on examination. A simple technique to easily evaluate for a leak is to perform a pelvic examination while an assistant fills the bladder through the suprapubic tube with normal saline colored with a dye such as methylene blue or indigo carmine. If a leak is present, it will be readily apparent when the blue-tinged fluid is noted leaking through the fistula site in the vagina. If the patient is concerned a leak is present but cannot come to the office for immediate evaluation, another option would be for her to do a pyridium pad test at home. If her pad turns orange after taking pyridium post-BNC, then that is strongly suggestive that a fistula is present.

Fistula Management

If a VVF develops between the vagina and bladder neck closure site despite appropriate surgical technique and peri-operative care, then several options are available. An attempt to maximize drainage with supravesical diversion using bilateral nephrostomy tubes could be attempted. This has primarily been used in the postoperative setting in patients with a urine leak at the ureteroileal anastamosis site after urinary diversion. With a mature fistula tract, it is unlikely this will allow for closure of the fistula, though this may theoretically help close a leak early in the postoperative period.

Once the fistula tract has matured, the patient is destined to undergo further surgery if repair is desired. For experienced vaginal surgeons, a second attempt at a transvaginal BNC could be considered. The technique is essentially the same as was attempted with the initial attempt at closure. However, use of an adjuvant flap or graft is highly recommended in a redo procedure, especially if one was not used in the initial procedure. If a graft/flap was used with the initial attempt at BNC, it is possible that it could be identified intra-operatively and reused if healthy.

For those surgeons not experienced with transvaginal surgery, an abdominal approach should be considered after a failed prior attempt at BNC. If an abdominal BNC is performed, an omental flap can be harvested and placed at the closure site to add an extra layer of repair [9]. If further evaluation finds that the bladder is not salvageable or the BNC cannot be done, then the surgeon and patient should also be prepared for possible cystectomy and either continent or incontinent diversion to the skin. This is certainly a much larger undertaking than BNC and, if it is thought that this might be a possibility, appropriate preoperative preparation is required including patient counseling, stoma site marking, and obtaining of an adequate informed consent.

References

1. Zimmern PE, Hadley RH, Leach GE, et al. Transvaginal closure of the bladder neck and placement of a suprapubic catheter for destroyed urethra after long-term indwelling catheterization. J Urol. 1985;134:554–6.
2. Andrews HO, Shah PJR. Surgical management of urethral damage in neurologically impaired female patients with chronic indwelling catheters. Br J Urol. 1998;82:820–4.
3. Levy JB, Jacobs JA, Wein AJ. Combined abdominal and vaginal approach for bladder neck closure and permanent suprapubic tube: urinary diversion in the neurologically impaired woman. J Urol. 1994;152:2081–2.
4. Ginger VA, Miller JL, Yang CC. Bladder neck closure and suprapubic tube placement in the debilitated patient population. Neurourol Urodyn. 2010;29:382–6.
5. Rovner ES, Goudelocke CM, Gilchrist A, et al. Transvaginal bladder neck closure with posterior urethral flap for devastated urethra. Urology. 2011;78:208–12.
6. Detsky AS, Baker JP, O'Rourke K. Perioperative parenteral nutrition: a meta-analysis. Ann Intern Med. 1987;107:195–203.
7. Hebbar R, Harte B. Do preoperative nutritional interventions improve outcomes in malnourished patients undergoing elective surgery? Cleve Clin J Med. 2007;74 Suppl 1:8–10.
8. Smith CP, Somogyi GT, Chancellor MB. Emerging role of botulinum toxin in the treatment of neurogenic and non-neurogenic voiding dysfunction. Curr Urol Rep. 2002;3:382–7.
9. Shpall AI, Ginsberg DA. Bladder neck closure with lower urinary tract reconstruction: technique and long-term followup. J Urol. 2004;172:2296–9.
10. Nielsen KT, Bruskewitz RC. Female urinary incontinence treated by transvaginal urethral closure and suprapubic tube. Int Urol Nephrol. 1989;21:603–8.
11. Eckford SB, Kohler-Ockmore J, Feneley RCL. Long-term follow-up of transvaginal urethral closure and suprapubic cystostomy for urinary incontinence in women with multiple sclerosis. Br J Urol. 1994;74:319–21.
12. Stoffel JT, McGuire EJ. Outcome of urethral closure in patients with neurologic impairment and complete urethral destruction. Neurourol Urodyn. 2006;25:19–22.

Bladder Augmentation

Sender Herschorn and Blayne K. Welk

Introduction

Bladder augmentation with an ileal patch was first described by Von Mickulicz [1]. Different gastrointestinal segments were subsequently reported, colon by Lemoine in 1912 [2], sigmoid by Bisgard [3], cecum by Couvelaire [4], and stomach by Leong [5]. In 1950, Couvelaire began augmentation cystoplasty to treat contracted bladders as a result of tuberculosis, and the technique started to gain acceptance [4]. Other attempts using organic tissues such as peritoneum, omentum, human dura, skin, pericardium, placenta, gallbladder, free fascial grafts, and preserved bladder tissue were unsuccessful as were efforts using synthetic materials [6]. In 1959, Goodwin described the modern operative technique of using a detubularized ileal patch [7].

Bladder augmentation is often done in conjunction with other surgical procedures, such as creation of a continent stoma, or bladder outlet procedures to reduce urinary incontinence. This chapter will outline the indications and techniques of bladder augmentation and focus on short- and long-term complications and their management.

S. Herschorn, BSc, MDCM, FACS (✉)
B.K. Welk, MD, FRCSC
Division of Urology, Sunnybrook Health
Sciences Centre, University of Toronto,
2075 Bayview Avenue, Suite MG408,
Toronto, ON, Canada M4N 3M5
e-mail: s.herschorn@utoronto.ca

Indications

In 1977, Smith et al. [8] reviewed augmentation cystoplasty and suggested that the procedure was "a successful long-term solution for patients with small contracted bladders of almost any etiology." Table 16.1 lists the current indications.

Congenital Conditions

Myelodysplasia, a form of spinal dysraphism, may lead to neurogenic bladder dysfunction. Approximately 1/3 of patients have sphincter dyssyngeria, and the urodynamic pattern often changes as the child ages [9]. The failure of conservative or medical therapy to adequately treat urinary incontinence, high detrusor leak point pressures, and renal dysfunction are indications for bladder augmentation. It has been estimated with data approximately 5% [10] to 30% [11] of patients with spina bifida may undergo an augmentation cystoplasty. Augmentation is often combined with other procedures such as a catheterizable abdominal stoma and bladder neck procedures or slings to increase urinary outlet resistance.

Posterior urethral valves in males can lead to bladder dysfunction and renal failure. Augmentation cystoplasty may be required prior to renal transplantation [12–15]. Patients with exstrophy/epispadias complex also require bladder augmentation when staged functional reconstruction is unsuccessful [16–19].

H.B. Goldman (ed.), *Complications of Female Incontinence and Pelvic Reconstructive Surgery*,
Current Clinical Urology, DOI 10.1007/978-1-61779-924-2_16, © Springer Science+Business Media, LLC 2013

Table 16.1 Indications for augmentation cystoplasty (usually with associated symptoms of urinary incontinence, high detrusor pressures, or renal dysfunction refractory to other management options)

	Indication
Congenital	Myelodysplasia
	Posterior urethral valves
	Exstrophy/epispadias complex
Acquired neurogenic bladder	Spinal cord injury
	Multiple sclerosis
Acquired non-neurogenic bladder	Overactive bladder
Infectious	Tuberculosis
	Schistosomiasis
Inflammatory	Radiation cystitis (interstitial cystitis)
Iatrogenic	Intraoperative loss of bladder wall
	Urinary undiversion

Other congenital anomalies include sacral agenesis, cloacal exstrophy, imperforate anus, and persistent urogenital sinus [20].

Acquired Neurogenic Bladder

Spinal cord injury can lead to severe detrusor overactivity, poor bladder compliance, and decreased capacity over time. The changes are frequently related to the level of injury. Suprasacral spinal cord lesions often lead to detrusor overactivity with sphincter dyssynergia. This antagonistic dysfunction of the bladder and the outlet can impair detrusor compliance, and over time lead to reduced bladder capacity [21]. Sacral spinal cord lesions often lead to detrusor areflexia with a fixed, nonrelaxing sphincter. Generally the bladder has normal compliance; however over time decreased compliance and reduced capacity can develop [21].

Bladder augmentation may be indicated if incontinence, high detrusor leak point pressures, severe autonomic dysreflexia, or renal dysfunction occur due to failure of the bladder to store urine at a low pressure. Usually augmentation is considered when other measures such as behavioral modifications, anticholinergics, intravesical botulinum toxin, or rarely anterior nerve root stimulation are ineffective [22–24].

Multiple sclerosis is another cause of neurogenic bladder dysfunction that may result in detrusor overactivity with sphincter dyssynergia [25]. Bladder dysfunction can worsen over time, and progressive neuromuscular deterioration can make intermittent self-catheterization difficult [26]. Medical therapy with anticholinergics and intravesical botulinum toxin is usually the preferred treatment. However, occasional cases may be amenable to augmentation cystoplasty.

Overactive Bladder

Overactive bladder is a syndrome or symptom complex of urinary urgency, with or without urgency incontinence, urinary frequency, and nocturia [27]. Bladder augmentation is a treatment of last resort for refractory symptoms associated with detrusor overactivity that cannot be controlled with behavioral therapy, anticholinergics, intravesical botulinum toxin, or sacral/peripheral neuromodulation [28].

Infection

Genitourinary tuberculosis occurs in 10–20% of patients with pulmonary tuberculosis [29]. Tuberculous cystitis causes velvety granulations, bladder ulceration, and bladder wall thickening and can progress to severely reduced bladder capacity [26]. Tuberculosis, once a common indication for augmentation [30], is now a rarity due to better therapies and decreased incidence in the developed world [31, 32].

Schistosomiasis, an endemic parasitic infection found primarily in the Middle East and Africa, may cause bladder wall fibrosis due to granulomatous inflammation [33]. Reduced bladder capacity may be improved by augmentation [34].

Inflammatory Causes

Radiation changes may follow external beam radiation therapy for treatment of pelvic malignancy. Acute cystitis symptoms usually resolve within a few months, however occasionally seen bladder wall fibrosis may reduce bladder capacity and impair function [35]. Patient comorbidities and further oncologic treatment may limit augmentation in this group [36].

Bladder augmentation has been used as treatment for interstitial cystitis in patients with contracted, small capacity bladders [37]. However, augmentation has shown only modest success as treatment for pain associated with interstitial cystitis [26, 38]. Its use in this population is controversial [26, 39–41].

Iatrogenic

Augmentation cystoplasty may be necessary in patients with significant loss of the bladder wall due to surgical resection. This may be from the resection of locally advanced nonurologic cancer, or benign bladder resections. For patients with previous urinary diversion who did not undergo a cystectomy, redirecting the ureters to an augmentation cystoplasty may be a reasonable method of undiversion in some patients [42].

Contraindications

Serious bowel dysfunction, such as inflammatory bowel disease or after radiotherapy, in which removal of a segment will compromise absorption, is a contraindication. In patients with short gut syndrome, ileum and colon should not be used, although stomach may be an alternative. Another contraindication is when a patient is unwilling or unable to do clean intermittent catheterization (CIC), performed either by himself/herself or a caregiver [43].

Poor baseline renal function may predispose patients to severe electrolyte abnormalities and worsening renal function, and is a relative contraindication [43, 44] (although in patients with continuing renal dysfunction as a direct result of bladder dysfunction, augmentation may still be appropriate, and can slow the decrease in renal function [43]).

Surgical Considerations

Preoperative workup usually involves renal and bladder imaging (to assess renal anatomy, obstruction, and presence of stone disease), video-urodynamics (with special attention to the appearance of the bladder neck in order to assess the need for concomitant bladder neck or incontinence surgery), cystoscopy (to assess lower urinary tract anatomy), urine culture, complete blood count, renal function, and electrolyte levels. A history of bowel disease or surgery may require preoperative bowel imaging studies or colonoscopy. A full bowel preparation is generally used for these patients preoperatively however questions have been raised recently regarding its safety and need [45, 46].

The bladder is usually exposed through a midline lower abdominal incision, and the bowel segment is assessed for its suitability for use. The surgeon assesses the ease of moving the segment down to the bladder combined with the possible nutritional and metabolic consequences that will be discussed below. The bowel segment is usually detubularized to maximize the surface area (and therefore the resulting bladder volume), and reduces bowel contractions and postoperative detrusor pressure [47].

Ileum is often the preferred segment due to its familiarity among urologists, low complication rate, and tolerable metabolic profile [26, 44]. It may result in lower postoperative maximal detrusor pressures, and may reduce uninhibited contractions more effectively than sigmoid [48]. A 20–40 cm segment is selected (depending on the need), at least 20 cm proximal to the ileocecal valve. It is detubularized and used in various configurations for augmentation (Figs. 16.1 [49] and 16.2).

Sigmoid is an alternative and has been reported to have a lower rate of bowel obstruction [50, 51]. A 15–20 cm detubularized segment can be used.

Another alternative is cecum and ascending colon that can be mobilized up to the hepatic flexure. Cecum can be detubularized and used alone or in conjunction with a 15–30 cm segment

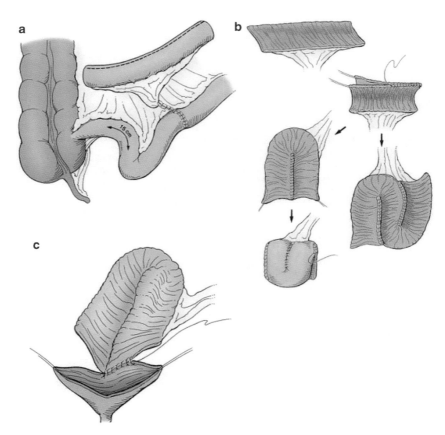

Fig. 16.1 (a) Ileocystoplasty. A 20–40-cm segment of ileum at least 15 cm from the ileocecal valve is removed and opened on its antimesenteric border. Ileoileostomy reconstitutes the bowel. (b) The opened ileal segment should be reconfigured. This can be done in a U, S, or W configuration. It can be further folded as a cup patch. (c) The reconfigured ileal segment is anastomosed widely to the native bladder (from Adams and Joseph in *Campbell-Walsh urology* [49])

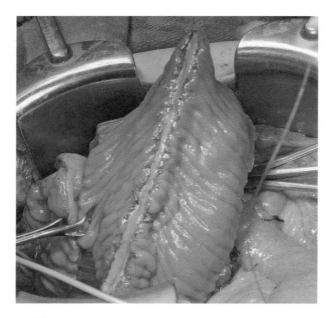

Fig. 16.2 A 40 cm length of ileum is shown. The segment has been isolated from the GI tract and reconfigured. The antimesenteric border was incised and the bowel segment was detubularized into an inverted U-shaped. It will be anastomosed to the bladder

of detubularized ileum to form the augment. Ileum or appendix can be used as a continent catheterizing channel with the ileocecal valve (or intravesical tunneling of the appendix) providing the continence mechanism. The ileal segment can also be used as a bladder "chimney" to reach resected or obstructed ureters for reimplantation if necessary.

Stomach is rarely used and jejunum should be avoided because of associated metabolic complications.

Alternative procedures for bladder augmentation include ureterocystoplasty (which is an option in patients with megaureter and an ipsilateral nonfunctional kidney [52, 53]) and autoaugmentation. Autoaugmentation involves performing a detrusor myectomy to create a large, low-pressure bladder diverticulum. Autoaugmentation avoids the complications associated with bowel, however it has poor reported long-term efficacy [54–58].

Once the bowel segment has been selected, the bladder is usually opened with a sagittal incision to bivalve it ("clam" cystoplasty [59]). An alternative is a wide U-shaped anterior or posterior incision that effectively creates a large flap for a wide anastomosis [60]. Supratrigonal bladder excision [61] can also be done. The ureteric orifices are identified to avoid damage. The bowel segment is sutured to the bladder with a wide anastomosis to ensure good drainage of the augmentation. A pelvic drain, suprapubic tube, and foley catheter may be placed for the postoperative period.

Reports of completely intraperitoneal laparoscopic, robotic-assisted, and single port augmentation cystoplasties in both adults and children have been published. These procedures require advanced laparoscopic skills and are not yet widely used [62–64].

Follow-Up

Close follow-up is necessary in the immediate postoperative period until indwelling catheters are removed, and the patient adjusts to CIC and bladder irrigations. The augmentation usually enlarges with time. Long-term follow-up consists of renal imaging, renal function tests, electrolyte measurements (to test for metabolic derangements), and complete blood count (to detect pernicious anemia). Some authors have advocated screening cystoscopy 5–10 years after augmentation to assess for bladder cancer; however this is controversial [65, 66]. Urodynamics may be done if there is a change in symptoms, onset of new hydronephrosis, or worsening renal function.

The overall complication rates in various series range from 3 to 41% depending on the duration of follow-up and completeness of reporting [67, 68].

Early Postoperative Complications

With any major abdominal surgery, there are associated cardiovascular, respiratory, and gastrointestinal complications. Postoperative mortality rates have been reported between 0 and 3.2% [43, 67, 69–76], and were generally the result of postoperative myocardial infarction (0–2.7%) and pulmonary embolus/deep vein thrombosis (0–7%) [39]. There have been a small number of reports of other severe complications, such as major bleeding requiring reoperation [39] and necrosis of the bowel segment [8, 76].

Small bowel obstruction requiring operative intervention may occur in 3–6% of patients, and approximately 5–6% of patients may develop a wound infection or dehiscence [43]. Anastomotic leak from the bladder occurs in 2–4% of patients. Postoperative ileus is common, and prolonged ileus occurs in approximately 5% of patients [43]. Severe postoperative complications are less frequent in contemporary case series [43].

Continence and Urodynamic Outcomes

Several groups have reported long-term functional outcomes in adult and pediatric populations. Blaivas et al. [60] reported on 65 adult patients who underwent augmentation cystoplasty (primarily with an ileocecal segment) with or without creation of an abdominal stoma (and included an additional 11 patients who had a continent diversion). At a mean follow-up of 5 years, 70% considered themselves cured, and 18% considered themselves improved. Failures consisted almost exclusively of interstitial cystitis patients. Mean bladder capacity increased from 166 to 572 mL, and mean maximal detrusor pressure fell from 53 to 14 cm H_2O. Flood et al. [36] reported on 122 augmentation cystoplasties (67% ileocystoplasty, 30% ileocecocystoplasty) with a mean follow-up of 3 years. They had a primarily adult population. They reported similar urodynamic improvements, a 75% cure rate, and a 20% improvement rate in incontinence.

Quek and Ginsberg [77] reported durability of the urodynamic improvements and 96% patient satisfaction among 24 patients with a mean follow-up of 8 years (range 4–13).

Herschorn and Hewitt [67] preformed a cross-sectional survey of 59 adults who underwent augmentation cystoplasty (usually with additional simultaneous reconstructive procedures) at a median follow-up of 6 years. Sixty-seven percent of patients reported complete continence, and 30% reported only mild incontinence (requiring on average 1–2 pads per day). Almost all patients were very satisfied with their urologic management.

Results in the pediatric populations are similar, although the majority of patients require additional reconstructive procedures such as ureteral reimplantation, bladder neck procedures, and creation of catheterizable channels. Lopez Pereira et al. reported on 29 children with a mean follow-up of 11 years [78]. Mean postoperative bladder capacity increased from 90 to 521 mL, and mean maximal detrusor pressure fell from 45 to 10 cm H_2O. Shekarriz et al. reported a 95% continence rate among 133 pediatric patients at a mean follow-up of 5 years [50].

A number of authors have compared the outcomes of ileum, ileocecal, and sigmoid segments, and have not shown any consistent advantages of any segment in terms of urinary continence or renal function [76, 79–81]. Urodynamically demonstrated contractions might persist postoperatively with colonic segments [48, 82].

Long-Term Consequences

The possible long-term consequences of augmentation are listed in Table 16.2 and discussed below. Complications requiring intervention may occur years after the original surgery [67, 68]. This underscores the necessity of long-term follow-up.

Growth Retardation and Decreased Bone Mineral Density

Small case series by Mundy and Nurse [83] and Wagstaff et al. [84] were the first to suggest there is a decrease in linear growth in children after augmentation cystoplasty. Since then, several additional studies have been published, of which two suggested there is approximately a 15% decrease in linear growth after augmentation, and six which did not demonstrate a significant change to linear growth [85, 86]. There is also contradictory evidence as to whether decreased bone mineral density or osteopenia is a result of the augmentation [86]. In a case series of 24 children followed for an average of 9 years after augmentation, Hafez et al. reported a 20% incidence of significant osteopenia [87]. The osteopenia is likely a result of buffering of the acidosis by the skeletal system, which leads to changes in bone mineralization [88]. Correction of this acidosis may improve bone density [89]. Other mechanisms of osteopenia include reduced renal tubular reabsorption of calcium and intestinal malabsorption of calcium [90]. The long-term impact of the osteopenia and how it affects children as adults is still unknown [86].

Management includes appropriate screening and treatment of postoperative metabolic acidosis. Patients with renal failure are more likely to have uncompensated acidosis and should be followed closely and treated for this complication. Some authors have advocated bone mineral density measurements after augmentation [87].

Table 16.2 Long-term consequences of augmentation cystoplasty and potential management strategies

	Description	Management
Growth retardation and osteopenia	Conflicting evidence on presence of linear growth reduction	Consider monitoring bone mineral density
	Chronic acidosis may lead to osteopenia	Treat acidosis
Electrolyte abnormalities		
Ileum/colon	Hyperchloremic, metabolic acidosis ± hypokalemia	Chloride restriction, bicarbonate, niacin, chlorpromazine
Stomach	Hypochloremic, hypokalemia, metabolic alkalosis ± hematuria-dysuria syndrome	IV fluids, potassium supplementation, histamine antagonists, proton pump inhibitors
Renal insufficiency	May occur as a result of complications associated with augmentation cystoplasty, especially in patients with poor preoperative renal function	Postoperative monitoring of renal function
Vitamin B12 deficiency	Due to ileal resection	Postoperative monitoring of complete blood count
		B12 supplementation
Bladder cancer	Increased risk of aggressive bladder cancer among patients with neurogenic bladder; controversial if the augmentation is an independent risk factor	Aggressive investigation of hematuria, frequent urinary infections, or penile/scrotal discharge
Bladder perforation	Consider if any patient with peritonitis, septic shock, abdominal pain and distension, nausea and vomiting, fever, referred shoulder pain, or intraperitoneal fluid	In stable patients, a trial of conservative therapy may be attempted.
		Standard treatment is laparotomy for surgical repair
Stone disease	Due to metabolic alterations, poor bladder emptying, mucus, and chronic infection	Endoscopic, percutaneous, or open surgical procedure
		Increased fluid intake and dietary modifications
Mucus	Produced by the bowel segment	Bladder irrigations
		Acetylcysteine/urea irrigations
Urinary tract infection	Asymptomatic bacteriuria is common	Antibiotic therapy for symptomatic infections
	Symptomatic urinary infection require treatment	Antibiotic prophylaxis or intravesical irrigations for frequent symptomatic infections
Bowel dysfunction	Due to alterations to bile acid metabolism; often exacerbates underlying neurogenic bowel or irritable bowel syndrome	Low fat diet
		Antidiarrheal medication
		Bile acid binders (cholestyramine)
Voiding dysfunction	Incomplete emptying or inability to void	CIC is commonly required postoperatively
	Incontinence may occur due to an incompetent outlet	Surgical treatment of incontinence is common
Bowel dysfunction	Due to alterations to bile acid metabolism; often exacerbates underlying neurogenic bowel or irritable bowel syndrome	Low fat diet
		Antidiarrheal medication
		Bile acid binders (cholestyramine)
Pregnancy		Vaginal delivery preferable
		Urologic assistance is helpful during elective cesarean sections

Electrolyte Abnormalities

The expected pattern of metabolic abnormality is dependent on the segment of bowel used in the augmentation cystoplasty. Other factors that influence the severity of the electrolyte imbalance include the surface area of the augmentation, urine pH, and the urine contact time [90].

Ileum and Colon

The classic electrolyte pattern is hyperchloremic metabolic acidosis. The symptoms associated with metabolic acidosis are fatigue, anorexia, weight loss, and polydipsia. There are several possible mechanisms: frequent pyelonephritis may lead to distal tubular acidification defect, urea in the urine may be metabolized by intestinal flora to ammonium which is then absorbed by the bowel, loss of bicarbonate from the bowel that can lead to metabolic acidosis, or chloride that is actively transported from the bowel into the urine leads to reabsorption of ammonium or hydrogen ions [91]. The most likely mechanism is ammonium substituting for sodium in a sodium-hydrogen ion antiport; this antiport is coupled with a bicarbonate-chloride exchanger, leading to a net reabsorption of hydrogen ion, ammonium, and chloride [92]. Hypokalemia can occur during treatment of an acidosis, which unmasks low total body potassium, or as a result of renal potassium wasting (seen more frequently with colonic segments) [92, 93]. Associated hypocalcemia and hypomagnesemia (usually restricted to patients with renal insufficiency, and more commonly seen in colonic augmentations) may be due to reduced renal reabsorption due to a high level of sulfate that is reabsorbed from the bowel, or due to chronic acidosis causing calcium mobilization and subsequent activation of parathyroid hormone [93, 94].

Normal renal function can often compensate for this acidosis; the majority of patients will have a measurable abnormality [95], however it will only be clinically relevant in approximately 10–20% of patients [43, 96]. The absorptive properties of the bowel may be attenuated with time due to mucosal atrophy [97, 98]. Treatment of the acidosis is usually considered once the base excess falls below −2.5 mmol/L [93, 96]. Therapy consists of dietary chloride restriction, bicarbonate supplementation (sodium bicarbonate, potassium citrate), and maximal urinary drainage [94]. Niacin or chlorpromazine inhibits active chloride transportation in the intestine, and may be useful, especially when the solute load of bicarbonate therapy is undesirable [98].

Stomach

The classic electrolyte pattern is hypochloremic, hypokalemic, metabolic alkalosis. Clinical symptoms associated include pelvic pain, fatigue, mental status changes, seizures, or cardiac arrhythmias [93]. Treatment of the electrolyte disturbance involves maximal bladder drainage, normal saline fluid resuscitation, and potassium replacement when necessary [93, 99]. Long-term

therapy with potassium chloride may be necessary [93]. Acid secretion can be suppressed with histamine antagonists, or proton pump inhibitors [93].

Hematuria-dysuria syndrome is characterized by excess acid secretion causing peptic ulcer disease, hematuria and dysuria; it occurs in up to 25% of patients, and treatment with a proton pump inhibitor is required intermittently or continuously in a small proportion of patients [100].

Hyperammonemia

The liver is responsible for metabolizing ammonium (absorbed from an augmentation cystoplasty) into urea. Impaired hepatic function or sepsis can lead to the inability of the liver to cope with the hyperammonemia; symptomatically this presents as ammoniagenic encephalopathy [94]. Treatment is maximal urinary drainage, low protein diet, ammonium binders (such as lactulose or neomycin), and in severe cases, intravenous arginine glutamate [93].

Renal Insufficiency

Deterioration of renal function may occur in 0–15% of patients after augmentation [43]. It is unknown whether this is a direct result of the augmentation or due to associated complications [101]. Renal insufficiency occurs, independent of the bowel segment selected [102, 103]. The etiology of renal dysfunction may be urinary stone disease, bacteriuria, high detrusor pressures, vesicoureteral reflux, unrecognized obstruction, and lack of compliance with catheterization [102]. One study suggests approximately 5% of patients will have renal dysfunction after augmentation without a clear etiology [102]. Some authors have demonstrated that baseline renal function is a significant predictor of renal deterioration after augmentation cystoplasty, with increased risk when creatinine clearance is <40 mL/min [8, 43, 104, 105]. Other studies in children and adults with baseline renal dysfunction did not appear to have accelerated renal failure after augmentation cystoplasty [67, 106]. There is no consensus on the order of a staged augmentation cystoplasty and a renal transplant [106].

Postoperatively, patients should have renal imaging and serum creatinine measurements to screen for renal insufficiency [94]. Serum creatinine can be difficult to interpret in this population, due to a low muscle mass in neurogenic patients, and increased reabsorption of urine creatinine by the ileum. Nuclear renograms may be better for definitive measurement.

Vitamin B12 Deficiency

Vitamin B12 is bound to intrinsic factor in the duodenum, which allows is to be absorbed in the terminal ileum. With ileocystoplasty, the most distal 15 cm of the ileum should be preserved to prevent this complication [94]. Vitamin B12 deficiency may cause megaloblastic anemia and neurologic changes [94]. In nutritionally normal individuals, it takes up to 3 years for the livers store of B12 to be depleted, and the resulting deficiency to manifest. The incidence of B12 deficiency related to ileal resection is 3–20% [94, 107].

This complication may be treated prophylactically with B12 supplementation if more than 50 cm of ileum is used for the bladder augmentation [108]. Otherwise, patients should have complete blood counts in follow-up to screen for pernicious anemia.

Bladder Cancer

Bladder cancer has been reported in young patients after augmentation [68, 109, 110]. It has also been reported that spinal cord injury patients and spina bifida patients develop bladder cancer at a young age (40–50 years), they have an increased risk of locally advanced disease, an increased number of adenocarcinomas and squamous cell carcinomas, and a short median survival after diagnosis [66, 111]. In a matched cohort study from a registry of patients with bladder dysfunction due to neurologic abnormalities, exstrophy, and posterior urethral valves, Higuchi et al. did not find a significant difference in the incidence of bladder cancer among patients with augmentation cystoplasty (using ileum or colon)

compared to patients managed with intermittent catheterization [65]. The authors did demonstrate that the incidence of bladder cancer was higher in both groups with congenital bladder anomalies independent of augmentation status when compared to the SEER database. Possible reasons for a higher rate of bladder cancer in patients with neurogenic bladder may be reduced intracellular antioxidant activity (leading to increased rates of DNA mutation) [112], impaired DNA repair in the bowel due to the hyperosmolar urine [113], and immunosuppressant use in patients after renal transplantation [65]. However, patients who have undergone a gastric augmentation may have a higher cancer risk compared to other bowel segments [65].

Urologists should have a particular awareness of the potential for aggressive bladder cancer in this population, whether or not they have had an augmentation cystoplasty. Symptoms such as hematuria, frequent urinary infections, or penile/scrotal discharge need to be aggressively investigated; visual changes in the bladder due to the augmentation, recent infections, or catheterization can make cystoscopy challenging, and biopsy or CT should be considered if there is any uncertainty [111].

Bladder Perforation

This is a potentially life-threatening complication that occurs in approximately 6–13% of patients [20, 114–118]. Patients with neurogenic bladders, those with competent bladder necks, those without a catheterizable channel, and those who abuse alcohol appear to be at an increased risk [20, 43, 119, 120]. Perforation can occur at any time postoperatively, even years later. It can present with fever, abdominal pain and distension with intraperitoneal fluid, nausea and vomiting, referred shoulder pain, peritonitis, and septic shock [50, 116]; because of neurological abnormalities of these patients, the presenting symptoms are often nonspecific. Diagnosis can be made with a CT cystogram; standard fluoroscopic cystography has a 10–20% false negative rate [50, 115, 121]. CT or US can demonstrate intraperitoneal fluid, which is an important sign that bladder perforation has occurred [122]. Due to the augmentation, extraperitoneal ruptures are rare [123]. The area of perforation is usually at the bowel-bladder anastomosis, or within the weaker bowel wall [115]. The etiology of bladder perforation is thought to be from traumatic catheterization, acute over distension, or increased intravesical pressure chronic over distension (from CIC noncompliance) or infection leading to localized areas of ischemia and necrosis [121, 124].

The treatment of patients with large perforations and clinical instability usually is laparotomy for surgical repair. In patients that are stable, (usually with a small perforation), a trial of conservative therapy (foley catheter and antibiotics) may be considered [124, 125]. Mortality is high in patients with clinical instability on presentation, and those with a delayed diagnosis; overall mortality has been estimated at up to 25% [114, 126, 127]. If clinical suspicion is high, and imaging is negative, the patient should still be treated as a possible bladder perforation [43]. There is a 25% rate of recurrence of bladder perforation after the initial episode [20, 121, 128].

Stone Disease

Patients are at increased risk for bladder and upper tract calculi. Urinary calculi have been reported in 9–15% of patients after augmentation [43, 67, 129–131], and in some series as high as 50% [132]. Many of the risk factors for stones are present in patients that undergo augmentation, and may not be directly related to the surgical procedure [133]. Patients with a continent catheterizable channel (which may not drain the bladder completely), those using urethral CIC (compared to those voiding spontaneous), and patients with urease splitting bacteriuria are at increased risk [43, 130]. Possible reasons for stone formation include chronic bacteriuria (a significant risk factor in multivariable analysis [134]), intravesical foreign bodies, elevated postvoid residuals, and mucus secretion from the bowel segment [135]. Similar to regular stone forming population, dietary choices, and inadequate fluid intake

increase the risk of stone disease [136]. Metabolic changes, such as hypercalciuria and hypocitraturia secondary to metabolic acidosis, water loss through the cystoplasty bowel segment, and mild enteric hyperoxaluria (from the bowel resection or antibiotic-related deficiency of oxalobacter formigenes) can predispose these patients to stone formation [132, 136, 137]. Most stones are struvite due to frequent bacteriuria, or calcium oxalate; they are usually mixed with calcium phosphate due to the alkalotic urine [132, 136, 138].

Treatment of stones includes endoscopic, percutaneous, or open surgical procedures depending on the stone size, location, and patient factors [43, 129]. Prevention of stones consists of bladder irrigation, which may [139] or may not [140] be preventive role, increased fluid intake, decreased salt, purine and oxalate intake, and medical therapy directed by 24 h urine and stone analysis.

Mucus

Ileal and colonic segments used in augmentations continue to produce mucus. Up to 40 g of mucus can be produced daily and continues over time despite villous atrophy [141]. Colonic bowel segments produce more mucus than ileal segments [143]. The mucus is thought to help reduce malignant changes [142], however it has been implicated as a causative factor in urinary tract infections, stone formation, poor bladder emptying, and bladder perforation [43].

Problematic mucus secretion can be treated with daily bladder irrigations. These can be augmented with acetylcysteine or urea irrigations which help dissolve mucus [143], or oral ranitidine which may help to reduce mucus production [144].

Urinary Tract Infection

Asymptomatic bacteriuria is nearly universal among augmentation enterocystoplasty patients and usually does not require treatment except in cases of urease splitting organisms (such as *Proteus* and *Klebsiella*) [145]. Studies in ileal conduits have shown that bacteria freely adhere to bowel mucosa, and do not incite an inflammatory reaction [146]. This chronic bacteriuria has been cited as a risk factor for stone disease, incontinence, and bladder cancer [43, 147]. The most common organism is *Escherichia coli* [148].

Symptomatic urinary tract infection, which occurs in 5–40% of patients [43, 76, 80], requires antibiotic treatment. Risk factors are similar to asymptomatic bacteriuria and include urinary stasis, mucus production, and intermittent catheterization [39]. Symptoms may be nonspecific if bladder sensation is absent and include incontinence, abdominal pain, hematuria, new onset foul urine, and lethargy.

Management of urinary tract infection consists of appropriate antibiotic therapy. In patients with frequent symptomatic infections despite oral antibiotic prophylaxis, intravesical irrigation with antibiotics may reduce symptomatic infections [149]. In a small pilot study of 15 patients after ileocystoplasty, cranberry extract reduced asymptomatic bacteriuria [150].

Bowel Dysfunction

Bowel dysfunction after bowel resection for augmentation or diversion occurs in approximately 20–50% of patients [67, 151, 152]. The most common symptom is diarrhea seen in about 25% of patients, however potentially more distressing symptoms of fecal urgency and incontinence and nocturnal bowel movements are also common [151]. Bowel dysfunction is more common among patients with a neurologic diagnosis as a result of associated neurogenic bowel dysfunction and among patients with previous radiation or bowel resections [151, 152]. Approximately 30% of patients with irritable bowel syndrome have detrusor overactivity; this may be due to an intrinsic disorder of smooth muscle calcium metabolism [152].

Specific surgical factors may contribute to postoperative changes in bowel function that lead to diarrhea. Bile acids, generated in the liver and secreted into the small intestine, are necessary for fat absorption. Bile acids are reabsorbed in the distal ileum, enter the liver, and participate in the feedback mechanism for regeneration. Resection

of long sections of the terminal ileum can lead to bile acid malabsorption. Bile acids entering the colon may cause diarrhea by inducing water and salt secretion and by promoting motility [153]. Ileal resection of more than 100 cm results in severe bile acid malabsorption that cannot be compensated for by increased hepatic synthesis. In such cases, steatorrhea results from impaired micelle formation due to decreased luminal concentrations of conjugated bile acids. In shorter ileal resections, bile acid malabsorption can usually be compensated for by an increase in hepatic synthesis; and malabsorbed bile acids cause the diarrhea rather than steatorrhea [154, 155]. Resection of the ileocecal valve leads to bacterial colonization of the distal ileum that destroys the bile acids. The lack of bile acids, which leads to unabsorbed fatty acids in the large bowel, stimulates the colon to secrete more water and mucus, increase motility, and prompt defecation [156].

Treatment of this complication involves a low fat diet and antidiarrheal medications. Bile acid-related diarrhea can be diagnosed with a selenium homocholic acid taurine test, or a therapeutic trial of bile acid binders such as cholestyramine [156] may be helpful.

Voiding Dysfunction and Incontinence

The interposition of bowel into the bladder usually prevents the efficient detrusor contractions that are necessary for voiding [157]. The urethral outlet resistance may be high due to neurologic disease, or concomitant surgery to treat incontinence. Some patients are able to void spontaneously with abdominal straining.

If the patient is unable to void, or has complications from incomplete emptying, he/she will need to use CIC to empty their bladder. This is necessary in 25–100% of neurogenic patients, and a lower proportion of neurologically intact patients [43].

Continence rates range from 60 to 100% [67, 77]. Nocturnal incontinence can occur due to failure of the urethral sphincter to respond to contractions of the augmented bowel, and increased urine output due to water loss from the augmented bowel segment. Daytime incontinence can be due to stress incontinence, detrusor overactivity, or from phasic contractions of the augmented bowel segment [158, 159]. These phasic contractions are usually <40 cm H_2O, and occur at higher volumes [77].

Treatment of incontinence in these patients includes behavioral modification (such as more frequent CIC), anticholinergics, and surgical procedures such as midurethral slings, bladder neck slings or bladder neck reconstruction, and artificial urinary sphincters [43, 160]. Occasionally repeat augmentation is necessary [131].

Pregnancy

While not a postoperative complication, pregnancy after augmentation cystoplasty is becoming more common [121]. Complications such as premature labor, urinary tract infection, renal dysfunction, and urinary tract obstruction are more prevalent [161]. Patients usually require antibiotic treatment of bacteriuria; screening urinalysis for infection or proteinuria is not accurate due to mucus from the augmentation cystoplasty [162].

Vaginal delivery is preferable [162, 163], however there is controversy as to whether cesarean section is necessary for patients with artificial sphincters and bladder neck procedures [43, 162]. If an elective cesarean section is scheduled for other reasons, urologic assistance during the surgery and a high segment section may help avoid damage to the bladder augmentation [43, 162]. The bowel segment can survive inadvertent damage to the vascular pedicle, however this may lead to eventual contraction of the bowel segment [164].

Conclusion

Bladder augmentation with intestine has been successfully used to treat various conditions that results in small capacity bladders. The surgical technique involves detubularization and reconfiguration of a segment of bowel (usually the ileum or colon) to create a patch. A successful clinical outcome is dependent upon creating a large capacity, low-pressure reservoir to store urine; additional procedures to aid in catheterization or continence are often necessary. Potential complications have been well described and are usually reported in case series. Medical and surgical treatments of complications are similarly well elucidated although some are still controversial. Since complications may occur at any time after surgery prolonged follow-up and monitoring are essential.

References

1. Mikulicz J. Zur Operation der angeborenen Blasenspalte. Zentralbl Chir. 1899;26:641–3.
2. Charghi A, Charbonneau J, Gauthier GE. Colocystoplasty for bladder enlargement and bladder substitution: a study of late results in 31 cases. J Urol. 1967;97:849–56.
3. Bisgard JD. Substitution of the urinary bladder with a segment of sigmoid: an experimental study. Ann Surg. 1943;117:106–9.
4. Couvelaire R. [The "little bladder" of genito-urinary tuberculosis; classification, site and variants of bladder-intestine transplants]. J Urol Medicale Chir. 1950;56:381–434.
5. Leong CH. Use of the stomach for bladder replacement and urinary diversion. Ann R Coll Surg Engl. 1978;60:283–9.
6. Elbahnasy AM, Shalhav A, Hoenig DM, Figenshau R, Clayman RV. Bladder wall substitution with synthetic and non-intestinal organic materials. J Urol. 1998;159:628–37.
7. Goodwin WE, Winter CC, Barker WF. Cup-patch technique of ileocystoplasty for bladder enlargement or partial substitution. Surg Gynecol Obstet. 1959;108:240–4.
8. Smith RB, van Cangh P, Skinner DG, Kaufman JJ, Goodwin WE. Augmentation enterocystoplasty: a critical review. J Urol. 1977;118:35–9.
9. Sidi AA, Dykstra DD, Gonzalez R. The value of urodynamic testing in the management of neonates with myelodysplasia: a prospective study. J Urol. 1986;135:90–3.
10. Lendvay TS, Cowan CA, Mitchell MM, Joyner BD, Grady RW. Augmentation cystoplasty rates at children's hospitals in the United States: a pediatric health information system database study. J Urol. 2006;176:1716–20.
11. Kaefer M, Pabby A, Kelly M, Darbey M, Bauer SB. Improved bladder function after prophylactic treatment of the high risk neurogenic bladder in newborns with myelomentingocele. J Urol. 1999;162:1068–71.
12. Aki FT, et al. Renal transplantation in children with augmentation enterocystoplasty. Transplant Proc. 2006;38:554–5.

13. Fisang C, Hauser S, Muller SC. Ureterocystoplasty: an ideal method for vesical augmentation in children. Aktuelle Urol. 2010;41 Suppl 1:S50–2.

14. Kajbafzadeh AM, Quinn FM, Duffy PG, Ransley PG. Augmentation cystoplasty in boys with posterior urethral valves. J Urol. 1995;154:874–7.

15. Peters CA, et al. The urodynamic consequences of posterior urethral valves. J Urol. 1990;144:122–6.

16. Amirzargar MA, et al. Reconstruction of bladder and urethra using ileocecal segment and appendix in patients with exstrophy-epispadias complex: the first report of a new surgical approach. Int Urol Nephrol. 2007;39:779–85.

17. De Castro R, Pavanello P, Domini R. Indications for bladder augmentation in the exstrophy-epispadias complex. Br J Urol. 1994;73:303–7.

18. Gearhart JP, Peppas DS, Jeffs RD. The failed exstrophy closure: strategy for management. Br J Urol. 1993;71:217–20.

19. Lund DP, Hendren WH. Cloacal exstrophy: a 25-year experience with 50 cases. J Pediatr Surg. 2001;36:68–75.

20. Metcalfe PD, et al. Spontaneous bladder perforations: a report of 500 augmentations in children and analysis of risk. J Urol. 2006;175:1466–70; discussion 1461–70.

21. Jeong SJ, Cho SY, Oh SJ. Spinal cord/brain injury and the neurogenic bladder. Urol Clin North Am. 2010;37:537–46.

22. Sidi A, Becher E, Reddy P, Dykstra D. Augmentation enterocystoplasty for the management of voiding dysfunction in spinal cord injury patients. J Urol. 1990;143:83–5.

23. Van Rey F, Heesakkers J. Applications of neurostimulation for urinary storage and voiding dysfunction in neurological patients [review] [33 refs]. Urol Int. 2008;81:373–8.

24. Lewis J, Cheng E. Non-traditional management of the neurogenic bladder: tissue engineering and neuromodulation [review] [77 refs]. Scientific World Journal. 2007;7:1230–41.

25. Litwiller S, Frohman E, Zimmern P. Multiple sclerosis and the urologist. J Urol. 1999;161:743–57.

26. Reyblat P, Ginsberg D. Augmentation cystoplasty: what are the indications? [review] [41 refs]. Curr Urol Rep. 2008;9:452–8.

27. Abrams P, et al. The standardisation of terminology in lower urinary tract function: report from the standardisation sub-committee of the International Continence Society. Urology. 2003;61:37–49.

28. Reyblat P, Ginsberg D. Augmentation enterocystoplasty in overactive bladder: is there still a role? Curr Urol Rep. 2010;11:432–9.

29. Wise G, Shteynshlyuger A. An update on lower urinary tract tuberculosis. Curr Urol Rep. 2008;9:305–13.

30. Abel B, Gow J. Results of caecocystoplasty for tuberculous bladder contracture. Br J Urol. 1978;50:511–6.

31. Wesolowski S. Late resuls of cystoplasty in chronic tuberculous cystitis. Br J Urol. 1970;42:697–703.

32. de Figueiredo A, Lucon A, Srougi M. Bladder augmentation for the treatment of chronic tuberculous cystitis. Clinical and urodynamic evaluation of 25 patients after long term follow-up. Neurourol Urodyn. 2006;25:433–40.

33. Kehinde E, Anim J, Hira P. Parasites of urological importance. Urol Int. 2008;81:1–13.

34. Badr M, Zaher M. Ileocystoplasty in the treatment of bilharzial contracted bladder. J Egypt Med Assoc. 1959;42:33–49.

35. Smit S, Heyns C. Management of radiation cystitis. Nat Rev Urol. 2010;7:206–14.

36. Flood H, et al. Long-term results and complications using augmentation cystoplasty in reconstructive urology. Neurourol Urodyn. 1995;14:297–309.

37. Webster G, Maggio M. The management of chronic interstitial cystitis by substitution cystoplasty. J Urol. 1989;141:287–91.

38. Nielsen K, Kromann-Andersen B, Steven K, Hald T. Failure of combined supratrigonal cystectomy and Mainz ileocecocystoplasty in intractable interstitial cystitis: is histology and mast cell count a reliable predictor for the outcome of surgery? J Urol. 1990;144:255–8; discussion 258–9.

39. Worth P. The treatment of interstitial cystitis by cystolysis with observations on cystoplasty. A review after 7 years. Br J Urol. 1980;52:232.

40. Nurse D, Parry J, Mundy A. Problems in the surgical treatment of interstitial cystitis. Br J Urol. 1991;68:153–4.

41. MacDermott J, Charpied G, Tesluk H, Stone A. Recurrent interstitial cystitis following cystoplasty: fact or fiction? J Urol. 1990;144:37–40.

42. Herschorn S, Rangaswamy S, Radomski SB. Urinary undiversion in adults with myelodysplasia: long-term followup. J Urol. 1994;152:329–33.

43. Greenwell T, Venn S, Mundy A. Augmentation cystoplasty [review] [166 refs]. BJU Int. 2001;88:511–25.

44. Kilic N, et al. Bladder augmentation: urodynamic findings and clinical outcome in different augmentation techniques. Eur J Pediatr Surg. 1999;9:29–32.

45. Matsou A, et al. Mechanical bowel preparation before elective colorectal surgery: is it necessary? Tech Coloproctol. 2011;15 Suppl 1:59–62.

46. Wells T, Plante M, McAlpine JN. Preoperative bowel preparation in gynecologic oncology: a review of practice patterns and an impetus to change. Int J Gynecol Cancer. 2011;21:1135–42.

47. Hinman FJ. Selection of intestinal segments for bladder substitution: physical and physiological characteristics. J Urol. 1988;139:519–23.

48. Radomski S, Herschorn S, Stone A. Urodynamic comparison of ileum vs. sigmoid in augmentation cystoplasty for neurogenic bladder dysfunction. Neurourol Urodyn. 1995;14:231–7.

49. Adams MC, Joseph DB. Urinary tract reconstruction in children. In: Wein A, Kavoussi LR, Novick AC, Partin AW, Peters CA, editors. Campbell-Walsh urology, vol. 4. Philadelphia, PA: Saunders Elsevier; 2007. p. 3656–702.

50. Shekarriz B, Upadhyay J, Demirbilek S, Barthold J, Gonzalez R. Surgical complications of bladder augmentation: comparison between various enterocystoplasties in 133 patients. Urology. 2000;55:123–8.

51. Gough D. Enterocystoplasty [review] [40 refs]. BJU Int. 2001;88:739–43.

52. Hitchcock R, Duffy P, Malone P. Ureterocystoplasty: the 'bladder' augmentation of choice. Br J Urol. 1994;73:575–9.

53. Anderson P, Dewan P. Ureterocystoplasty: an alternative reconstructive procedure to enterocystoplasty in suitable cases. J Pediatr Surg. 2001;36:962.

54. MacNeily A, Afshar K, Coleman G, Johnson H. Autoaugmentation by detrusor myotomy: its lack of effectiveness in the management of congenital neuropathic bladder. J Urol. 2003;170:1643–6; discussion 1646.

55. Stohrer M, et al. Bladder autoaugmentation in adult patients with neurogenic voiding dysfunction. Spinal Cord. 1997;35:456–62.

56. Skobejko-Wlodarska L, Strulak K, Nachulewicz P, Szymkiewicz C. Bladder autoaugmentation in myelodysplastic children. Br J Urol. 1998;81 Suppl 3:114–6.

57. Duel B, Gonzalez R, Barthold J. Alternative techniques for augmentation cystoplasty [review] [134 refs]. J Urol. 1998;159:998–1005.

58. Cartwright P, Snow B. Bladder autoaugmentation: early clinical experience. J Urol. 1989;142:505–8.

59. Bramble F. The clam cystoplasty [review] [21 refs]. Br J Urol. 1990;66:337–41.

60. Blaivas J, et al. Long-term followup of augmentation enterocystoplasty and continent diversion in patients with benign disease. J Urol. 2005;173:1631–4.

61. Gil Vernet SG. [Neurogenic bladder, neuromuscular bladder and intestinal bladder]. Acta Urol Belg. 1962;30:405–20.

62. Traxel E, Minevich E, Noh P. A review: the application of minimally invasive surgery to pediatric urology: lower urinary tract reconstructive procedures [review] [38 refs]. Urology. 2010;76:115–20.

63. Noguera R, et al. Laparoscopic augmentation enterocystoplasty through a single trocar. Urology. 2009;73:1371–4.

64. Challacombe B, Dasgupta P. Reconstruction of the lower urinary tract by laparoscopic and robotic surgery. Curr Opin Urol. 2007;17:390–5.

65. Higuchi T, Granberg C, Fox J, Husmann D. Augmentation cystoplasty and risk of neoplasia: fact, fiction and controversy. J Urol. 2010;184: 2492–6.

66. Austin J. Long-term risks of bladder augmentation in pediatric patients. Curr Opin Urol. 2008;18:408–12.

67. Herschorn S, Hewitt R. Patient perspective of long-term outcome of augmentation cystoplasty for neurogenic bladder. Urology. 1998;52:672–8.

68. Metcalfe PD, Rink RC. Bladder augmentation: complications in the pediatric population. Curr Urol Rep. 2007;8:152–6.

69. Fontaine E, et al. Combined modified rectus fascial sling and augmentation ileocystoplasty for neurogenic incontinence in women. J Urol. 1997;157:109–12.

70. Cheng C, Hendry W, Kirby R, Whitfield H. Detubularisation in cystoplasty: clinical review. Br J Urol. 1991;67:303–7.

71. Sethia KK, Webb RJ, Neal DE. Urodynamic study of ileocystoplasty in the treatment of idiopathic detrusor instability. Br J Urol. 1991;67:286–90.

72. Kockelbergh R, et al. Clam enterocystoplasty in general urological practice. Br J Urol. 1991;68:38–41.

73. George V, Russell G, Shutt A, Gaches C, Ashken M. Clam ileocystoplasty. Br J Urol. 1991;68:487–9.

74. Gonzalez R, Sidi A, Zhang G. Urinary undiversion: indications, technique and results in 50 cases. J Urol. 1986;136:13–6.

75. Gearhart J, Albertsen P, Marshall F, Jeffs R. Pediatric applications of augmentation cystoplasty: the Johns Hopkins experience. J Urol. 1986;136:430–2.

76. Mitchell M, Kulb T, Backes D. Intestinocystoplasty in combination with clean intermittent catheterization in the management of vesical dysfunction. J Urol. 1986;136:288–91.

77. Quek M, Ginsberg D. Long-term urodynamics followup of bladder augmentation for neurogenic bladder. J Urol. 2003;169:195–8.

78. Lopez Pereira P, et al. Enterocystoplasty in children with neuropathic bladders: long-term follow-up. J Pediatr Urol. 2008;4:27–31.

79. Kreder K, Webster G. Management of the bladder outlet in patients requiring enterocystoplasty. J Urol. 1992;147:38–41.

80. Khoury J, Timmons S, Corbel L, Webster G. Complications of enterocystoplasty. Urology. 1992;40:9–14.

81. Lockhart J, Bejany D, Politano V. Augmentation cystoplasty in the management of neurogenic bladder disease and urinary incontinence. J Urol. 1986;135:969–71.

82. Goldwasser B, Barrett DM, Webster GD, Kramer SA. Cystometric properties of ileum and right colon after bladder augmentation, substitution or replacement. J Urol. 1987;138:1007–8.

83. Mundy A, Nurse D. Calcium balance, growth and skeletal mineralisation in patients with cystoplasties. Br J Urol. 1992;69:257–9.

84. Wagstaff K, Woodhouse C, Duffy P, Ransley P. Delayed linear growth in children with enterocystoplasties. Br J Urol. 1992;69:314–7.

85. Taskinen S, Makitie O, Fagerholm R. Intestinal bladder augmentation at school age has no adverse effects on growth. J Pediatr Urol. 2008;4:40–2.

86. Mingin G, Maroni P, Gerharz E, Woodhouse C, Baskin L. Linear growth after enterocystoplasty in children and adolescents: a review [review] [14 refs]. World J Urol. 2004;22:196–9.

87. Hafez A, et al. Long-term evaluation of metabolic profile and bone mineral density after ileocystoplasty in children. J Urol. 2003;170:1639–41; discussion 1632–41.

88. Vajda P, et al. Metabolic findings after colocystoplasty in children. Urology. 2003;62:542–6; discussion 546.

89. Abes M, Sarihan H, Madenci E. Evaluation of bone mineral density with dual x-ray absorptiometry for osteoporosis in children with bladder augmentation. J Pediatr Surg. 2003;38:230–2.

90. McDougal W. Metabolic complications of urinary intestinal diversion. J Urol. 1992;147:1199–208.

91. Koch M, McDougal W, Reddy P, Lange P. Metabolic alterations following continent urinary diversion through colonic segments. J Urol. 1991;145:270–3.

92. Stein R, Schroder A, Thuroff J. Bladder augmentation and urinary diversion in patients with neurogenic bladder: non-surgical considerations. J Pediatr Urol. 2011;8(2):145–52.

93. Tanrikut C, McDougal W. Acid-base and electrolyte disorders after urinary diversion. World J Urol. 2004;22:168–71.

94. Gilbert S, Hensle T. Metabolic consequences and long-term complications of enterocystoplasty in children: a review [review] [71 refs]. J Urol. 2005;173:1080–6.

95. Mitchell M, Piser J. Intestinocystoplasty and total bladder replacement in children and young adults: followup in 129 cases. J Urol. 1987;138:579–84.

96. Poulsen A, Steven K. Acid-base metabolism after bladder substitution with the ileal urethral Kock reservoir. Br J Urol. 1996;78:47–53.

97. Hall M, Koch M, Halter S, Dahlstedt S. Morphologic and functional alterations of intestinal segments following urinary diversion. J Urol. 1993;149:664–6.

98. Akerlund S, Forssell-Aronsson E, Jonsson O, Kock N. Decreased absorption of 22Na and 36Cl in ileal reservoirs after exposure to urine. An experimental study in patients with continent ileal reservoirs for urinary or fecal diversion. Urol Res. 1991;19:249–52.

99. Plawker M, Rabinowitz S, Etwaru D, Glassberg K. Hypergastrinemia, dysuria-hematuria and metabolic alkalosis: complications associated with gastrocystoplasty. J Urol. 1995;154:546–9.

100. Kurzrock E, Baskin L, Kogan B. Gastrocystoplasty: long-term followup [review] [32 refs]. J Urol. 1998;160:2182–6.

101. Jonsson O, Olofsson G, Lindholm E, Tornqvist H. Long-time experience with the Kock ileal reservoir for continent urinary diversion. Eur Urol. 2001;40:632–40.

102. Fontaine E, Leaver R, Woodhouse C. The effect of intestinal urinary reservoirs on renal function: a 10-year follow-up. BJU Int. 2000;86:195–8.

103. Whitmore III WF, Gittes RF. Reconstruction of the urinary tract by cecal and ileocecal cystoplasty: review of a 15-year experience. J Urol. 1983;129:494–8.

104. Decter R, Bauer S, Mandell J, Colodny A, Retik A. Small bowel augmentation in children with neurogenic bladder: an initial report of urodynamic findings. J Urol. 1987;138:1014–6.

105. Kuss R, Bitker M, Camey M, Chatelain C, Lassau J. Indications and early and late results of intestinocystoplasty: a review of 185 cases. J Urol. 1970;103:53–63.

106. Ivancic V, et al. Progression of renal insufficiency in children and adolescents with neuropathic bladder is not accelerated by lower urinary tract reconstruction. J Urol. 2010;184:1768–74.

107. Matsui U, Topoll B, Miller K, Hautmann R. Metabolic long-term follow-up of the ileal neobladder. Eur Urol. 1993;24:197–200.

108. Pannek J, Haupt G, Schulze H, Senge T. Influence of continent ileal urinary diversion on vitamin B12 absorption. J Urol. 1996;155:1206–8.

109. Shaw J, Lewis MA. Bladder augmentation surgery—what about the malignant risk? Eur J Pediatr Surg. 1999;9 Suppl 1:39–40.

110. Carr LK, Herschorn S. Early development of adenocarcinoma in a young woman following augmentation cystoplasty for undiversion. J Urol. 1997;157:2255–6.

111. Kalisvaart J, Katsumi H, Ronningen L, Hovey R. Bladder cancer in spinal cord injury patients. Spinal Cord. 2010;48:257–61.

112. Barrington J, Jones A, James D, Smith S, Stephenson T. Antioxidant deficiency following clam enterocystoplasty. Br J Urol. 1997;80:238–42.

113. Dixon B, Chu A, Henry J, Kim R, Bissler J. Increased cancer risk of augmentation cystoplasty: possible role for hyperosmolal microenvironment on DNA damage recognition. Mutat Res. 2009;670:88–95.

114. Couillard D, Vapnek J, Rentzepis M, Stone A. Fatal perforation of augmentation cystoplasty in an adult [review] [22 refs]. Urology. 1993;42:585–8.

115. Braverman R, Lebowitz R. Perforation of the augmented urinary bladder in nine children and adolescents: importance of cystography. AJR Am J Roentgenol. 1991;157:1059–63.

116. Fontaine E, Leaver R, Woodhouse C. Diagnosis of perforated enterocystoplasty. J R Soc Med. 2003;96:393–4.

117. DeFoor W, Tackett L, Minevich E, Wacksman J, Sheldon C. Risk factors for spontaneous bladder perforation after augmentation cystoplasty [review] [15 refs]. Urology. 2003;62:737–41.

118. Bauer S, et al. Perforation of the augmented bladder. J Urol. 1992;148:699–703.

119. Novak T, Salmasi A, Mathews R, Lakshmanan Y, Gearhart J. Complications of complex lower urinary tract reconstruction in patients with neurogenic versus nonneurogenic bladder—is there a difference? J Urol. 2008;180:2629–34.

120. Fox J, Husmann D. Continent urinary diversion in childhood: complications of alcohol abuse developing in adulthood. J Urol. 2010;183:2342–6.

121. Kurzrock E. Pediatric enterocystoplasty: long-term complications and controversies. World J Urol. 2009;27:69–73.

122. Malone T, Lisle D, McNabb C, Ryan G. Traumatic rupture of an augmented bladder: computed tomography appearances. J Trauma. 2009;67:E85–7.

123. Glass R, Rushton H. Delayed spontaneous rupture of augmented bladder in children: diagnosis with sonography and CT. AJR Am J Roentgenol. 1992;158:833–5.

124. Slaton J, Kropp K. Conservative management of suspected bladder rupture after augmentation enterocystoplasty. J Urol. 1994;152:713–5.

125. Wolff J, Boeckmann W, Jakse G. Spontaneous bladder rupture following enterocystoplasty can be treated conservatively. Urol Int. 1994;52:113–4.

126. Rushton H, Woodard J, Parrott T, Jeffs R, Gearhart J. Delayed bladder rupture after augmentation enterocystoplasty. J Urol. 1988;140:344–6.

127. Elder J, Snyder H, Hulbert W, Duckett J. Perforation of the augmented bladder in patients undergoing clean intermittent catheterization. J Urol. 1988;140:1159–62.

128. Rink R. Bladder augmentation. Options, outcomes, future. Urol Clin North Am. 1999;26:111–23.

129. Kronner K, et al. Bladder calculi in the pediatric augmented bladder. J Urol. 1998;160:1096–8.

130. Nurse D, McInerney P, Thomas P, Mundy A. Stones in enterocystoplasties. Br J Urol. 1996;77:684–7.

131. Metcalfe P, et al. What is the need for additional bladder surgery after bladder augmentation in childhood? J Urol. 2006;176:1801–5.

132. Palmer L, et al. Urolithiasis in children following augmentation cystoplasty. J Urol. 1993;150:726–9.

133. Barroso U, Jednak R, Fleming P, Barthold J, Gonzalez R. Bladder calculi in children who perform clean intermittent catheterization. BJU Int. 2000;85:879–84.

134. DeFoor W, et al. Bladder calculi after augmentation cystoplasty: risk factors and prevention strategies. J Urol. 2004;172:1964–6.

135. Khoury A, et al. Stone formation after augmentation cystoplasty: the role of intestinal mucus. J Urol. 1997;158:1133–7.

136. Hamid R, Robertson W, Woodhouse C. Comparison of biochemistry and diet in patients with enterocystoplasty who do and do not form stones. BJU Int. 2008;101:1427–32.

137. Woodhouse C, Robertson W. Urolithiasis in enterocystoplasties [review] [29 refs]. World J Urol. 2004;22:215–21.

138. Robertson W, Woodhouse C. Metabolic factors in the causation of urinary tract stones in patients with enterocystoplasties. Urol Res. 2006;34:231–8.

139. Hensle T, Bingham J, Lam J, Shabsigh A. Preventing reservoir calculi after augmentation cystoplasty and continent urinary diversion: the influence of an irrigation protocol. BJU Int. 2004;93:585–7.

140. Brough R, O'Flynn K, Fishwick J, Gough D. Bladder washout and stone formation in paediatric enterocystoplasty. Eur Urol. 1998;33:500–2.

141. Murray K, Nurse D, Mundy A. Secreto-motor function of intestinal segments used in lower urinary tract reconstruction. Br J Urol. 1987;60:532–5.

142. Iannoni C, et al. Abnormal patterns of colorectal mucin secretion after urinary diversion of different types: histochemical and lectin binding studies. Hum Pathol. 1986;17:834–40.

143. Gillon G, Mundy A. The dissolution of urinary mucus after cystoplasty. Br J Urol. 1989;63:372–4.

144. George V, et al. The effect of ranitidine on urine mucus concentration in patients with enterocystoplasty. Br J Urol. 1992;70:30–2.

145. Akerlund S, Campanello M, Kaijser B, Jonsson O. Bacteriuria in patients with a continent ileal reservoir for urinary diversion does not regularly require antibiotic treatment. Br J Urol. 1994;74:177–81.

146. Bruce A, Reid G, Chan R, Costerton J. Bacterial adherence in the human ileal conduit: a morphological and bacteriological study. J Urol. 1984;132:184–8.

147. Greenwell T, Woodhams S, Smalley T, Mundy A. Effect of antibiotics on enterocystoplasty urinary nitrosamine levels. Urology. 2001;58:660–4.

148. Wagstaff K, Woodhouse C, Rose G, Duffy P, Ransley P. Blood and urine analysis in patients with intestinal bladders. Br J Urol. 1991;68:311–6.

149. van Nieuwkoop C, den Exter P, Elzevier H, den Hartigh J, van Dissel J. Intravesical gentamicin for recurrent urinary tract infection in patients with intermittent bladder catheterisation. Int J Antimicrob Agents. 2010;36:485–90.

150. Botto H, Neuzillet Y. Effectiveness of a cranberry (Vaccinium macrocarpon) preparation in reducing asymptomatic bacteriuria in patients with an ileal enterocystoplasty. Scand J Urol Nephrol. 2010;44:165–8.

151. Singh G, Thomas D. Bowel problems after enterocystoplasty. Br J Urol. 1997;79:328–32.

152. N'Dow J, Leung H, Marshall C, Neal D. Bowel dysfunction after bladder reconstruction. J Urol. 1998;159:1470–4; discussion 1474–5.

153. Jacobsen O, et al. Effect of enterocoated cholestyramine on bowel habit after ileal resection: a double blind crossover study. Br Med J (Clin Res Ed). 1985;290:1315–8.

154. Hofmann AF, Poley JR. Role of bile acid malabsorption in pathogenesis of diarrhea and steatorrhea in patients with ileal resection. I. Response to cholestyramine or replacement of dietary long chain triglyceride by medium chain triglyceride. Gastroenterology. 1972;62:918–34.

155. Fromm H, Malavolti M. Bile acid-induced diarrhoea. Clin Gastroenterol. 1986;15:567–82.

156. Pattni S, Walters J. Recent advances in the understanding of bile acid malabsorption. Br Med Bull. 2009;92:79–93.

157. Strawbridge L, Kramer S, Castillo O, Barrett D. Augmentation cystoplasty and the artificial genitourinary sphincter. J Urol. 1989;142:297–301.

158. Robertson A, Davies J, Webb R, Neal D. Bladder augmentation and replacement. Urodynamic and clinical review of 25 patients. Br J Urol. 1991;68:590–7.

159. McInerney PD, DeSouza N, Thomas PJ, Mundy AR. The role of urodynamic studies in the evaluation of patients with augmentation cystoplasties. Br J Urol. 1995;76:475–8.

160. Lopez Pereira P, Somoza Ariba I, Martinez Urrutia M, Lobato Romero R, Monroe E. Artificial urinary sphincter: 11-year experience in adolescents with congenital neuropathic bladder. Eur Urol. 2006;50:1096–101.

161. Hill D, Kramer S. Management of pregnancy after augmentation cystoplasty. J Urol. 1990;144:457–9.

162. Niknejad K, Atala A. Bladder augmentation techniques in women. Int Urogynecol J Pelvic Floor Dysfunct. 2000;11:156–69.

163. Fenn N, Barrington J, Stephenson T. Clam enterocystoplasty and pregnancy. Br J Urol. 1995;75: 85–6.

164. Kearse WJ, St Clair S, Hixson C, Ritchey M. Functional characteristics of enterocystoplasty after interruption of the mesenteric blood supply. J Urol. 1993;150:593–6.

Anal Sphincteroplasty

Patricia C. Alves-Ferreira and Brooke Gurland

Introduction

Direct sphincter trauma or neuropathic injuries from vaginal deliveries are the principal causative factors in the development of fecal incontinence in women less than 40 years old [1]. Treatment options for the incontinent woman include anal sphincteroplasty, sacral nerve stimulation (SNS), artificial anal sphincter, posterior anal repair, and dynamic graciloplasty. Anal sphincteroplasty has been the preferred surgical treatment for the symptomatic female with an anatomically disrupted external anal sphincter (EAS) muscle. Short-term results report improved bowel incontinence as high as 90% [2, 3] with decreasing continence on long-term follow-up studies. Over the past decade, SNS has been utilized as a treatment modality with good results for patients with fecal incontinence with or without an anal sphincter defect [4–7], but SNS has only recently approved in the USA for this indication. The artificial anal sphincter, a silastic band surgically placed around the lower rectum, has been shown to improve bowel control.

However, infection rates are reported at 33% [8, 9] leading to device failure or extrusion. Posterior anal repair is indicated for neuropathic incontinence and not very popular as its earlier results could not be duplicated. At best, only about 30% of the patients report improvement [10–12]. However, several long-term studies have shown favorable results [13, 14]. Dynamic graciloplasty is a complex procedure that involves gracilious muscle transposition and stimulation. This requires expertise; it is associated with a high morbidity and it is expensive [15–20]. This procedure is not an option in the United States since the stimulator used for muscle contraction is not commercially available. Other options include injectable bulking agents [21–24] into the anal sphincter which have shown to be effective in some studies, but are not presently approved in the USA for treatment of fecal incontinence. Transobturator insertion of a rectal sling has been reported with some success [25] and ongoing USA studies are in progress.

Unlike many of the alternatives mentioned, anal sphincteroplasty does not require expensive devices or postoperative maintenance required with implantable devices.

Sphincteroplasty can be performed in conjunction with other pelvic organ prolapse and urinary incontinence procedures without additional morbidity [26].

The complications associated with anal sphincteroplasty are low and will be discussed in this chapter.

P.C. Alves-Ferreira, PT • B. Gurland, MD, FACS (✉)
Department of Colorectal Surgery A30,
Cleveland Clinic, 9500 Euclid Avenue,
Cleveland, OH 44195, USA
e-mail: gurlanb@ccf.org

H.B. Goldman (ed.), *Complications of Female Incontinence and Pelvic Reconstructive Surgery*,
Current Clinical Urology, DOI 10.1007/978-1-61779-924-2_17, © Springer Science+Business Media, LLC 2013

Patient Evaluation

The following considerations are important when evaluating a patient with fecal incontinence for sphincteroplasty:

1. Bowel habits
2. Age
3. Obesity
4. Severity of symptoms
5. Local physical findings
6. Anal physiology and endoanal ultrasound

1. Bowel habits: Loose or watery stools may results in fecal incontinence. Bulking agents and antidiarrheals to thicken and decrease frequency of bowel movements remain the first line therapies. Sphincteroplasty will not be effective in patients with loose and irregular stools.
2. Age of the patient: Aging tissues are less likely to recover and maintain good quality over time. Several retrospective analyses suggest that older women have anorectal function that deteriorates over time [27, 28]. Advancing age may be associated with other pelvic floor defects including increased fibrosis and collagen deposition [29]. Other studies have found that age does not affect outcomes [2, 30]. Each case should individually take into consideration factors such as tissue quality and anal muscle contractility rather than biologic age alone.
3. Obesity: A high body mass index has been associated with poorer outcome after sphincteroplasty [27]. Obese women may have other factors that can contribute to the incontinence such as excessive pelvic floor descent and diabetes.
4. Severity of symptoms: Mild fecal symptoms or gas incontinence may persist even after successful sphincter repair. Patients should be counseled preoperatively regarding realistic postsurgical expectations. Nikiteas et al. [27] found that patients with severe symptoms undergoing primary repair reported the best outcomes.
5. Local physical findings: Lax anal sphincter muscles or a patulous anus may be associated with mucosal or full thickness rectal prolapse. Decreased or no anal sphincter contractility noted on physical examination is a poor prognostic sign for sphincter repair as it represents a poorly functioning anal sphincter. Good muscle bulk was reported by Vaizey et al. [31] as an important selection criterion for best results.
6. Anal physiologic testing: includes endoanal ultrasound and anal manometry. Low-squeeze pressure on anal manometry in conjunction with an anterior sphincter defect on endoanal ultrasound is the primary indication for sphincteroplasty. Other sonographic findings may include a variegated appearance of the EAS-indicating atrophic muscles, a very thin internal anal sphincter (IAS), or a large (more than 120°) defect of the EAS muscle. Pudendal nerve terminal latencies (PNTML) have also been used to evaluate the neurologic function of the anal sphincters, but the significance of prolonged PNTML are debated. In some studies, bilateral prolonged pudendal nerve latencies have been shown to be an important prognostic factor in patients undergoing anal sphincter repair [32].

Preoperative Management

Preoperative management includes:
– Appropriate patient selection
– Setting realistic postoperative continence expectations
– Mechanical bowel preparation 24 h before the onset of surgery
– A single dose of intravenous antibiotics administered prior to the surgery

Fecal diversion prior to sphincteroplasty has not been shown to improve outcomes and is not recommended. Hasegawa et al. [33] demonstrated equivalent sphincter reported outcomes between groups randomized to sphincteroplasty with or without diverting stoma. Patients in the stoma group suffered stoma-related complications.

Postoperative Management

Postoperative management requires keeping the stools soft, the area clean, and pain tolerable. Patients are kept overnight and discharged the following morning. There is no consensus on the routine administration of postoperative oral antibiotics at discharge. The patient is discharged on stool softeners.

Operative Management

Operative Technique and Results

A number of techniques have been described for sphincteroplasty and the choice is operator-dependant. Some authors advocate direct muscle apposition verses overlapping sphincteroplasty. Tjandra et al. [34] studied 36 patients with fecal incontinence caused by obstetric injuries, 12 underwent direct repair and 11 overlapping sphincter repair. At a median follow-up of 18 months, the functional results were significantly improved in both groups irrespective of the technique with improvement in incontinence in 75% and 73%, respectively.

For surgeons preferring overlapping sphincteroplasty, this can be performed *en bloc* thus avoiding separating the internal and external sphincters [35]. An anterior 120° curvilinear incision is made along the perineum to allow dissection and mobilization of the sphincter muscle and scar. It is important to preserve all scar tissue in order to anchor the sutures. *En bloc* repair involves mobilization of the EAS and IAS as a unit with overlap of the muscles complex. Other authors advocate anterior levatorplasty, IAS imbrication, and overlapping EAS repair [30]. The EAS is overlapped and mattress sutures are used to approximate the ends 2.0 PDS (Figs. 17.1, 17.2 and 17.3).

The edges of the wound are approximated in a V shape or longitudinally with interrupted 3.0 Vicryl mattress sutures. The center of the wound can be left open, a small drain inserted, or the wound can be closed. There are no studies that compare the functional results of *en bloc* compared to layered sphincteroplasty.

For patients with recurrent fecal incontinence after sphincteroplasty reevaluation and repeat repair is an alternative.

The rate of acceptance of the repeat sphincter repair is the same as that after a primary repair [31] and hence should be considered for selected patients with failed primary repairs.

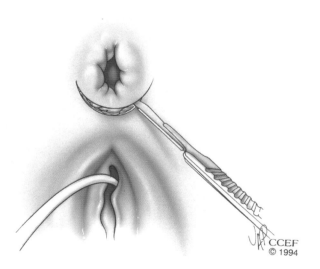

Fig. 17.1 A transverse incision along the perineum

Fig. 17.2 The external sphincter is identified and grasped with the Allis clamp

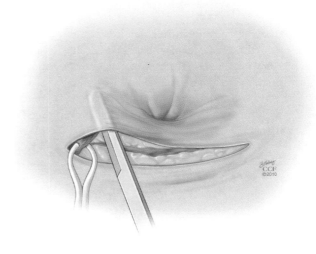

Fig. 17.3 The external sphincter is overlapped and sutured into place

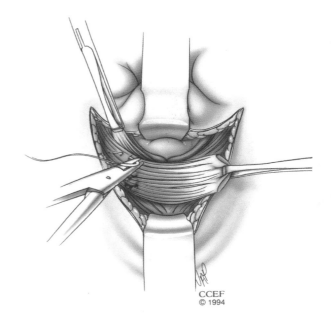

Complications

Complications that can occur in the early postoperative period include hematoma or seroma formation. This can be treated by opening the wound and evacuating the contents. Warm soaks in a bathtub or sitz bath for 5–10 min help with pain relief by promoting relaxation of the pelvic floor muscles. Directing a handheld shower or peribottle at the wound facilitates hygiene and gently debrides the perineum. Nonsteroidal medications are encouraged over narcotics for pain relief to avoid the constipating side effects associated with narcotics. Antibiotics with gram positive,

Table 17.1 Previous studies and complications after sphincteroplasty surgery

References	N	Age, mean (ranges)	Repair	Complications	FU, mean (ranges)	Outcomes, good/excellent N (%)
Gibbs [36]	36	47 (20–74)	OSR	Total: 11 (31%) Urinary alteration: 8 Anal stenosis: 3 Congestive heart failure: 1	43 (4–114)	24 (73)
Rothbarth [37]	39	51 (29–74)	Anterior sphincter repair	Total: 5 (12.8%) UTI: 1 Pneumonia: 1 Wound infection: 3	39.3 (12–114)	24 (62%)
Halverson and Hull [26]	44	38.5 (22–80)[a]	OSR	Wound infection: 4 (9%)	62.5 (47–141)[a]	30 (68)
Mevik [38]	29	45 (6–77)	Anterior sphincteroplasty	Total: 7 (24%) Wound complications: 4 UTI: 2 Pudendal damage: 1	84 (74–185)[a]	9 (53%)
Oom et al. [42]	172	58 (30–85)[a]	OSR	Total: 39 (23%) Wound complications: 35 Ileus: 2 DVT: 1 Lung embolism: 1	111 (12–207)[a]	44 (37)
Johnson et al. [43]	33	36 (22–75)[a]	OSR	Wound infection: 6 (18%)	103 (62–162)[a]	21 (64)

OSR overlapping sphincter repair; *UTI* urinary tract infection
[a]Results reported as median

negative, and anaerobic coverage are selectively prescribed in the setting of wound cellulitis.

Late complications include abscess formation and wound dehiscence. Abscesses require drainage; wound breakdown usually heals secondarily and rarely requires secondary suturing. The patient's main complaint after surgery is pain from the perineal wound. Table 17.1 reports previous studies and complications after sphincteroplasty surgery. Among the studies analyzed, the overall complications rate ranged from 9 to 31%. The outcomes are reported using different endpoints making comparisons difficult.

Early symptom improvement is noted after sphincteroplasty [2, 3, 30, 39]. However, there is a deterioration of fecal incontinence over time with return to baseline in 10 years. Long-term 5 and 10 year follow-up reveals [3] a decline in continence and increasing fecal accidents [28, 40]. Barisic et al. [41] reported that 48% of their patients had good or excellent results, with patients totally continent or continent to solid and liquid feces after a median follow-up of 6.7 years, while Oom et al. [42] reported 37% after 9 years. Johnson et al. [43] reported improved results in 55% of patients and excellent results in just 9%

of patients after 8.6 years. Halverson and Hull [26] reported 17% of patients totally continent after 5 years and 41% continent to liquid and solid stools.

Conclusion

Despite criticism regarding long-term functional results, sphincteroplasty is a viable option for women with sphincter trauma and associated fecal incontinence. Improvement after sphincteroplasty is noted but it is not to the level that it was before the sphincter injury. Complication rates are low and this procedure can be offered with limited morbidity.

References

1. Sultan AH, Kamm MA, Bartram CI, Hudson CN. Anal sphincter trauma during instrumental delivery. Int J Gynaecol Obstet. 1993;43(3):263–70.
2. Simmang C, Birnbaum EH, Kodner IJ, Fry RD, Fleshman JW. Anal sphincter reconstruction in the elderly: does advancing age affect outcome? Dis Colon Rectum. 1994;37(11):1065–9.

3. Grey BR, Sheldon RR, Telford KJ, Kiff ES. Anterior anal sphincter repair can be of long term benefit: a 12-year case cohort from a single surgeon. BMC Surg. 2007;7:1.

4. Jarrett ME, Dudding TC, Nicholls RJ, Vaizey CJ, Cohen CR, Kamm MA. Sacral nerve stimulation for fecal incontinence related to obstetric anal sphincter damage. Dis Colon Rectum. 2008;51(5):531–7.

5. Chan MK, Tjandra JJ. Sacral nerve stimulation for fecal incontinence: external anal sphincter defect vs. intact anal sphincter. Dis Colon Rectum. 2008;51(7):1015–24; discussion 1024–5.

6. Leroi AM, Parc Y, Lehur PA, et al. Efficacy of sacral nerve stimulation for fecal incontinence: results of a multicenter double-blind crossover study. Ann Surg. 2005;242(5):662–9.

7. Wexner SD, Coller JA, Devroede G, et al. Sacral nerve stimulation for fecal incontinence: results of a 120-patient prospective multicenter study. Ann Surg. 2010;251(3):441–9.

8. Wong WD, Jensen LL, Bartolo DC, Rothenberger DA. Artificial anal sphincter. Dis Colon Rectum. 1996;39(12):1345–51.

9. Christiansen J, Rasmussen OO, Lindorff-Larsen K. Long-term results of artificial anal sphincter implantation for severe anal incontinence. Ann Surg. 1999;230(1):45–8.

10. Engel AF, van Baal SJ, Brummelkamp WH. Late results of postanal repair for idiopathic faecal incontinence. Eur J Surg. 1994;160(11):637–40.

11. Jameson JS, Speakman CT, Darzi A, Chia YW, Henry MM. Audit of postanal repair in the treatment of fecal incontinence. Dis Colon Rectum. 1994;37(4):369–72.

12. Setti Carraro P, Kamm MA, Nicholls RJ. Long-term results of postanal repair for neurogenic faecal incontinence. Br J Surg. 1994;81(1):140–4.

13. Abbas SM, Bissett IP, Neill ME, Parry BR. Long-term outcome of postanal repair in the treatment of faecal incontinence. ANZ J Surg. 2005;75(9):783–6.

14. Mackey P, Mackey L, Kennedy ML, et al. Postanal repair—do the long-term results justify the procedure? Colorectal Dis. 2010;12(4):367–72.

15. Sielezneff I, Malouf AJ, Bartolo DC, Pryde A, Douglas S. Dynamic graciloplasty in the treatment of patients with faecal incontinence. Br J Surg. 1999;86(1):61–5.

16. Eccersley AJ, Williams NS. Dynamic graciloplasty for severe anal incontinence. Br J Surg. 1998;85(8):1158–9.

17. Rosen HR, Novi G, Zoech G, Feil W, Urbarz C, Schiessel R. Restoration of anal sphincter function by single-stage dynamic graciloplasty with a modified (split sling) technique. Am J Surg. 1998;175(3):187–93.

18. Christiansen J, Rasmussen OO, Lindorff-Larsen K. Dynamic graciloplasty for severe anal incontinence. Br J Surg. 1998;85(1):88–91.

19. Baeten CG, Geerdes BP, Adang EM, et al. Anal dynamic graciloplasty in the treatment of intractable fecal incontinence. N Engl J Med. 1995;332(24):1600–5.

20. Mander BJ, Wexner SD, Williams NS, et al. Preliminary results of a multicentre trial of the electrically stimulated gracilis neoanal sphincter. Br J Surg. 1999;86(12):1543–8.

21. Chan MK, Tjandra JJ. Injectable silicone biomaterial (PTQ) to treat fecal incontinence after hemorrhoidectomy. Dis Colon Rectum. 2006;49(4):433–9.

22. Davis K, Kumar D, Poloniecki J. Preliminary evaluation of an injectable anal sphincter bulking agent (Durasphere) in the management of faecal incontinence. Aliment Pharmacol Ther. 2003;18(2):237–43.

23. Kenefick NJ, Vaizey CJ, Malouf AJ, Norton CS, Marshall M, Kamm MA. Injectable silicone biomaterial for faecal incontinence due to internal anal sphincter dysfunction. Gut. 2002;51(2):225–8.

24. Vaizey CJ, Kamm MA. Injectable bulking agents for treating faecal incontinence. Br J Surg. 2005;92(5):521–7.

25. Yamana T, Takahashi T, Iwadare J. Perineal puborectalis sling operation for fecal incontinence: preliminary report. Dis Colon Rectum. 2004;47(11):1982–9.

26. Halverson AL, Hull TL. Long-term outcome of overlapping anal sphincter repair. Dis Colon Rectum. 2002;45(3):345–8.

27. Nikiteas N, Korsgen S, Kumar D, Keighley MR. Audit of sphincter repair. Factors associated with poor outcome. Dis Colon Rectum. 1996;39(10):1164–70.

28. Zutshi M, Tracey TH, Bast J, Halverson A, Na J. Ten-year outcome after anal sphincter repair for fecal incontinence. Dis Colon Rectum. 2009;52(6):1089–94.

29. Keighley M, Williams N. Fecal incontinence. In: Keighley M, editor. Surgery of the anus, colon and rectum, vol. 1. Philadelphia: WB Saunders; 2001.

30. Evans C, Davis K, Kumar D. Overlapping anal sphincter repair and anterior levatorplasty: effect of patient's age and duration of follow-up. Int J Colorectal Dis. 2006;21(8):795–801.

31. Vaizey CJ, Norton C, Thornton MJ, Nicholls RJ, Kamm MA. Long-term results of repeat anterior anal sphincter repair. Dis Colon Rectum. 2004;47(6):858–63.

32. Gilliland R, Altomare DF, Moreira Jr H, Oliveira L, Gilliland JE, Wexner SD. Pudendal neuropathy is predictive of failure following anterior overlapping sphincteroplasty. Dis Colon Rectum. 1998;41(12):1516–22.

33. Hasegawa H, Yoshioka K, Keighley MR. Randomized trial of fecal diversion for sphincter repair. Dis Colon Rectum. 2000;43(7):961–4; discussion 964–5.

34. Tjandra JJ, Han WR, Goh J, Carey M, Dwyer P. Direct repair vs. overlapping sphincter repair: a randomized, controlled trial. Dis Colon Rectum. 2003;46(7):937–42; discussion 942–3.

35. Galandiuk S, Roth LA, Greene QJ. Anal incontinence-sphincter ani repair: indications, techniques, outcome. Langenbecks Arch Surg. 2009;394(3):425–33.

36. Gibbs DH, Hooks VW. Overlapping sphincteroplasty for acquired anal incontinence. South Med J. 1993;86(12):1376–80.

37. Rothbarth J, Bemelman WA, Meijerink WJ et al. Dig Surg 2000;17(4):390–3.
38. Mevik K, Nordervals S, Kileng H, Johansen M, Vonen B. Long-term results after anterior sphincteroplasty for anal incontinence. Scand J Surg 2009;98(4):234–8.
39. Karoui S, Leroi AM, Koning E, Menard JF, Michot F, Denis P. Results of sphincteroplasty in 86 patients with anal incontinence. Dis Colon Rectum. 2000; 43(6):813–20.
40. Bravo Gutierrez A, Madoff RD, Lowry AC, Parker SC, Buie WD, Baxter NN. Long-term results of anterior sphincteroplasty. Dis Colon Rectum. 2004;47(5): 727–31; discussion 731–2.
41. Barisic GI, Krivokapic ZV, Markovic VA, Popovic MA. Outcome of overlapping anal sphincter repair after 3 months and after a mean of 80 months. Int J Colorectal Dis. 2006;21(1):52–6.
42. Oom DM, Gosselink MP, Schouten WR. Anterior sphincteroplasty for fecal incontinence: a single center experience in the era of sacral neuromodulation. Dis Colon Rectum. 2009;52(10):1681–7.
43. Johnson E, Carlsen E, Steen TB, Backer Hjorthaug JO, Eriksen MT, Johannessen HO. Short- and long-term results of secondary anterior sphincteroplasty in 33 patients with obstetric injury. Acta Obstet Gynecol Scand. 2010;89(11):1466–72.

Complications of Cosmetic Gynecologic Surgery

18

Dani Zoorob and Mickey Karram

Whether called cosmetogynecology or genito-plasty, the desire for enhancement of the genitalia is becoming more prevalent. As this field grows and is more in demand, surgeons have devised various techniques in the hopes of generating better outcomes. In the recent past, there has been a tremendous amount of direct to consumer marketing of these modalities by individual surgeons, promising improved sexual function.

The objective of this chapter will be to briefly discuss these various techniques and how to best avoid and manage complications when they occur.

Labioplasty

Labioplasty, also known as labial rejuvenation, is a term used to indicate surgical enhancement of the labia minora.

The documented origin of labioplasty dates back to the Pharos in Egypt [1]. This practice, although modified, has persisted in the African continent with variations as minor as modification of the labia minora up to extensive resection of

all external female genital organs including both labia majora and minora as well as the clitoris.

Amongst the earliest modern medical references discussing labioplasty is that of Hodgkinson and Hait [2] where they discuss the functional and aesthetic standpoints. Over the years, multiple procedures by Alter [3], Rouzier [4], Choi [5] and others were devised with varied outcomes and complications inherent to the different techniques used. Although less commonly used, the term labioplasty may encompass the augmentation or reduction of the labia majora.

A common nonaesthetic indication for labioplasty is dyspareunia, which usually occurs in women with labial hypertrophy due to the labia being pulled inward during intercourse. Other indications include vulvar irritation and discomfort with the use of underclothes or during ambulation or exercise. Some patients report an inimical impact on hygiene, especially when menstruating. The negative psychological impact of the "unnatural" or abnormally appearing labia, even if subjective, is also a frequent reason to consult a physician.

When performing a labioplasty, the essential goals [6, 7] should include the reduction of the hypertrophied labia minora with maintenance of the neurovascular supply, preservation of the introitus, optimal color/texture match, and minimal invasiveness.

While many systems to stage the severity of this condition exist, there is still no consensus on how best to define and classify labial hypertrophy. One system divides the classification into

D. Zoorob, MD • M. Karram, MD (✉)
Division of Female Pelvic Medicine & Reconstructive Surgery, The Christ Hospital, University of Cincinnati, 2123 Auburn Avenue, Suite 307, Cincinnati, OH 45219, USA

Department of Obstetrics/Gynecology, University of Cincinnati, Cincinnati, OH, USA
e-mail: mickey.karram@thechristhospital.com

H.B. Goldman (ed.), *Complications of Female Incontinence and Pelvic Reconstructive Surgery*, 197
Current Clinical Urology, DOI 10.1007/978-1-61779-924-2_18, © Springer Science+Business Media, LLC 2013

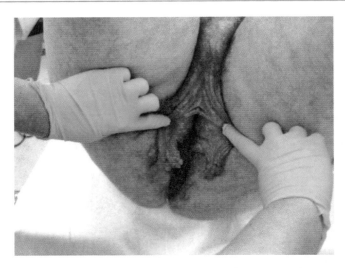

Fig. 18.1 Massive hypertrophy of the labia minor in a young woman with cerebral palsy

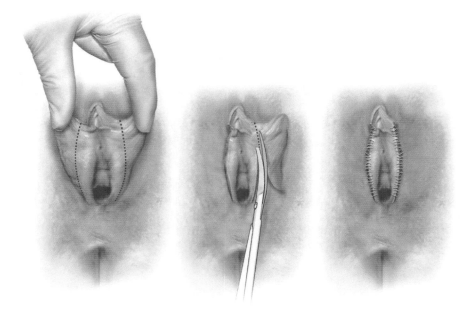

Fig. 18.2 The technique for simple excision of enlarged or hypertrophied labial skin. (**a**) Excess skin to be removed is marked. (**b**) Skin is excised. (**c**) Interrupted sutures reap proximate the edges of the labia

three stages: none (no edges protruding beyond the labia majora), mild (1–3 cm beyond the labia majora edges), severe (>3 cm). Another system described by Felicio [8] divides labial hypertrophy into four stages: I (<2 cm), II (2–4 cm), III (4–6 cm), IV (>6 cm). Franco and Franco [9] describe a similar classification. However, Rouzier et al. [4] considered that the normal maximal length of the labia minora should not exceed 4 cm whereas Radman [10] considers it to be 5 cm (Fig. 18.1).

A myriad of surgical techniques have been reported in the literature, including simple resection, wedge resection with modification of excisions, VY and Z-plasties, and de-epithelialization (Figs. 18.2 and 18.3).

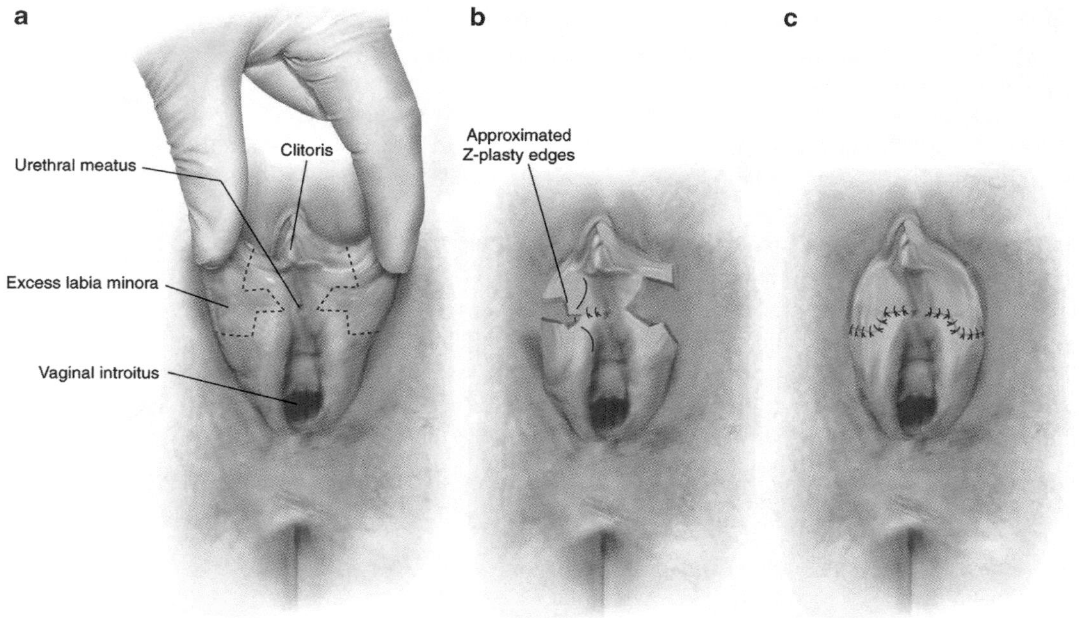

a   b   c

Fig. 18.3 Technique for Z-plasty. (**a**) Skin is to be excised. (**b**) Skin is excised and to be reapproximated transversely with fine interrupted sutures. (**c**) Completed repair

In simple resection, the excess or protuberant labial tissue is removed using scissors, a scalpel, or even a laser [11], in an elliptical or straight line. The edges are thereafter reapproximated with sutures, preferably simple interrupted, to ensure appropriate healing while maintaining the new contour. Depending on the defect or abnormality, the resection is preferably made while preserving a regular labia minora edge. Hodgkinson and Hait [2] and Maas and Hage [12] suggested a remnant minimal depth/length of 1 cm of labia minora. A novel technique called "Lazy S" reported by Warren [13] is reported to assist in reducing the likelihood of contractures and phimosis of the labia minora. This technique involves marking the area to be resected in an S shape—rather than an ellipse or straight line—prior to infiltration with local anesthetic and then resecting along the broadly wavy tract. It is reported that once healing occurs, the wavy line would take a relaxed appearance with little tension at the periphery of the tissue, giving a more "natural" and esthetic look.

Another technique is wedge resection, which is reported to reduce hypersensitivity and contour irregularities upon healing. The wedge system targets the most hypertrophied region in the labia minora and resects it all the way to its base in a V or wedge form. This in turn allows for a smaller exposed healing area; however, depending on the resection required, it might be deep enough that it reaches the proximity of the labia majora. Multiple variants of this procedure have been devised including Z-plasty and VY and the Matarasso modification/Star wedge resection [6]. The initial description of the technique was by Alter [3]. It involved a V-shaped wedge resection of the area with the most excess tissue identifiable. Maas and Hage [12] reported the wedge technique to strictly involve a W-shaped resection margin in the labia minora with no involvement of the clitoral dorsal hood, prepuce or fourchette. The advantage of this technique (also known as the Zig-Zag technique) was reported to be less likelihood of dyspareunia and introital obliteration. This technique is reported by some to induce loss of the pigmentation along the border of the labia minora despite the more natural contour being generated. In 2008, Alter [14] published the extended central wedge technique, a modification of his previous wedge resection, producing a more esthetic look, with the possibility of resection of excess tissue in the clitoral hood. This was based on the follow-up of previously operated patients. Among the modifications was one reported by Munhoz et al. [15] where the wedge is resected from the inferior aspect of the labia minora and a superior pedicle flap is developed. This is reported to provide a better esthetic look due to a more homogenous tinting of the labia.

In 2000, a novel technique devised by Choi and Kim [5] was reported to preserve tint, texture, sensation, and the neurovascular supply to the labia minora. This technique involved the central de-epithelialization of both labia minora on both sides with suturing of the new edges together.

In 2011, Alter [16] described the use of YV advancement flaps for the reconstruction of either absent, abruptly terminated, distorted, or scalloped labial edges. Being the closest match to labial tissue, clitoral hood tissue is mobilized in such a manner as to release two parallel folds—including the Dartos fascia and blood supply—from around the clitoris and rotating them on each side to form the labia minora.

Relative to the labia majora, Salgado et al. [17] reported that grafts of fat pads as well as fat injections could improve the atrophied look in some patients. Felicio [18] reported up to a maximum of 60 mL of fat injected into each labia majora per session, while requiring a drain if more is to be implanted or a continuation of the procedure 6 months later. Labia minora injections are also possible. Labia majora augmentation is reported to assist in increased comfort and sexual satisfaction, possibly due to acting as a shock absorber and possibly due to increased fullness and firmness of the labial tissues. Relative to hypertrophied labia majora, the option of resection in an elliptical or S-shaped incision may be necessary. However, the closer the final incisional edge to the labia minora, the more inconspicuous the scar is. Miklos and Moore [19] reported use of a semilunar incision on the medial

border of the labia majora. The possibility of lipoplasty could assist in avoiding large incisions and shorten the recovery period and reduce postoperative pain, however, the need for repeat or touch-up surgery may be required.

Labioplasty Complications

A variety of complications have been reported with labioplasty surgery. As a multitude of different techniques and modifications have been described, it is essential that the surgeon undertaking these procedures be intimately familiar with the anatomy of the external genitalia and its surrounding structures.

Infection: The perineal area seems less susceptible to infection compared to other regions of the body but the potential for abscess formation does exist and it is mandatory to follow the universal guidelines for surgical site cleansing prior to initiating surgery. Although no definitive recommendations for labioplasty have been set by any society, the routine gynecologic surgical antibiotic prophylaxis is advisable.

Surgical site breakdown: The possibility of contractures, tissue breakdown along the suture line, flap necrosis, edge necrosis, irregular resorption, phimosis of the clitoral hood, new onset of dyspareunia, loss of sensation or hyperalgesia may occur in the resection areas.

Care following surgery whether immediately postoperatively or few weeks out is mandatory. No set criteria is available in the literature denoting particular postoperative wound care. However, it is advisable that postoperative patients observe pelvic rest for a minimum of 4–6 weeks to ensure adequate healing with time and avoid trauma to the surgical site. Felicio [18] reports that ice packs and NSAIDs are ideal for postoperative edema and swelling. He also recommends ensuring that labioplasty is not concurrently performed with perineoplasty due to the intense swelling resulting in prolonged discomfort persisting up to 6 months. In addition to the discomfort, the likelihood of suture-line breakdown is much higher with the swelling. Thus staging the enhancement procedure would be advisable for both patient care and outcome.

Whether preceded by a wound hematoma or not, the development of a wound dehiscence is particularly ominous. Generalized flap degeneration or necrosis is more commonly seen in patients with sutures that have been placed tightly across the edges or when there is excessive traction on the attached tissue or flaps. It is crucial that when a flap is to be mobilized, the surgeon needs to ensure the persistence of the blood supply to allow the flap to survive as well as incorporate appropriately into the transposition site. Distal flap necrosis and subsequent gap formation in the labia may ensue if the vascular supply is not preserved. Additionally, in YV advancement flaps, the de-vascularization due to extensive undermining or extreme skinning prior to mobilization particularly endangers the survival of the transposed flap. Thus, ensuring minimal vessel distortion when mobilizing tissue with the least possible rotation/torque applied allows for better tissue survival.

Bleeding: Hemorrhage and the possibility of hematomas may be encountered based on the vessels severed. Arterial blood vessels usually require active control by cautery or suture ligation, whereas venous bleeders may need less aggressive management including pressure applied to the area involved or simple application of hemostatic agents.

The acute worsening of pain postoperatively may indicate the expansion of a hematoma, specifically if the labioplasty involved the labia majora. In addition to the psychological impact on a patient, the formation of a hematoma could potentially require drainage as well as prolonged courses of antibiotics, and ultimately exploration to control the bleeding vessel. This can be attempted initially by freeing the suture line and then evacuating the hematoma. Since not all hematomas are associated with arterial bleeding, the use of fibrin clotting agents could be useful at times when persistent minimal venous oozing is noted. While multiple agents exist, there are no studies identifying the benefit of one vs. another in the setting of labial hematomas.

Dyspareunia: Postoperative dyspareunia is known to occur more with wedge excisions as well as simple resection due to the newly formed exposed labial edge. Multiple studies [20–22] have been done to assess the innervations in hypertrophied labia compared to normal sized ones with no evidence of variability relative to size. However, postoperative hyperalgesia has been noted to occur, especially with associated infection, severe inflammation, or severe edema ensuing postoperatively. If swelling occurs and the tissue perfusion is impacted, the possibility of labial retraction and contracture (called phimosis if involving the clitoral hood) may occur as the healing process continues. This contracture may in turn cause severe dyspareunia that may require reoperation due to inability to achieve penetration.

Suture granulomas and scarring: The use of running sutures may predispose to contracture formation. Compared to simple interrupted sutures, the use of running locked sutures at the edges may predispose to a rugged or irregular labial edge due to localized necrosis or skin retraction. The use of simple interrupted sutures is preferred in simple excision procedures. The various studies available in the literature report the use of a variety of suture material with none proven to be superior to the other. When using absorbable sutures, the use of vicryl and monocryl would be ideal, although the use of chromic sutures in the study by Choi and Kim [5] also had good outcomes. Use of nonabsorbable sutures is theoretically associated with the least reaction at the suture site with possibly better cosmesis; however, it is less convenient to use due to the discomfort endured by the patient upon removal of the sutures. To ensure better outcomes, it is advisable to inquire preoperatively about any history of vicryl-associated suture granulomas. The removal of any permanent sutures should be carried out within 1 week of surgery to assist in healing while ensuring the pressure on the incision site is lower since the edema will have partially receded by then. When left too long, the sutures can potentially develop epithelialized tracts and this may have an unsightly appearance.

Maas and Hage [12] reported that simple amputation of the protuberant labium will generate a stiff and weakly healed edge along which irritation and potential retraction. The stiff edge formation is mostly due to extensive local fibrosis developing when healing. A technique called "Lazy S" reported by Warren [13] is reported to assist in reducing the likelihood of contractures and phimosis. This technique involves marking the area to be resected in an S shape. With healing, the wavy line takes a relaxed appearance with little tension at the margin. The homogenous or gradual labial pigmentary changes need to be preserved in order to ensure esthetic outcomes. The sudden change from dark pigmented folds to lightly pigmented labial folds is not advisable. The de-epithelialization and zig-zag techniques preserve this best.

Postoperative labial asymmetry: A complication that has been reported is inability to perceive the length of labial tissue necessary to be resected once they have been infiltrated with local anesthetic. The distortion incurred intra-operatively by the solution injected could render the margins irregular and not easily identifiable and thus it is imperative to mark the area for excision prior to any local injection. This helps prevent over-resection and provides the appropriate aesthetic result. It would be prudent that the delineation be done immediately preoperatively while the patient is awake, as well as preferably initially in the office during the surgical scheduling appointment so the appropriate change in labial size that is medically advisable compared to the patient's expectations can be determined.

Vaginoplasty

Vaginoplasty refers to modifications in the vagina to incur visual, sexual, or functional improvement. Its indications remain vague but usually include the desire for enhancement of vaginal aesthetics and improvement and augmentation of the sexual experience. Ostrzenski [23] considers

it a transformation involving both anatomy and function to allow for heightened sensation in intercourse. Typically, aesthetic vaginoplasty is primarily a perineoplasty. It involves restoring the normal visual anatomy of the region of the perineum/and posterior fourchette.

At all times, the vaginal canal should have a perpendicular relationship relative to the perineum. Having had an episiotomy or laceration during parturition, many women have been inadequately repaired and end up with an introitus that has a large membranous portion covering the posterior fourchette. This membrane often causes dyspareunia due to friction and stretching. This is usually due to an iatrogenic mal-approximation of musculature and overlying skin resulting in the perineum not having sufficient support and thus dyspareunia develops due to significant stretching and pulling of the thinned-out portion of this vulvovaginal structure (Fig. 18.4). The "membrane" itself does not have any physiologic purpose and thus it is advisable to have the "membrane" resected when restoring normal anatomy to the perineum.

Moving deeper into the vagina, the presence of significantly redundant tissue inside, whether following any surgical procedure or even if present naturally, could be reported as unappealing to the sexual partner. In rejuvenation and vaginoplasties, this may be considered as a potential repair site, where excess rugae may be excised, cauterized, or lasered. Certain areas to be targeted while resurfacing are episiotomy skin/mucosal tags or laceration repair sites, areas of previous colporrhaphies where dog-ears/tags have developed, as well as possible breakdowns in the repairs.

Another form of rejuvenation, called mucosal tightening/lateral colporrhaphy, involves excision of a wedge of vaginal mucosa after which the raw edges are sutured together. A case series by Adamo and Corvi [24] showed a 95% improvement in sensation after such a procedure.

At times, band-like adhesions may be noted extending across the vagina due to varied resorption and healing after any kind of repair (Fig. 18.5). Sometimes strictures may be seen

Fig. 18.4 The skin of the labia minor has been previously sewn across the midline, most likely at the time of the repair of a midline episiotomy

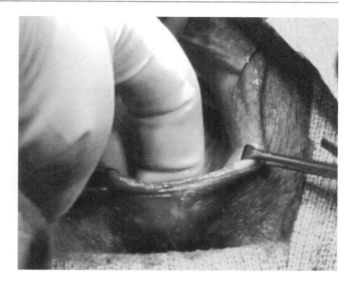

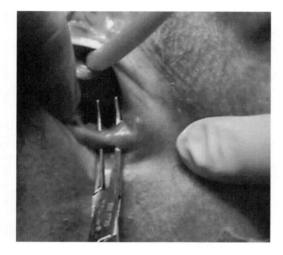

Fig. 18.5 Band of perineal scar tissue in a young patient following the repair of a perineal laceration

across the vagina. Severing these adhesion bands may be accomplished by using a cautery that is allowed to go deep into the vaginal wall—releasing the adhesion at its base if possible.

This typically allows for restoration of the normal vaginal caliber. Healing in such cases

may require secondary intention closure rather than surgical mucosal overlay. Recent studies have aimed at the regeneration of vaginal rugae to effect augmentation of sensory-coital pleasure. Loss of this rugation may occur with age as estrogen production dwindles, as well as in areas with site-specific defects. Studies have also shown that the anterior vaginal wall has denser innervation relative to the posterior wall [25–27] particularly distally. Attempts at regenerating rugae using linear laser stratification with vaporization up to the vaginal fascia was noted to improve sexual satisfaction in a prospective observational study but in only 20% of the test subjects [23].

Typically occurring postpartum, many women develop a widened genital hiatus as well as vaginal laxity. Prior to surgical repair aimed at tightening of the vagina itself, pelvic floor rehabilitation should be initiated to ensure adequate muscular toning of the vagina. In general, only a perineoplasty is required for tightening the genital hiatus but some may consider doing a posterior colporrhaphy (Fig. 18.6). Studies done to assess dyspareunia following colporrhaphy show that it is less frequent if perineorrhaphy involving the levators is avoided.

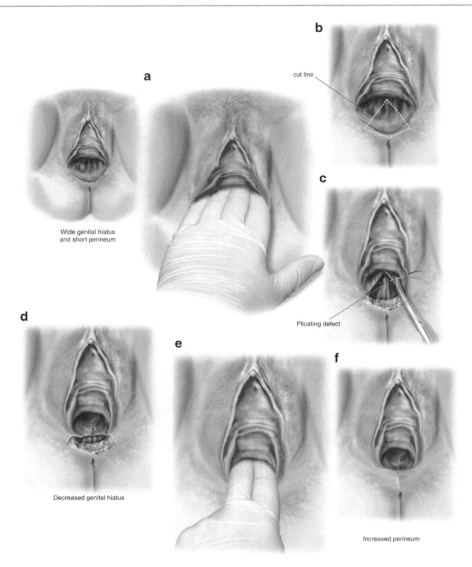

Fig. 18.6 The technique of vaginoplasty and reconstruction with the sole aim of tightening the vaginal introits. (**a**) Note the wide genital hiatus, which easily allows the insertion of four fingers. (**b**) A diamond-shaped piece of tissue to be excised is marked. (**c**) The tissue has been removed, and deep stitches are taken through the perirectal fascia and levitator muscles to build up the posterior vaginal wall. Great care is taken to avoid the creation of a posterior vaginal wall ridge. (**d**) The upper portion of the posterior vaginal wall is closed in preparation for perineal reconstruction. (**e**) After perineal reconstruction, the introits allows the insertion of only two fingers. (**f**) Completed repair; note the perpendicular relationship between the posterior vaginal wall and the perineum

Complications of Vaginoplasty

Depending on the procedure used for vaginoplasty, a myriad of complications may occur.

Laser and cautery-related complications—If the laser is used to create rugae, the avoidance of damage to the fascial layers is important. Currently, there are no recommendations for the depth of vaporization but it is best to avoid reaching the glistening fascial layer so as to avoid iatrogenic development of site-specific defects. The laser vaporization, if not used judiciously, may incur damage to any of the underlying tissues including the bowels, bladder, and urethra. Furthermore, it is advisable to avoid prolonged tissue exposure—of the same spot—to avoid peripheral damage by heat conduction. As with the laser and due to significant peripheral heating of adjacent tissues, caution is advised with extensive use of monopolar cautery. In procedures of resurfacing where the extra rugae or skin tags in vagina are removed, it is best to brush rather than attempt to cut or shave the rugae. The brushing technique, as its name implies, involves rapid and superficial back and forth cautery tip motion. This modality will result in removal of only the necessary tissue particularly since the extent of the cautery is well visualized and controlled. If the cautery tip is placed on the vaginal mucosal tag and activated continuously until the tag shrivels, the underlying tissue may be damaged by the heat generated from the tag degeneration and accordingly may result in a potential area of necrosis that could impact the integrity of vaginal walls. This in turn may predispose for vesicovaginal or rectovaginal fistulas. If reporting new onset fluid leakage or foul odor on intercourse, then a detailed pelvic exam with assessment for fistulas should ensue. Furthermore, it is important to inform the patient of the significant discharge that will develop after surgery which could last for weeks as the sloughing occurs. Pain should be absent to minimal with this type of procedure and the patient should recover rapidly. If the patient develops worsening pain or if pain develops days after surgery, then the likelihood of damage to an adjacent structure is very high. The development of fever is unlikely unless an infection has occurred. The use of the cautery to create relaxing incision when vaginal strictures exist is highly successful in resolving the constrictions as long as bleeding is controlled and vessels are avoided. Being familiar with the vascular anatomy of the vagina prior to any surgery is crucial. It is advisable to use simple interrupted sutures to control hemorrhage of actively bleeding tissues since cautery may sometimes make further suturing difficult, especially if retraction of the vessel occurs with unsuccessful cautery. The sutures applied should preferably be placed perpendicular to the band that was released so as to maintain the newly developed caliber. The use

of any form of energy in the vagina increases the risk of stricture and fibrotic band formation, even if the initial surgery was for the release of strictures.

Persistent postoperative dyspareunia—The vaginal innervation is densest anteriorly and distally. If colporrhaphy is primarily performed for rejuvenation and not defect repair, then the risk of dyspareunia is lower but is least when a perineoplasty is not performed. Severe superficial dyspareunia has been reported when the perineoplasty involved levator muscle plication. The discomfort classically occurs when the introitus is tightened significantly. The pain is usually muscular-related and not neurogenic in nature, but the dyspareunia can be quite significant at times, resulting in abstinence instead of enhancement of the sexual experience.

Pelvic muscle dyssynergia—The use of Botox described by some for alleviation of Levator ani spasm has been reported in the literature with notable results. It has been described for the rejuvenation process as well; however, the associated complications, although rarely encountered, can potentially last for a few months until the medication wears off. Judicious injection could help avoid the development of retroperitoneal hematomas and internal bleeding, pelvic muscle dyssynergia, urinary and fecal incontinence and obstruction, pelvic abscess formation, permanent neural damage, leg and pelvic weakness, and new onset of referred pain. Careful assessment and application of Botox are necessary while ensuring an injection that is not too deeply placed.

Site-specific augmentation complications—To increase sensation to both partners, injections of fat or fillers into the vagina, and even grafts, have been described. The placement of grafts is potentially associated with erosions and dyspareunia as well as bowel and bladder perforation. Despite it being typically injected into the labia majora in vaginal rejuvenation, some have used fat to create ring formations within the vagina with the hope of providing an enhanced sexual experience. The complication that may ensue is severe edema that could potentially impact urination as well as abscess formation and vaginal mucosal wall breakdown with ulcer formation—with the breakdown developing immediately postoperatively or potentially during intercourse. Another potentially injectable and often topical form of treatment for vaginal rejuvenation is mesotherapy which uses herbs and chemicals to induce lipolysis or change tissue consistency and thus theoretically enhance vaginal sensation. Since these compounds have not been tested adequately for vaginal use, they should be avoided as they may create irritative and potentially damaging effects resulting in sclerosis and significant sloughing of the epithelium causing pain and copious discharge.

Clitoroplasty

The first well-documented corrective clitoral surgery dates back to 1934 where Young [28] described a clitoridectomy. As time passed, studies in the mid- to late-1960s ascertained the need and importance of the clitoris in the sexual experience.

Clitoroplasty can involve the increased exposure of clitoral tissue which may augment sexual enjoyment. It may also involve the removal of tissues to assist in an enhanced visual genital appearance, especially when combined with labioplasty and possibly vaginoplasty. Furthermore, clitoroplasty may involve the repositioning and resizing of the clitoris especially in women with evidence of hypertrophy—particularly if afflicted with hyperandrogenism.

Various techniques have been described to surgically manage clitoromegaly. One technique involves resecting the excess tissue from the clitoral hood and then reapproximating the edges with concurrent reduction in the clitoral size by resecting part of its corpora then attaching it to the periosteum [29].

With the desire for increased sexual pleasure, a procedure for exposing the clitoris has been devised. Clitoral unhooding involves resection of tissue covering the clitoral tip, at times circumferentially, thus exposing it more, much like circumcision in males. A similar procedure is the reduction of the clitoral hood which involves repositioning of the tissues overlying the clitoris with the help of sutures rather than actual tissue resection. This usually allows for increased stimulation during intercourse and accordingly heightened sexual pleasure.

Complications of Clitoroplasty

Hemorrhage and necrosis of the clitoris—When reducing, advancing, or repositioning, the clitoris, the likelihood of severing of the vascular supply is high. Undiagnosed, this could result in withering and death of the reattached clitoral tip. Partial resection of the clitoris, which is often done in certain types of female genital mutilation (sometimes misleadingly called "circumcision"), will usually have a marked negative impact on intercourse and is associated with significant blood loss. The blood supply to the labia minora as well as the clitoris arises from the posterior labial, perineal, and dorsal clitoral branches of the pudendal artery. The neurovascular bundle lies at the dorsal side of the clitoris, covered with fatty tissue padding and with the suspensory ligament of the clitoris lying beneath it. Ensuring appropriate dissection is crucial to avoiding these complications.

New-onset clitoral pain—When reduction of the clitoris involves resection or repositioning of the clitoris, it is crucial to safeguard the neurovascular connection between the tip of the clitoris and the body [30]. The interruption of the neural pathway could render the clitoris insensitive and its contribution to the sexual experience rendered absent, thus nerve sparing techniques have been devised and their use is advised.

The posterior labial and perineal branches of the pudendal nerve (S2–S4) predominantly supply sensation to the labia minora with the clitoris receiving additional autonomic innervation from the hypogastric and pelvic plexuses. Anecdotally, the entity of persistent postoperative pain generated at the periosteal clitoral insertion site as well as throughout the clitoris occurring with arousal has been reported.

Contractures around the clitoris—Contracture of the incision line may result in phimosis and theoretically strangulation of the clitoral tip especially if multiple gynecoplasty procedures are done simultaneously. Due to the edema that develops postoperatively, it is advisable to avoid using a running suture line and use widely spaced interrupted sutures instead.

In cases of clitoral reduction, development of contractures along the suture lines as well as long standing pain are risks the patient needs to know about preoperatively—these develop more often in association with infection and hematomas. In clitoral unhooding, both the amount of tissue excised as well as the closure techniques are crucial. The complete exposure of the clitoris causing hypersensitivity could become bothersome due to the continuous friction with the patient's clothes. Furthermore, the appearance of the clitoris, if excessively unhooded, might be unsightly.

Conclusion

As women become more aware of the their genital appearance in comparison to what is publicized as normal or ideal, more women turn to surgical alternatives for cosmetic or perceived sexual enhancement. This is an evolving field with different techniques continuously being developed to achieve both better outcomes and reduced risks. Since cosmetogynecology deals with improvement of quality of life, it is crucial that the enhancements are what the patient desires and are within the limits of safe surgical practice. Patients who are considering such procedures should be fully aware of the various potential complications discussed in this chapter.

References

1. Hosken FP. The epidemiology of female genital mutilations. Trop Doct. 1978;8:150–6.
2. Hodgkinson DJ, Hait G. Aesthetic vaginal labioplasty. Plast Reconstr Surg. 1984;74(3):414–6.
3. Alter GJ. A new technique for aesthetic labia minora reduction. Ann Plast Surg. 1998;40(3):287–90.
4. Rouzier R, Louis-Sylvestre C, Paniel BJ, Haddad B. Hypertrophy of labia minora: experience with 163 reductions. Am J Obstet Gynecol. 2000;182(1 Pt 1): 35–40.
5. Choi HY, Kim KT. A new method for aesthetic reduction of labia minora (the deepithelialized reduction of labioplasty). Plast Reconstr Surg. 2000;105(1): 419–22; discussion 423–4.
6. Tepper OM. Labioplasty: anatomy, etiology, and a new surgical approach. Aesthet Surg. 2011;31:511.
7. Assaad MB. Female circumcision in Egypt: social implications, current research, and prospects for change. Stud Fam Plann. 1980;11:3–16.
8. Felicio Y. Chirurgie Intime. La Rev Chir Esth Lang Franc. 1992;XVII(67):37–43.
9. Franco T, Franco D. Hipertrofia de Ninfas. J Bras Ginecol. 1993;103:163–5.
10. Radman HM. Hypertrophy of the labia minora. Obstet Gynecol. 1976;48:78S–9.
11. Pardo J, Solà V, Ricci P, Guilloff E. Laser labioplasty of labia minora. Int J Gynaecol Obstet. 2006;93(1): 38–43.
12. Maas SM, Hage JJ. Functional and aesthetic labia minora reduction. Plast Reconstr Surg. 2000;105: 1453–6.
13. Warren AE. Techniques for labia minora reduction: an algorithmic approach. Aesthetic Plast Surg. 2010;34: 105–10.
14. Alter GJ. Aesthetic labia minora and clitoral hood reduction using extended central wedge resection. Plast Reconstr Surg. 2008;122:1780–9.
15. Munhoz AM, Filassi JR, Ricci MD, et al. Aesthetic labia minora reduction with inferior wedge resection and superior pedicle flap reconstruction. Plast Reconstr Surg. 2006;118:1237–47; discussion 1248–50.
16. Alter GJ. Labia minora reconstruction using clitoral hood flaps, wedge excisions, and YV advancement flaps. Plast Reconstr Surg. 2011;127(6):2356–63.
17. Salgado CJ, Tang JC, Desrosiers III AE. Use of dermal fat graft for augmentation of the labia majora. J Plast Reconstr Aesthet Surg. 2012;65(2):267–70.
18. Felicio Y. Labial surgery. Aesthetic Surg J. 2007;27: 322–8.
19. Miklos JR, Moore RD. Simultaneous labia minora and majora reduction: a case report. J Minim Invasive Gynecol. 2011;18(3):378–80.
20. Sommerova J, Malinovsky L, Martincik J. Sensory nerve endings in hypertrophy of the human labium minus pudenda. Folia Morphol (Praha). 1974;22: 266–7.
21. Malinovsky L, Sommerova J. Sensory nerve endings in the human labia pudenda and their variability. Folia Morphol (Praha). 1973;21:351–3.
22. Malinovsky L, Sommerova J, Martincik J. Quantitative evaluation of sensory nerve endings in hypertrophy of labia minora pudenda in women. Acta Anat (Basel). 1975;92:129–44.
23. Ostrzenski A. Vaginal rugation rejuvenation (restoration): a new surgical technique for an acquired

sensation of wide/smooth vagina. Gynecol Obstet Invest. 2012;73(1):48–52.

24. Adamo C, Corvi M. Cosmetic mucosal vaginal tightening (lateral colporrhaphy): improving sexual sensitivity in women with a sensation of wide vagina. Plast Reconstr Surg. 2009;123(6):212e–3.

25. Hilliges M, Falconer C, Ekman-Ordeberg G, Johansson O. Innervation of the human vaginal mucosa as revealed by PGP 9.5 immunohistochemistry. Acta Anat. 1995;153:119–26.

26. Alzate H, Londono ML. Vaginal erotic sensitivity. J Sex Marital. 1984;10:49–56.

27. Hoch Z. Vaginal erotic sensitivity by sexual examination. Acta Obstet Gynecol Scand. 1986;5:767–73.

28. Young HH. Genital abnormalities, hermaphroditism and related adrenal disease. Baltimore, MD: Williams and Wilkins; 1937. p. 103–5.

29. Sayer RA, Deutsch A, Hoffman MS. Clitoroplasty. Obstet Gynecol. 2007;110(2 Pt 2):523–5.

30. Papageorgiou T, Hearns-Stokes R, Peppas D, Segars JH. Clitoroplasty with preservation of neurovascular pedicles. Obstet Gynecol. 2000;96 (5 Pt 2):821–3.

Martius Fat Pad Construction

19

Sunshine Murray and Philippe E. Zimmern

Introduction

The Martius labial fat pad is a pedicle graft of fatty tissue from the labia majora which can be used as an interposition layer during a variety of vaginal procedures. First described by Martius [1], the procedure is fairly simple and quick, allowing the surgeon to harvest a well-vascularized fat pad of variable length (typically 8–12 cm) and transfer it where needed to enhance the repair of complex or recurrent urethral or vesical pathology. However, as with any surgical technique, complications can occur including hematoma, infection, pain or numbness, sexual dysfunction, and labial distortion. We aim to describe these complications as well as provide what information is available from the literature and our own experience on how to avoid them and manage them when necessary. To this end, we will also briefly cover the indications and technique for this versatile procedure.

S. Murray, MD • P.E. Zimmern, MD (✉)
Department of Urology, UT Southwestern
Medical Center, 5323 Harry Hines Boulevard,
Dallas, TX 75390-9110, USA
e-mail: philippe.zimmern@utsouthwestern.edu

Indications

The Martius fat pad is quite versatile and therefore has been used as an adjunct in many complex vaginal reconstructive surgeries to improve outcomes. It can be used as an additional tissue interposition layer in closure of vesico- or urethrovaginal fistulas and may be most important in those fistulas associated with radiation and/or recurrent fistulas that have failed to close after prior attempt at repair [2–6]. It has been reported in the closure of ano- and rectovaginal fistulas [6–8] as well as in the transvaginal repair of bladder injury during vaginal hysterectomy to prevent fistula formation [9]. Martius flap can be used in transvaginal bladder neck closures as well as urethral diverticulectomy and can also be useful in transvaginal artificial urinary sphincter placement although most authors recommend a retropubic approach for placement of cuffs. Another rare indication is in the postcystectomy patient with a peritoneovaginal fistula [10] or neobladder-vaginal fistula [11]. It can also be used in construction of a neovagina after pelvic exenteration or other rare cases requiring vaginal construction or reconstruction [12]. The most common indication in our practice is as an adjunct to urethrolysis to prevent rescarring to the back of the pubic symphysis [13–15].

Technique

An 8–10 cm long vertical incision is made over the labia majora from the level of the mons pubis down towards the level of the fourchette. This is a typical incision for a high vault vesico-vaginal fistula because the length of the fat pad must be sufficient to reach the vaginal apex. When the procedure is indicated for urethral or bladder neck pathology, the incision can be shorter and may start midway over the labia majora, still extending down to the level of the posterior fourchette. The side, left or right, depends on the location of the pathology being repaired, and at times should be done from the side opposite to where the fat pad will ultimately be placed because of the need for it to cross over.

The labia majora incision is deepened to the level of the labial fat pad. The fat pad can be gently grasped with a Babcock clamp and mobilized on an inferior pedicle providing a postero-inferior blood supply to the graft based on branches from the internal pudendal artery. To facilitate the dissection of the flap, the skin edges can be held retracted by the hooks of a Lonestar retractor. To avoid medial labial skin distortion or retraction after the fat pad harvest has been completed, we recommend leaving some fat medially beneath the labial skin and carrying the fat pad dissection slightly obliquely and away from the inner labial folds. Once a sufficient length has been dissected laterally and medially, the flap is gradually divided superiorly. Large veins can supply the apex of the flap coming from the mons pubis and they may require careful ligature to avoid retraction and a secondary labial hematoma. Next, the Martius fat pad graft dissection continues by detaching the fat pad posteriorly off the underlying ischiocavernosus and bulbocavernosus muscles, taking care once again to leave a broad base inferiorly to protect the blood supply.

Historically, the Martius labial fat pad included the bulbocavernosus muscle vascularized by the labial artery, a branch of the internal pudendal artery, as well as the fat pad of the labia majora vascularized by the obturator artery and the internal and external pudendal arteries. Currently, most specialists use the labial fat pad without excising the bulbocavernosus muscle. However, in situations involving a vaginal wall defect after extensive mesh removal or large vesico-vaginal fistulae, the labial fat pad graft can be harvested with a segment of skin to close both defects.

After having completed the mobilization of the fat pad, a figure of eight absorbable suture can be placed at the extremity of the flap to help with its tunnelling alongside the vaginal wall later on. The fat pad graft can be harvested ahead of any upcoming steps in the repair which can involve significant bleeding. By doing so, the fat pad is ready for use and can help decreasing the overall blood loss, thus reducing the likelihood for blood transfusion. The fat pad can be wrapped in a moist gauze until its use later on. Once the fistula repair or other procedure for which the fat pad graft was selected is completed, a tunnel should be created alongside the lateral vaginal wall toward the destination of the flap. This tunnel is created with long Metzenbaum scissors and/or a ring forceps. The tunnel should be widened to accept at least two fingers in order to prevent compression of the blood supply of the fat pad which could compromise its survival. The suture at the extremity of the fat pad can then be grasped at the end of a right angle clamp or long Kelly clamp, which can be slid through the pre-established tunnel alongside the vagina. The suture can be retrieved easily on the vaginal side and pulled out to direct the fat pad into its tunnel and ultimately into position over the intended area of coverage. The pedicle graft once passed through the tunnel can be secured in place with a few absorbable sutures over the suture line which it is intended to protect.

Although the dissection of the tunnel can sometime provoke bleeding, once the fat pad is in place the bleeding will typically decrease or stop. However, to avoid a secondary labial hematoma, it is recommended to place a labial drain (small

Penrose or #7 Jackson-Pratt). The incision is closed in two layers, a running subcutaneous deep absorbable suture over the drain, and then interrupted absorbable sutures on the skin. In case of a secondary infection or hematoma, some of these interrupted sutures at the lower extremity of the skin incision closure can be easily removed to facilitate a drain placement. In the absence of bleeding, swelling, or infection, the labial drain can be removed within 24–48 h postoperatively.

Complications

Hematoma or Seroma

As is the case with most surgical procedures, there is a risk of bleeding and hematoma formation. The fat pad is mobilized on an inferior pedicle based on branches of the internal pudendal vessels as discussed earlier. One of the benefits of this graft as a tissue interposition is its vascularity, but this also contributes to the risk of bleeding and hematoma formation. Thus, maintaining and ensuring achievement of hemostasis at the site of harvest as well as on the pedicle graft itself is of utmost importance in preventing hematoma formation. In addition to meticulous hemostasis at the time of surgery, the use of a drain (penrose or Jackson-pratt) postoperatively may also decrease the likelihood of hematoma formation. Although incidence of hematoma is not reported in the literature, Songne et al. [8] described a seroma formation in 3 of 14 patients (21%) undergoing repair of anovaginal or rectovaginal fistulas with Martius interposition. Seroma formation may also be prevented or decreased by the use of a drain postoperatively. Typically, seromas and hematomas when they occur will resolve on their own over time without any intervention. However, if either becomes infected as would be indicated by erythema surrounding and/or purulent drainage from the incision, then prompt drainage is indicated.

Infection

Although the incidence of wound infection for a Martius fat pad graft is not well studied or reported, the risk of such a complication appears to be relatively small. McNevin et al. [7] reported one (6%) superficial labial wound breakdown among 16 patients undergoing repair of complex rectovaginal fistulas with the use of Martius as tissue interposition whereas Songne et al. [8] reported no wound infections in their retrospective series of 14 patients. Just as with hematoma and seroma, the use of a drain postoperatively may decrease the risk of infection as may appropriate perioperative antibiotic usage. This has been a very rare occurrence in our practice over the past 25 years. Yeast infection can also easily develop in the groin or over the incision, and should be treated by the use of antifungal ointment or oral medications. This can sometimes be prevented by the preoperative treatment of infections present prior to surgery and by keeping the groin and perineum clean and dry postoperatively. When they occur, postoperative wound infections can be treated with antibiotics and when necessary, incision and debridement.

Pain and/or Numbness

Pain in the immediate postoperative period is expected and typically lasts a few days until the drain is removed and the swelling decreases. Ice packs are recommended initially. Loose underwear or garments allow for avoidance of direct skin contact and irritation. Likewise, a urethral Foley catheter when necessary is taped to the leg opposite the involved labia, or, when not critically needed, it is removed early on, trusting a suprapubic tube for bladder drainage. Following showering or bathing, direct contact with a towel can be avoided by using a blow dryer.

Chronic pain at the harvest site appears to be a rare complication of the procedure and might be a result of nerve injury during the harvesting. Intermittent discomfort and labial sensitivity was found in a retrospective review by Petrou et al. [13], in 3 of 8 women undergoing a Martius flap at the time of suprameatal urethrolysis for bladder outlet obstruction up to 1 year postoperatively. However, 5 (62%) reported self-perceived decreased sensation or numbness at the harvest site. A few other reports had similar findings, including Webster et al. [15], where 2/12 (17%) women undergoing Martius in combination with urethrolysis reported decreased sensation at the site of harvest, and Carey et al. [14], where 2/23 (9%) reported transient labial numbness. However, Carr and Webster reported on four women who underwent full-thickness cutaneous Martius flap for vaginal reconstruction [16] and all patients reported reduced sensation at the harvest site suggesting that when a skin island of the labia majora is harvested with the fatty pedicle flap the incidence of decreased sensation may be increased.

Sexual Dysfunction

Sexual dysfunction secondary to a Martius fat pad graft appears related to the labial pain and/or numbness, as well as sometimes to skin retraction medially. Sexual function typically resumes within 2–3 months after the original procedure once the labial and vaginal incisions are completely healed. Sexual dysfunction is uncommon even in series reporting initial pain and/or numbness. For example, Petrou et al. [13] noted 38% of pain at the harvest site and 62% with decreased sensation or numbness at 1 year, yet only 1 of 8 patients (12.5%) reported sexual dysfunction due to pain. Elkins et al. [6] in a retrospective review of patients undergoing Martius flap along with vesico- and rectovaginal fistula repairs reported a 25% incidence of dyspareunia.

Since the Martius is used in complex vaginal surgery where scarring can be expected and this scarring could potentially lead to a high rate of secondary dyspareunia, it has been suggested that its use will lead to lesser scarring and therefore possibly less vaginal discomfort or dyspareunia. In fact, in one series by Rangnekar et al. [5], 38 patients underwent successful urinary-vaginal fistula repair (20 with Martius and 18 without). No patients undergoing repair with Martius reported dyspareunia postoperatively whereas 6 (33%) of those repaired without Martius did. The authors proposed that the increased blood supply and lymphatic drainage afforded by the flap interposition might have lessened vaginal scarring thereby leading to the lower rates of dyspareunia.

Labial Distortion

Due to the removal of underlying fatty tissue from the labia majora on one side, labial distortion can raise cosmetic concerns. A few reports comment on the incidence of this complication, but all are retrospective reviews and the numbers reported are quite variable. McNevin et al. [7] reported no complaints related to cosmesis among 16 patients undergoing Martius in combination with low rectovaginal fistula repair. However, in eight women who underwent Martius in combination with suprameatal urethrolysis, Petrou et al. [13] reported 2 (25%) felt the harvest site appeared no different from preoperative appearance, 2 (25%) that it was almost normal and 1 (12%) noted it was markedly different. The remaining three patients (38%) had never examined the harvest site. In an attempt to prevent or limit this secondary distortion due to labial skin healing and outward retraction at the superior medial edge of the labia majora, we have changed our practice to a more lateral incision over the bulge of the labia majora. In addition, we purposely leave fat medially over the inner portion of the labia majora. The surgical outcome of this technique is shown with intraoperative and postoperative images in Fig. 19.1. In addition, an in situ technique for Martius harvesting has been described by Rutman et al. [17] which avoids a

Fig. 19.1 Martius fat pad harvested through an incision on the lateral side of the labial bulge. Fat was left medially to avoid any postoperative distortion or retraction (**a**). Same patient seen 1 year later. The incision is barely visible and there is no asymmetry (**b**)

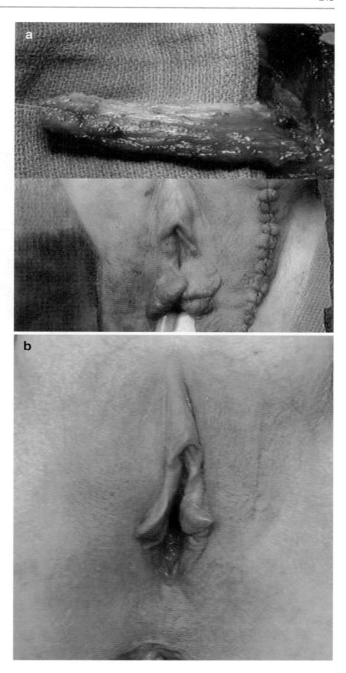

labial incision entirely by dissecting a tunnel under the vaginal wall and harvesting the pedicle graft through the vaginal incision. Although potentially useful, no reports on these technical variants regarding cosmetic outcomes can be found in the literature thus far.

In case of symptomatic labial distortion, a labial fat injection to remodel the labia can be considered. In a single patient (pre- and postoperative views seen in Fig. 19.2), autologous fat was harvested and injected with good cosmetic and functional outcomes.

Fig. 19.2 Pre- (**a**) and postoperative (**b**) images of a patient with labial distortion after a Martius who underwent autologous fat injection into the right labia majora for cosmetic repair

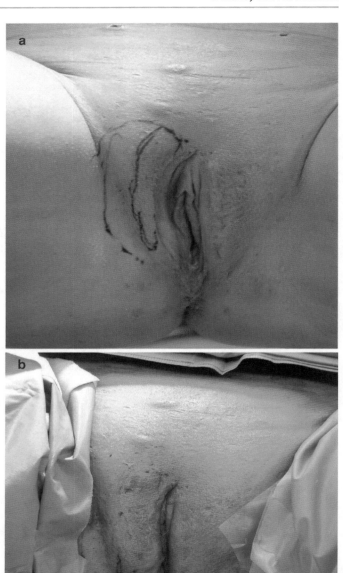

Conclusions

The Martius labial fat pad is a pedicle graft which can be used as an additional layer of tissue interposition when needed in complex vaginal reconstructive cases. It is relatively simple to harvest and use, but does have a few known associated complications, including hematoma or seroma formation, wound infection, pain or numbness at the site of harvest, sexual dysfunction, and labial distortion. The true incidence of these complications is not well documented, but believed to be overall low based on the limited evidence found in the literature as well as the opinion and experience of these authors. Solutions to avoid these complications or treat them after the fact are predominantly based on the authors' experience with very little discussion of such techniques in the literature. Overall the Martius labial fat pad graft is a relatively safe adjunct to complex vaginal reconstruction which can improve rates of successful outcome in some difficult situations.

References

1. Martius H. Die operative Widerherstellung der vollkommen fehlenden Harnrohre und des Schliessmuskels derselben. Zentralbl Gynakol. 1928;52:7.
2. Patil U, Waterhouse K, Laungani G. Management of 18 difficult vesicovaginal and urethrovaginal fistulas with modified Ingelman-Sundberg and Martius operations. J Urol. 1980;123(5):653–6.
3. Ezzat M, Ezzat MM, Tran VQ, Aboseif SR. Repair of giant vesicovaginal fistulas. J Urol. 2009;181(3): 1184–8.
4. Eilber KS, Kavaler E, Rodriguez LV, Rosenblum N, Raz S. Ten-year experience with transvaginal vesicovaginal fistula repair using tissue interposition. J Urol. 2003;169(3):1033–6.
5. Rangnekar NP, Imdad Ali N, Kaul SA, Pathak HR. Role of the Martius procedure in the management of urinary-vaginal fistulas. J Am Coll Surg. 2000;191(3): 259–63.
6. Elkins TE, DeLancey JO, McGuire EJ. The use of modified Martius graft as an adjunctive technique in vesicovaginal and rectovaginal fistula repair. Obstet Gynecol. 1990;75(4):727–33.
7. McNevin MS, Lee PY, Bax TW. Martius flap: an adjunct for repair of complex, low rectovaginal fistula. Am J Surg. 2007;193(5):597–9; discussion 599.
8. Songne K, Scotte M, Lubrano J, et al. Treatment of anovaginal or rectovaginal fistulas with modified Martius graft. Colorectal Dis. 2007;9(7):653–6.
9. Hernandez RD, Himsl K, Zimmern PE. Transvaginal repair of bladder injury during vaginal hysterectomy. J Urol. 1994;152(6 Pt 1):2061–2.
10. Blander DS, Zimmern PE, Lemack GE, Sagalowsky AI. Transvaginal repair of postcystectomy peritoneovaginal fistulae. Urology. 2000;56(2):320–1.
11. Tunuguntla HS, Manoharan M, Gousse AE. Management of neobladder-vaginal fistula and stress incontinence following radical cystectomy in women: a review. World J Urol. 2005;23(4):231–5.
12. Green AE, Escobar PF, Neubaurer N, Michener CM, Vongruenigen VE. The Martius flap neovagina revisited. Int J Gynecol Cancer. 2005;15(5):964–6.
13. Petrou SP, Jones J, Parra RO. Martius flap harvest site: patient self-perception. J Urol. 2002;167(5):2098–9.
14. Carey JM, Chon JK, Leach GE. Urethrolysis with Martius labial fat pad graft for iatrogenic bladder outlet obstruction. Urology. 2003;61(4 Suppl 1):21–5.
15. Webster GD, Guralnick ML, Amundsens CL. Use of the Martius labial fat pad as an adjunct in the management of urinary fistulae and urethral obstruction following antiincontinence procedures. J Urol. 2000; 163(Suppl):76.
16. Carr LK, Webster GD. Full-thickness cutaneous Martius flaps: a useful technique in female reconstructive urology. Urology. 1996;48(3):461–3.
17. Rutman MP, Rodriguez LV, Raz S. Vesicovaginal fistula: vaginal approach. In: Raz S, Rodriguez LV, editors. Female urology. 3rd ed. Philadelphia: Saunders Elsevier; 2008. p. 798.

Complications of Soft Tissue Bulking Agents Used in the Treatment of Urinary Leakage

20

Deborah J. Lightner and John J. Knoedler

Introductory Comments

Why are bulking agents used for stress urinary incontinence? Meatally-based urinary incontinence occurring with increases in intra-abdominal pressure is the sign qua non of stress urinary incontinence and results from urethral failure to resist increases in intra-abdominal pressure. The proximate cause may be related to poor anatomic support of the urethra and bladder neck; this generally responds well to pelvic floor resuspension procedures of various types. Urethral failure, however, may be also intrinsic, meaning the urethral closure pressure is inefficient at resisting increases in intra-abdominal pressures; this is generally treated with sphincter augmentation procedures, which include periurethral bulking agents [1]. Of course, while there is considerable overlap between these two causes of stress urinary incontinence, treatment success with bulking agents used in the patient with predominantly poor anatomic support do not differ markedly from the treatment success in the patient with predominantly intrinsic sphincteric deficiency (ISD) [2, 3]. Conventionally, however, the use of bulking agents is more widely applied if the urinary loss related to poor urethral function without hypermobility.

Due to the low long-term efficacy of these agents in the treatment of urinary incontinence, these agents are not frequently chosen as first line therapy. It is in the nuanced or more difficult clinical situation where these agents are considered: in the elderly [4], in the denervated sphincter of a spinal cord injured [5, 6] or neobladder patient [7] who is leaking between catheterizations and/or is a Valsalva voider, in the multiply-operated urethra of a patient [8] who has failed multiple prior attempts at treatment, or has had partial urethrectomy [9], in the frozen pelvis and pipestem urethra after radiation therapy or for the patient in whom continence procedures have largely ameliorated his or her symptoms, but who still desires moderate improvement over his or her current level of continence [8]. Male patients with postprostatectomy incontinence may choose a bulking agent, carefully informed that the success rates are low [10]. Complications in each of these patient groups are of more consequence as appropriate and acceptable alternatives are few.

Bulking agents are used for soft tissue augmentation in many other specialties, including plastic surgery, dermatology, otolaryngology, and within urologic subspecialties, pediatric urology for ureteric reflux, in reconstructive urology for male sphincteric incontinence [11–14] and in restoration of continence in catheterizable stomas [15]. There is renewed interest in bulking agents for fecal incontinence [16] and for GERD [17]. These soft tissue bulking agents continue to improve over their 70 year history. The commercially available agents currently are potentially

D.J. Lightner, MD (✉) • J.J. Knoedler, MD
Department of Urology, Mayo Clinic,
200 First Street, SW, Rochester, MN 55905, USA
e-mail: lightner.deborah@mayo.edu

H.B. Goldman (ed.), *Complications of Female Incontinence and Pelvic Reconstructive Surgery*,
Current Clinical Urology, DOI 10.1007/978-1-61779-924-2_20, © Springer Science+Business Media, LLC 2013

more durable [18], generally safe, inducing a minimal local inflammatory reaction and with a low prevalence of significant adverse events.

The discussions herein will concentrate on the currently available FDA-approved bulking agents for periurethral use: calcium hydroxylapatite (Coaptite®, Merz Aesthetics, Inc., formerly BioForm Medical, Inc., Frankfurt, DE), pyrolytic carbon-coated zirconium beads (Durasphere® EXP, Carbon Medical Technologies, Inc., Saint Paul, MN, USA), and vulcanized silicone micro-implant (Macroplastique®, Uroplasty, Inc., Minneapolis, MN, USA), each material purportedly forms a scaffold promoting secondary tissue infiltration with variable degrees of inflammatory reaction [19, 20] rather than the less desirable encapsulation [21], which risks extrusion [22]. The discontinuation of several older injected materials, including tetrafluoroethylene, autologous fat, and ethylene vinyl alcohol copolymer resulted from unreliable safety reports as well as the failure to deliver satisfactory rates of success [23]. They should not be used. Off-label use of other soft tissue bulking agents will be discussed to decry the practice.

Given these caveats of experience, the evaluation of future bulking agents, autologous myoblasts [24], or cartilage [25], or polyacrylamide hydrogel [26] (Bulkamid®, currently undergoing investigational studies, Contura International A/S, Soeborg, Denmark) should be subject to the same high degree of scrutiny regarding the unique complications related to the material as previous soft tissue bulking agents.

Of note, the complications seen in one surgical discipline generally mirror the experience of bulking agents across the spectrum of care. Polytetrafluoroethylene is one well-known example of granulomata formation [27–30]. Local migration with radio-opaque carbon-coated zirconium beads is another [31–33], although without clinical consequences. When considering newer periurethral agents, these should therefore be cross-linked for complications across specialties, as similar adverse events might occur in alternative applications.

Parenthetically, the discontinuation of Contigen (Bard™, Covington, GA, USA) was related to the lack of a primary supplier of the bovine product and neither due to lack of efficacy, nor significant complications with the material.

Complications from soft tissue bulking agents will be presented as local or systemic, acute or delayed in presentation, with emphasis on the extremely low risk of significant complications of any type.

Acute local complications of the current bulking agents used in a periurethral application are associated with very low rates of repetition complications. In 5–10% of patients, an uncomplicated or urinary tract infection from instrumentation, transient hematuria from the mucosal injection, transient urinary retention from periurethral edema can occur. A small French catheter is used if retention occurs, and applied for either intermittent catheterization or a short period of indwelling catheterization until resolution of this infrequent complication. Anecdotal concerns regarding the possible deformation of the injected bulking agents, leading to decreased efficacy, has lead to the recommendation that only a small French-sized catheter be used with acute transient urinary retention. As with any periurethral procedure for incontinence, there is an acceptable low incidence of de novo urge incontinence. In patients with either persistent acute urinary retention or secondary obstruction-related urge incontinence, the remote possibility of overbulking leading to obstruction should be considered. This can be treated early with simple aspiration [34, 35] with most agents. A transurethral approach is favored due to the theoretical, albeit never reported, risk of a secondary urethrovaginal fistula.

The type of complication is reported with periurethral bulking agents appear to be partially independent of the material used, in so far that *local chronic* complications of urethral prolapse, periurethral pseudoabscesses are reported in extremely low prevalence and are, at least, theoretically possible with each of these FDA-approved agents. This implies that some of these adverse events may be characteristic of the procedure and location and less likely resultant of the material.

Long-term local complications with the current commercially available bulking agents are also acceptably low and are reported only as small case series. A periurethral collection variously described as a pseudocyst [36] or pseudoabscess [37] or a noncommunicating diverticulum [38] each appear to reflect the same process and present with a palpable well circumscribed mass and secondary obstructive or irritative voiding symptoms. The mass may be tender or not. Several authors have reported that these collections may be infected [39], although the microbiological reports have not been conclusive. Imaging can be definitive [40] if clinically needed. Aspiration alone may lead to recurrence of the pseudoabscess, whereas transurethral unroofing of these periurethral masses is invariably associated with reoccurrence of their presenting symptom of stress urinary incontinence. The periurethral pseudocyst is thick-walled, containing cystic or loculated cavities which may or may not communicate with the urethral lumen; none have been associated with malignant or premalignant changes on explorations occurring up to 19 months postinjection [41]. Historically, pseudoabscess formation was thought secondary to delayed hypersensitivity to the bovine dermal product [42]; however, repeated skin tests do not show conversion [37]. Furthermore, pseudoabscesses can be reported with low prevalence with each of the bulking agents applied either peri- or transurethrally, suggesting that the etiology may be partially related to the specific urethral application. Consistent with this is the fact that pseudoabscess as described is not reported with either ureteral or dermatologic applications, although rarely, other local complication of overlying skin or mucosal erosion, and granulomata formation are common to each application site. Hence, the etiology of pseudoabscess remains enigmatic.

Pseudoabscess is described with virtually all bulking agents used in a periurethral application for stress urinary incontinence. This is not to discount that some agents are associated with this complication in an unacceptable percentage of those treated; dextranomer-hyaluronic acid is an agent particularly associated with granulomata [43, 44] and/or pseudoabscess formation [45].

The classical presentation of a pseudoabscess is outlined in this case: a otherwise healthy female with mixed urinary incontinence but without prior operative management opted for treatment of her stress urinary incontinence component with an injectable bulking agent; bovine glutaraldehyde-cross-linked collagen was chosen. After a negative skin test for bovine collagen allergy, a periurethral injection of a total of 5 cc was performed uneventfully. Six weeks later, she complained of terminal dysuria, her symptoms progressing rapidly to obstructive symptoms with straining to void, and increasing urethral discomfort and dysuria. Her physical examination demonstrated a large nonexpressible periurethral fluctuance. Urine analysis and urine culture were both negative for infection. Imaging demonstrated a large fluid collection periurethrally (Figs. 20.1, 20.2, and 20.3).

Parenthetically, in this case, there was no pointing of the pseudoabscess towards the urethral lumen on cystoscopy as the cystoscopic presence of obvious thinning of the urethral luminal mucosa over pseudoabscess can facilitate performing a complete transurethral drainage of the pseudoabscess.

Pseudoabscess formation and subsequent drainage of the submucosal space into the true urethral lumen is the presumptive mechanism for another small set of chronic local complications: pseudodiverticulum formation [38].

Urethral prolapse has also been reported in case reports with several agents of both current and historic interest [46–48]. Theoretically, this could occur with any bulking agent if it is causes separation of the supporting periurethral stroma. Treatment is local excision, if symptomatic.

Misdiagnosis of periurethral and bladder masses can occur if the history is not available [49]; imaging can be definitive [40].

Local tissue necrosis and subsequent erosion of the overlying mucosa has been described with a bulking agent leading to its removal from the market [22, 50]. Most currently available agents are rarely associated with this in small case series, as the submucosal injection may reduce blood supply to the thin overlying mucosal leading to erosion prior to tissue ingrowth. Fistulation to the

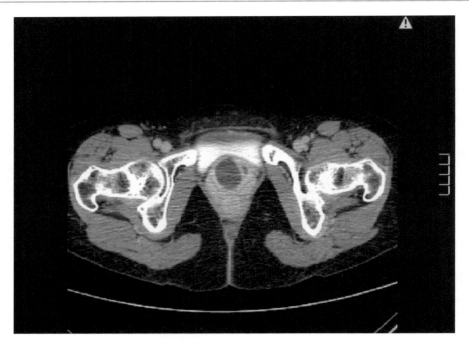

Fig. 20.1 CT imaging reveals a large periurethral fluid collection, Collagen pseudoabscesses can be challenging to diagnose on unenhanced CT imaging, the avascular fluid collection becomes readily apparent after administration of contrast agents. Also, the pseudoabscess is always considerably larger than the injected total bulking agent volume; these cases do not result from obstruction due to overbulking. Due to the acute nature of the process, the pseudoabscess was vaginally drained through a inverted-U incision, taking care to preserve the periure-thral fascia. A simple longitudinal incision is made directly into the pseudoabscess, in order to establish complete drainage. The pseudoabscess fluid here is typical: nonodiferous viscous toothpaste-appearing fluid compresses adjacent tissues, with negative gram stains for bacteria and negative cultures even for fastidious organisms. The high pressures on the surrounding tissues are putatively the cause of the urethral pain, and reoccurrence of the pain should precipitate an evaluation for recurrence of the pseudoabscess (Image courtesy of Howard B. Goldman)

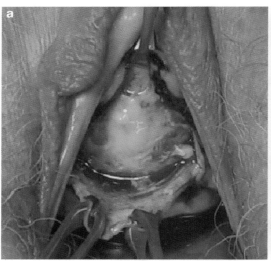
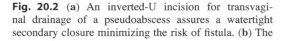
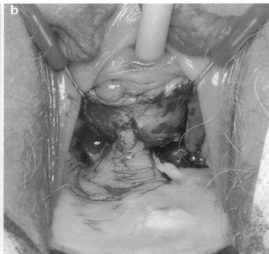

Fig. 20.2 (a) An inverted-U incision for transvaginal drainage of a pseudoabscess assures a watertight secondary closure minimizing the risk of fistula. (b) The pseudoabscess should be expressed and drained completely; loculations can occur and should be adequately drained (Image courtesy of Howard B. Goldman)

Fig. 20.3 Coronal image of a large periurethral pseudoabscess associated with obstructive voiding symptoms

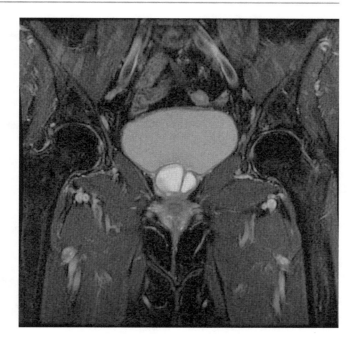

vagina has been described [51, 52] as might occur rarely with any soft tissue expansion occurring in a limited space.

Chronic urinary retention may develop secondary to overbulking [53, 54]. The necessity of transurethral aspiration, or failing this, resection will lead to the reoccurrence of stress urinary incontinence. However, in the elderly, the author has seen the late development of urinary retention due to progressive loss of detrusor power, without intervening outlet obstruction or other complication of the outlet. These rare patients require treatment as clinically indicated for their detrusor failure; the bulking agent itself does not require other management.

Acute systemic complications are exceedingly rare. Any injected agent—injected at any pressure in juxtaposition to lymphatics or vessels—could be potentially migratory or embolic. Construction of bulking agents above a threshold size of 80 μm reduces but does not eliminate that potential risk [33]. There have been no reports of symptomatic embolic phenomenon with the currently available agents, in contradistinction to older agents, particularly dangerous is autologous fat [37]. The embolic and migratory potentials of agents injected adjacent to lymphatics and blood vessels

has been a concern since the initial investigations of these agents [28]: it is generally accepted that bulking agents be larger than 80 μm in diameter to reduce the risk of these occurrences [55]. The injection of agents under pressure into a highly vascular area with abundant lymphatics is likely associated with migration and/or embolism, but clinical consequences have not been reported with Durasphere® EXP, Coaptite® or Macroplastique®. Asymptomatic particle migration, presumptively into lymphatics and submucosal tissues, has been described with those agents which are radiographically visible [33]. Submucosal urethral migration clearly occurs in men with traumatically injured sphincters treated with radiographically visible bulking agents, but these have a low therapeutic efficacy in this setting, limiting their use. Particle size is also directly related to phagocytic activity, with larger particle (herein, of Macroplastique) less likely to be phagocytosed [56]; there have been no clinically reported sequelae of this phenomenon.

There are no chronic systemic complications of soft tissue bulking agents reported, in large part because of the care taken to ensure that these agents are nonimmunogenic, hypoallergenic and biocompatible [21].

This is not to dismiss that fact that several agents are simply unsafe! Agents producing high-grade complications such as obstruction from the granulomata (as in polytetrafluoroethylene), truly embolic phenomenon (as in autologous fat [37]) should simply not be used. Likewise, agents with a high prevalence of adverse reactions (as in ure-thral erosion with ethylene vinyl alcohol copoly-mer [22], or pseudoabscess formation with dextranomer-hyaluronic acid [45]) should not be used, as has occurred with the use of these off-label.

In summary, the judicious use of the currently approved bulking agents, Coaptite, Durasphere, and Macroplastique, in the treatment of sphinc-teric incontinence are associated with an extremely low prevalence of local complications, the most serious of which occur chronically in the form of pseudoabscess formation and/or out-let obstruction. The treatment of these two com-plications is invariably associated with the reoccurrence of the urinary incontinence. The reader is cautioned that other bulking agents may not have the same clinical safety profile particu-larly when applied in the urethra; off-label use of other soft tissue bulking agents is specifically discouraged.

References

1. Klarskov N, Lose G. Urethral injection therapy: what is the mechanism of action? Neurourol Urodyn. 2008;27(8):789–92.
2. Bent AE, Foote J, Siegel S, Faerber G, Chao R, Gormley EA. Collagen implant for treating stress uri-nary incontinence in women with urethral hypermo-bility. J Urol. 2001;166(4):1354–7.
3. Zullo MA, Plotti F, Bellati F, Muzii L, Angioli R, Panici PB. Transurethral polydimethylsiloxane implantation: a valid option for the treatment of stress urinary incontinence due to intrinsic sphincter deficiency without urethral hypermobility. J Urol. 2005;173(3):898–902.
4. Zullo MA, Ruggiero A, Montera R, et al. An ultra-miniinvasive treatment for stress urinary incontinence in complicated older patients. Maturitas. 2010;65(3): 292–5.
5. Hamid R, Arya M, Khastgir J, Patel HRH, Shah PJR. The treatment of male stress urinary incontinence with polydimethylsiloxane in compliant bladders following spinal cord injury. Spinal Cord. 2003;41(5):286–9.
6. Bennett JK, Green BG, Foote JE, Gray M. Collagen injections for intrinsic sphincter deficiency in the neu-ropathic urethra. Paraplegia. 1995;33(12):697–700.
7. Wilson S, Quek ML, Ginsberg DA. Transurethral injection of bulking agents for stress urinary inconti-nence following orthotopic neobladder reconstruction in women. J Urol. 2004;172(1):244–6.
8. Appell RA, Davila GW. Treatment options for patients with suboptimal response to surgery for stress urinary incontinence. Curr Med Res Opin. 2007;23(2):285–92.
9. Plotti F, Zullo MA, Palaia I, Angioli R, Panici PB. Urinary incontinence after radical vulvectomy treated with macroplastique implantation. J Minim Invasive Gynecol. 2008;15(1):113–5.
10. Comiter CV. Surgery insight: surgical management of postprostatectomy incontinence—the artificial uri-nary sphincter and male sling. Nat Clin Pract Urol. 2007;4(11):615–24.
11. Brown JA, Elliott DS, Barrett DM. Postprostatectomy urinary incontinence: a comparison of the cost of con-servative versus surgical management. Urology. 1998;51(5):715–20.
12. Imamoglu MA, Tuygun C, Bakirtas H, Yigitbasi O, Kiper A. The comparison of artificial urinary sphinc-ter implantation and endourethral macroplastique injection for the treatment of postprostatectomy incontinence. Eur Urol. 2005;47(2):209–13.
13. Kylmala T, Tainio H, Raitanen M, Tammela TLJ. Treatment of postoperative male urinary incontinence using transurethral macroplastique injections. J Endourol. 2003;17(2):113–5.
14. Westney OL, Bevan-Thomas R, Palmer JL, Cespedes RD, McGuire EJ. Transurethral collagen injections for male intrinsic sphincter deficiency: the University of Texas-Houston experience. J Urol. 2005;174(3):994–7.
15. Roth CC, Donovan BO, Tonkin JB, Klein JC, Frimberger D, Kropp BP. Endoscopic injection of submucosal bulking agents for the management of incontinent catheterizable channels. J Pediatr Urol. 2009;5(4):265–8.
16. Maeda Y, Laurberg S, Norton C. Perianal injectable bulking agents as treatment for faecal incontinence in adults. Cochrane Database Syst Rev. 2010(5): CD007959.
17. Ganz RA, Fallon E, Wittchow T, Klein D. A new injectable agent for the treatment of GERD: results of the Durasphere pilot trial. Gastrointest Endosc. 2009;69(2):318–23.
18. Ghoniem G, Corcos J, Comiter C, Westney OL, Herschorn S. Durability of urethral bulking agent injec-tion for female stress urinary incontinence: 2-year mul-ticenter study results. J Urol. 2010;183(4):1444–9.
19. Stenberg A, Larsson E, Lackgren G. Endoscopic treat-ment with dextranomer-hyaluronic acid for vesi-coureteral reflux: histological findings. J Urol. 2003;169(3):1109–13.
20. Radley SC, Chapple CR, Lee JA. Transurethral implantation of silicone polymer for stress inconti-nence: evaluation of a porcine model and mechanism of action in vivo. BJU Int. 2000;85(6):646–50.

21. Dmochowski RR, Appell RA. Injectable agents in the treatment of stress urinary incontinence in women: where are we now? Urology. 2000;56(6 Suppl 1): 32–40.

22. Hurtado EA, McCrery RJ, Appell RA. Complications of ethylene vinyl alcohol copolymer as an intraurethral bulking agent in men with stress urinary incontinence. Urology. 2008;71(4):662–5.

23. Haab F, Zimmern PE, Leach GE. Urinary stress incontinence due to intrinsic sphincteric deficiency: experience with fat and collagen periurethral injections [Erratum appears in J Urol. 1997;158(1):188]. J Urol. 1997;157(4):1283–6.

24. Mitterberger M, Marksteiner R, Schwaiger W, et al. Can autologous myoblasts be used as a potential bulking agent? BJU Int. 2008;102(11):1731–6.

25. Bent AE, Tutrone RT, McLennan MT, Lloyd LK, Kennelly MJ, Badlani G. Treatment of intrinsic sphincter deficiency using autologous ear chondrocytes as a bulking agent. Neurourol Urodyn. 2001;20(2):157–65.

26. Lose G, Sorensen HC, Axelsen SM, Falconer C, Lobodasch K, Safwat T. An open multicenter study of polyacrylamide hydrogel (Bulkamid) for female stress and mixed urinary incontinence. Int Urogynecol J Pelvic Floor Dysfunct. 2010;21(12):1471–7.

27. Aragona F, D'Urso L, Scremin E, Salmaso R, Glazel GP. Polytetrafluoroethylene giant granuloma and adenopathy: long-term complications following subureteral polytetrafluoroethylene injection for the treatment of vesicoureteral reflux in children. J Urol. 1997;158(4):1539–42.

28. Malizia Jr AA, Reiman HM, Myers RP, et al. Migration and granulomatous reaction after periurethral injection of polytef (Teflon). JAMA. 1984;251(24):3277–81.

29. Hubmer MG, Hoffmann C, Popper H, Scharnagl E. Expanded polytetrafluoroethylene threads for lip augmentation induce foreign body granulomatous reaction. Plast Reconstr Surg. 1999;103(4):1277–9.

30. Toth G, Rubeiz H, Macdonald RL. Polytetrafluoroethylene-induced granuloma and brainstem cyst after microvascular decompression for trigeminal neuralgia: case report. Neurosurgery. 2007;61(4):E875–7; discussion E877.

31. Altomare DF, La Torre F, Rinaldi M, Binda GA, Pescatori M. Carbon-coated microbeads anal injection in outpatient treatment of minor fecal incontinence. Dis Colon Rectum. 2008;51(4):432–5.

32. Tjandra JJ, Chan MKY, Yeh HCH. Injectable silicone biomaterial (PTQ) is more effective than carbon-coated beads (Durasphere) in treating passive faecal incontinence—a randomized trial. Colorectal Dis. 2009;11(4):382–9.

33. Pannek J, Brands FH, Senge T. Particle migration after transurethral injection of carbon coated beads for stress urinary incontinence. J Urol. 2001;166(4):1350–3.

34. Petrou SP, Pak RW, Lightner DJ. Simple aspiration technique to address voiding dysfunction associated with transurethral injection of dextranomer/hyaluronic acid copolymer. Urology. 2006;68(1):186–8.

35. Hartanto VH, Lightner DJ, Nitti VW. Endoscopic evacuation of Durasphere. Urology. 2003;62(1): 135–7.

36. Wainstein MA, Klutke CG. Periurethral pseudocyst following cystoscopic collagen injection. Urology. 1998;51(5):835–6.

37. Sweat SD, Lightner DJ. Complications of sterile abscess formation and pulmonary embolism following periurethral bulking agents. J Urol. 1999;161(1): 93–6.

38. Clemens JQ, Bushman W. Urethral diverticulum following transurethral collagen injection. J Urol. 2001;166(2):626.

39. McLennan MT, Bent AE. Suburethral abscess: a complication of periurethral collagen injection therapy. Obstet Gynecol. 1998;92(4 Pt 2):650–2.

40. Bridges MD, Petrou SP, Lightner DJ. Urethral bulking agents: imaging review. AJR Am J Roentgenol. 2005;185(1):257–64.

41. Leonard MP, Canning DA, Epstein JI, Gearhart JP, Jeffs RD. Local tissue reaction to the subureteral injection of glutaraldehyde cross-linked bovine collagen in humans. J Urol. 1990;143(6):1209–12.

42. Hanke CW, Higley HR, Jolivette DM, Swanson NA, Stegman SJ. Abscess formation and local necrosis after treatment with Zyderm or Zyplast collagen implant. J Am Acad Dermatol. 1991;25(2 Pt 1): 319–26.

43. Bedir S, Kilciler M, Ozgok Y, Deveci G, Erduran D. Long-term complication due to dextranomer based implant: granuloma causing urinary obstruction. J Urol. 2004;172(1):247–8.

44. Abdelwahab HA, Ghoniem GM. Obstructive suburethral mass after transurethral injection of dextranomer/hyaluronic acid copolymer. Int Urogynecol J Pelvic Floor Dysfunct. 2007;18(11):1379–80.

45. Lightner DJ, Fox J, Klingele C. Cystoscopic injections of dextranomer hyaluronic acid into proximal urethra for urethral incompetence: efficacy and adverse outcomes. Urology. 2010;75(6):1310–4.

46. Ko EY, Williams BF, Petrou SP. Bulking agent induced early urethral prolapse after distal urethrectomy. Int Urogynecol J Pelvic Floor Dysfunct. 2007;18(12): 1511–3.

47. Khalil A, Ghazeeri G, Chammas M, Usta I, Awwad J, Seoud M. Teflonoma presenting as a cystourethrocele. Clin Exp Obstet Gynecol. 2001;28(1):58–9.

48. Harris RL, Cundiff GW, Coates KW, Addison WA, Bump RC. Urethral prolapse after collagen injection. Am J Obstet Gynecol. 1998;178(3):614–5.

49. Kulkarni S, Davies AJW, Treurnicht K, Dudderidge TJ, Al-Akraa M. Misplaced macroplastique injection presenting as a vaginal nodule and a bladder mass. Int J Clin Pract Suppl. 2005;147(Suppl):85–6.

50. Hurtado E, McCrery R, Appell R. The safety and efficacy of ethylene vinyl alcohol copolymer as an intra-urethral bulking agent in women with intrinsic urethral deficiency. Int Urogynecol J Pelvic Floor Dysfunct. 2007;18(8):869–73.

51. Carlin BI, Klutke CG. Development of urethrovaginal fistula following periurethral collagen injection. J Urol. 2000;164(1):124.

52. Pruthi RS, Petrus CD, Bundrick Jr WS. New onset vesicovaginal fistula after transurethral collagen injection in women who underwent cystectomy and orthotopic neobladder creation: presentation and definitive treatment. J Urol. 2000;164(5):1638–9.

53. Bernier PA, Zimmern PE, Saboorian MH, Chassagne S. Female outlet obstruction after repeated collagen injections. Urology. 1997;50(4):618–21.

54. McKinney CD, Gaffey MJ, Gillenwater JY. Bladder outlet obstruction after multiple periurethral polytetrafluoroethylene injections. J Urol. 1995; 153(1):149–51.

55. Henly DR, Barrett DM, Weiland TL, O'Connor MK, Malizia AA, Wein AJ. Particulate silicone for use in periurethral injections: local tissue effects and search for migration. J Urol. 1995;153(6):2039–43.

56. Solomon LZ, Birch BR, Cooper AJ, Davies CL, Holmes SA. Nonhomologous bioinjectable materials in urology: 'size matters'? BJU Int. 2000;85(6):641–5.

Index

Printed by Printforce, the Netherlands